D1783985

THE DEVELOPMENT OF THE PERSON

The Development of the Person

The Minnesota Study of Risk and Adaptation from Birth to Adulthood

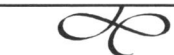

L. ALAN SROUFE
BYRON EGELAND
ELIZABETH A. CARLSON
W. ANDREW COLLINS

THE GUILFORD PRESS
New York   London

© 2005 The Guilford Press
A Division of Guilford Publications, Inc.
72 Spring Street, New York, NY 10012
www.guilford.com

All rights reserved

No part of this book may be reproduced, translated, stored in
a retrieval system, or transmitted, in any form or by any means,
electronic, mechanical, photocopying, microfilming, recording,
or otherwise, without written permission from the Publisher.

Printed in the United States of America

This book is printed on acid-free paper.

Last digit is print number: 9 8 7 6 5 4 3 2

Library of Congress Cataloging-in-Publication Data
The development of the person : the Minnesota study of risk and adaptation
from birth to adulthood / by L. Alan Sroufe ... [et al.].
    p. cm.
  Includes bibliographical references and index.
  ISBN 1-59385-158-8 (alk. paper)
  1. Child development—Longitudinal studies. 2. Child psychology—
Longitudinal studies. 3. Adolescent psychology—Longitudinal
studies. 4. Maturation (Psychology)—Longitudinal studies. 5. Adjustment
(Psychology)—Longitudinal studies. 6. Child psychopathology—Longitudinal
studies. 7. Adolescent psychopathology—Longitudinal studies. 8. Parent and
child—Longitudinal studies. 9. Minnesota Longitudinal Study of Parents and
Children. I. Sroufe, L. Alan.
  HQ767.9.D477 2005
  305.231—dc22

                               2004026206

To the parents, children, and now their children,
of the Minnesota Parent–Child Project—
for your commitment and generosity
in sharing your lives with us

About the Authors

L. Alan Sroufe, PhD, is the William Harris Professor of Child Psychology in the Institute of Child Development and Adjunct Professor in the Department of Psychiatry at the University of Minnesota. He is a member of the Society for Research in Child Development and is on the editorial boards of three professional journals. An internationally recognized expert on early attachment relationships, emotional development, and developmental psychopathology, Dr. Sroufe has published six books and more than 100 articles on these and related topics.

Byron Egeland, PhD, is the Irving B. Harris Professor of Child Development at the University of Minnesota and Codirector of the Irving B. Harris Training Center for Infant and Toddler Development. He is a Fellow of the American Psychological Association, the American Psychological Society, and the American Association of Applied and Preventive Psychology; is on the board of directors of a number of national organizations, including Prevent Child Abuse America; and is on the Youth Advisory Board of the Boy Scouts of America. Dr. Egeland has published articles and book chapters in the areas of child maltreatment, high-risk children, developmental psychopathology, and preventative intervention programs with high-risk families.

Elizabeth A. Carlson, PhD, is a Research Associate and Instructor in the Institute of Child Development at the University of Minnesota. She has published numerous papers on the influence of early experience on emotional and behavioral disturbance, the internalization of experience, and the mutual influence of representation and experience. Dr. Carlson is internationally recognized as a trainer in infant attachment assessment.

W. Andrew Collins, PhD, is Morse-Alumni Distinguished Teaching Professor of Child Development and Psychology in the Institute of Child Development at the University of Minnesota. He has written widely about processes of mass media influence, parent–adolescent relationships and influences during adolescence, and peer and romantic relationships during adolescence and early adulthood. A Fellow of both the American Psychological Association and the American Psychological Society, Dr. Collins currently serves as Chair of the Scientific Advisory Board for the NICHD Study of Early Child Care and Youth Development.

Preface

For the last three decades we have been conducting a comprehensive study of children in their families, from birth to adulthood. It is a dream of developmental psychologists to know what children experience and to know their circumstances at each age, and to watch them unfold. This book is the story of what we learned about children as they progressed from one age to the next and what we came to understand about the development of individuals—how they became the persons they are.

We studied 180 children born into poverty in order to track the courses of their lives. Direct assessments of the children and the care they received were made at multiple times, and information was gathered from interviews and other procedures with parents, teachers, and, ultimately, the young people themselves, usually at the same ages. All aspects of development and the developmental context were examined, many times in the first 4 years, then yearly into elementary school, and every 2 or 3 years thereafter. Settings for the study included the home, the laboratory, the school, and the peer group. We examined parenting, peer relationships, temperament, and cognitive functioning, and we examined the interplay of all of these factors age by age in detail, beginning at the beginning. Moreover, the study included ongoing assessments of the entire range of contextual factors, from child and parent IQ and personality, to family-life stress, disruptions, and social support, to socioeconomic conditions. Finally, the study relied on multiple measures and multiple sources of information, including ample direct observation of children and parents. Rather than relying on what someone said had occurred in the past, or what the child was like as an infant, we directly assessed such things at the time.

Our goals were to outline the general trends in development, as well as to describe the course of individual lives. At each age, we were able to coordinate our measures of the nature and characteristics of individual children as these emerged and changed over time, as well as the quality of care the child was receiving and critical features of the context surrounding each family. Because the information on many features of development was comprehensive, we were able to evaluate the potential critical influences on individual development. For example, we looked at the influence of temperament, attachment, and other aspects of care; intelligence of children and parents; the peer group; and the stress families were experiencing. We evaluated not only the relative predictive power of these factors but also how they worked together to shape development. Because the children we followed were born into poverty, their lives were often challenging, and some experienced harsh circumstances. Not surprisingly, a number of them had difficulties. Others, however, had social assets that offset this adversity and did very well indeed. This was a study of competence, as well as a study of developmental problems.

The comprehensiveness and longitudinal nature of the study allowed us to ask three kinds of questions. The first questions concerned the conditions that promoted competent functioning across development or, alternatively, that led to developmental difficulties. How well could outcomes such as dropping out of school, aggression, or attention problems, to name just a few, be predicted? What were the predictors of such problems? We found that dropping out, for example, could be predicted even prior to school entry, and that other problems also followed an understandable course. Second, we were able to answer questions about "exceptions"; that is, some children developed well despite experiencing early risks for problems (were "resilient"), and other children showed problems even though early predictors were not present. We were able to account for and explain such changes in adaptation and show that they, too, were lawful. Finally, we were able to answer complex developmental questions: What was the fate of early experience following developmental change? In the face of different later circumstances, is early experience erased?

Thus, the study was much more than an investigation of the predictability of who did well and who struggled. Rather, our central focus was the very nature and process of development. We wanted to understand both continuity and change in adaptation, the ongoing transaction between the developing child and the environment, and the child's changing role with development. We illustrate a particular viewpoint in which the child is seen as emerging through a process of development. At each point the child is shaped by the history of experience and current circumstances, but at each point the child also contributes to the circumstances and creates the experience that will be part of the new history.

In the introductory part of the book, we first lay out these questions (Chapter 1) and present the conceptual background for our viewpoint on development (Chapter 2). These chapters make clear why the study was conducted as it was. The nature of the questions required a prospective, longitudinal study of the kind we did. Then, in Chapters 3 and 4, we describe in some detail the study itself, including the inception of the study and the measures and methods we employed. We wrote the book so that readers with particular interests could skip ahead and find their way, and be referred back to discussion of particular methods as required. But we urge most readers to read the methods chapters first. What distinguishes our work from others who make claims about forces that shape development is that our comprehensive measurement allows us to control for other factors when we claim the importance of one factor or another. When we make claims about the impact of temperament or IQ, or a particular pattern of care or maltreatment at a particular time, or the consequences of family disruption or of witnessing abuse, or the stress the family experienced during any particular period, we take into account each of these other factors (and more).

In the second section of the book (Chapters 5–10), we describe the emergence of the person, attained patterns of adaptation, and their origins and course, age by age. We not only predict individual outcomes but also account for changes in trajectories. There are chapters on infancy, toddlerhood, the preschool period, middle childhood, early adolescence, and late adolescence/early adulthood. In each case, the age is first described in terms of its salient developmental issues, and variations in patterns of adaptation with regard to those issues are described and explained.

The third section is devoted to development and psychopathology. Chapter 11 describes the developmental process, what we have learned about the interplay of experience, representation of experience, and surrounding circumstances over time. We account for the fate of early experience following change and the development of individual constructs such as resilience. This is a backdrop for understanding disturbance. In Chapter 12, we present a developmental model of disturbance and provide data on the development and course of disturbed patterns of behavior, including attention/hyperactivity problems, dissociation, depression and anxiety, and conduct disturbance. Implications for assessment, classification, and treatment of problems follow in Chapter 13.

In the final chapter, we discuss current directions of our work and present very recent data on adult disturbance, adult relationships and relationship representation, and continuity of parenting across generations, based on the beginning study of the children of our grown-up participants. We point to the new level of process-oriented questions that can now be addressed.

This was a large, comprehensive study that we could not have carried out without a great deal of help. We would like to thank first of all the parents, children, and now their children who participated in the Minnesota Parent–Child Study. You gave of your time, you shared your lives with us, and we were inspired by you. We greatly appreciate your commitment to this project, and this book is dedicated to you.

We also are indebted to the many people who contributed their time and talent to this project. First, we thank the more than 200 graduate and undergraduate students who contributed both effort and creativity to this study. This remarkable group of students were the backbone of this project, and readers will see their work throughout this book. We also mention in particular staff who, over the years, maintained contact with our families—Michele Dodds, Julie Johnson, Hunter Roe, and Anne List—for their work in the early years of the project, and Judy Cook, who is our core staff person now. Peter Clark and Jane Love were our primary preschool teachers. Robert Weigand directed our summer camps. They created humane and nurturing environments for our participants. We could not have done this without you, literally. In addition, we acknowledge the school administrators and more than 1,000 teachers who gave of their time, because of their commitment to the improved well-being of children.

Finally, we acknowledge the generous financial support of foundations and federal agencies that allowed us to carry on this work. Over the years, we have been funded by the Office of Child Abuse, the Department of Maternal and Child Health, the National Science Foundation, the Office of Education, the William T. Grant Foundation, the Spencer Foundation, the Irving B. Harris Foundation, and, for more than 20 consecutive years, the National Institute of Mental Health (MH-48064). In this regard, we would also like to thank the numerous peer review panels that deemed our work worthy of support.

Contents

PART I. UNDERSTANDING DEVELOPMENT

PART II. DEVELOPMENT AND ADAPTATION

PART I

Understanding Development

CHAPTER 1

The Challenge

The premiere developmental question is, of course, the nature of the transition from one developmental stage to another—the emergence of new forms. How does a system retain continuity and yet produce discontinuous manifestations?
—THELEN (1989)

The question of how individuals become the persons they are has intrigued developmental researchers and clinicians alike, and no wonder. It is the most complicated and important question in all of psychology. Not only are there myriad potential influences that must be taken into account simultaneously, but we must also consider them in action over time.

Consider briefly three 10-year-old children that we observed at a summer camp as part of our research. The first, SM, was popular with other children and well liked by counselors. This child had close friendships and functioned very smoothly in the larger peer group, coordinating friendships and group functioning. SM also negotiated well the other major tasks of middle childhood—doing well in school, developing special talents, enthusiastically engaging challenges, and abiding by rules even when not under direct supervision. Everyone found SM to be thoughtful, engaging, and empathic.

The second child, TJ, who attended a public school in a tough neighborhood, was not well liked by peers or counselors at our camp, largely because of physically aggressive and disruptive behavior. School was going very poorly, and rules seemed to be made to be broken. When a challenge arose, explosive behavior followed. TJ's parents reported at this time that TJ "just can't be controlled."

Finally, our third child, SJ, presents another contrast. This child was not disliked by other children but was hardly noticed. SJ was very dependent on counselors and teachers, some of whom accepted this, while others found it annoying. Schoolwork was inconsistent, depending on the guidance that was provided. Almost everything seemed to be a challenge at our camp or at school, and quickly giving up was SJ's predominant reaction.

How did these children get to be the way they were at age 10? Could we recognize these same patterns at an earlier age? Surely, they would not have been exactly the same, so what would we have seen? What would have been the developmental issues in the toddler or preschool periods that would have been appropriate comparisons for predicting close friendships and doing well in school at the later age? In fact, are these the best foci at age 10? How would we know? And does what we saw at age 10 forecast later functioning? Would children like SM always be free from problems? How likely is TJ to show disordered conduct as a teenager? Are children like SJ at risk for depression? We address each one of these questions in this book, and although each turns out to be extraordinarily complex, we have been able to provide answers for all of them.

With regard to the question of the origins of these profiles at age 10, psychologists have suggested a substantial list of potential influences. Some have pointed to temperament, IQ, academic aptitude, genetic "predispositions," or other things that are commonly considered "child characteristics." Others would emphasize experiences in the family or the peer group, or the school itself. Still others would suggest the importance of surrounding factors, such as degree of poverty, stress, and chaotic life circumstances. Each of these can readily be shown to be worthy of consideration, and most researchers would now say that they are all important. But having such a list would be the bare beginning of understanding.

Thus, for example, determining that some child characteristic is associated with a certain outcome raises as many questions as it answers. As an illustration, one seemingly clear child characteristic is gender, and it is of obvious importance in a certain sense. What gender came to mind when you read the example of TJ, the aggressive, disruptive child? Likely, a male, and it is indeed the case that this profile, as described, is much more common among boys. But why is this so? How does gender exert its influence in development? Surely, being a boy does not directly cause TJ's problems, because most boys do not have these problems.

Certain characteristics of SM also would seem to play an important role. The capacity to respond well to challenge (referred to as "resilience") and the talent for schoolwork would promote subsequent positive adaptation. As described, these are characteristics of this child at age 10, and they are important. Having said this, we can quickly see that even more important questions are raised by such assertions. How do these characteristics arise in the first place? How did the child develop the capacity to respond well to challenge? Was he or she born to be that way? How would we know? As it turns out, resilience and scholastic aptitude develop and change in response to a variety of influences. We have conducted a major study of both developmental constructs and report our findings later in this book.

Another finding from our work is that children's influences on their own development appear to increase over time. Children play increasingly active roles in their own development as they grow older, likely because of deepening attitudes and expectations, and the reactions their established patterns of behavior draw from others. This is another complexity. The influences of particular ingredients in the developmental equation are not static; they may change over time. Nor are they linear; that is, in combination with another factor, their impact may be disproportional to either influence acting alone.

Other complexities may be illustrated by considering the roles of experience and context. It is well established that experience and surrounding context are important features of development. For example, changes in family stress; changes in parents' characteristics, such as depression; and changes in parenting practices all are associated with changes in child behavior (e.g., Dishion & Bullock, 2002; Egeland, Kalkoske, Gottesman, & Erickson, 1990; Embry & Dawson, 2002). However, this does not tell us whether these factors were responsible for child behavior in the first place. Moreover, even if demonstrated, it is not enough to know that parenting or peer experiences play some role in later social functioning. We would need to understand why they do and how experiences are carried forward. It cannot simply be a matter of transferring practices from one context to another. What babies do with caregivers would not be a useful pattern for interacting with peers in preschool or middle childhood. Somehow, the transfer must be at the level of expectations and attitudes, or in underlying emotional capacities, and these are the processes we need to understand.

Likewise, we seek more than just the knowledge that both parents and peers are important, which, as it turns out, they are (see, e.g., Chapter 8). We need to understand the specifics of their influences and how they work together *over time*. We especially want to understand their reciprocal, mutual, or transactional influences (e.g., Sameroff & Chandler, 1975). How does what you experience with your parents promote your relationships with peers and siblings and how do the latter feed back on, supplement, amplify, or counterbalance the former? Our work is concerned with each of these questions.

In the same way, it is not enough to know that the child's pattern of adaptation at one age forecasts functioning at the next. As we report, it often clearly does, but it does not always do so. Thus, the more critical questions concern the processes of continuity and change. How does adaptation at one age contribute to adaptation at the next, and when change occurs, why and how does this happen? These are some of the questions we need to answer, and all are questions that we address.

In summary, to fully understand how we become the persons we are—the complex, step-by-step evolution of our orientations, capacities, and behavior over time—requires more than a list of ingredients, however important any one of them might be. It requires an understanding of the process of development, how all of these factors work together in an ongoing way over time. Such an understanding can come only from a certain kind of study, what is referred to as prospective, longitudinal research.

For three decades, we have been conducting a study of 180 children and their families. We began 3 months before the children were born and followed each case closely through all of the years of childhood and adolescence, and into adulthood, measuring all major aspects of the child's functioning and surrounding circumstances. Such a detailed study permits tracking of not only general trends in development but also the twists and turns of individual life courses. By comparing groups of children with similar or dissimilar histories, or challenges and supports across time, one gains understanding of the struggles and successes of individuals as they develop.

As we describe in this book, this study has allowed us to document the coherence and lawfulness of both continuity and change. When individuals struggle and continue to struggle, or succeed and continue to succeed, there are cumulative reasons for this. There is no magic characteristic and no bad seed that accounts for why some do well and others have a difficult time. Likewise, change for the better and change for the worse are describable, understandable outcomes of development.

This type of longitudinal study, in which children are followed forward through time, allows important questions to be addressed in a way that other types of studies do not. In much research, when one notes, for example, a correspondence between harsh discipline and child aggression, one cannot say which came first. Was the child always difficult and aggressive, with the parental discipline escalating over time in reaction, or is the child's aggression a reaction to a history of rejection and harsh discipline? In a prospective study one can uncover the ordering. It is also possible to learn something about the particular role of various influences and how they work together. The same parenting practice may be associated with different outcomes depending on the prior history of the child (as we discuss in Chapter 11).

Our particular viewpoint on development, which is laid out in some detail in Chapter 2, dictated that we conduct a comprehensive study. In brief, we believe that the explanation for why individual children and adults are the way they are lies in the entire cumulative history *and* the current circumstances surrounding the persons. The history includes the transactions between the child and significant others across each preceding developmental period, the surrounding stresses and supports, and the child's experiences of success and failure in a variety of contexts. Our concept of current circumstances includes not only external challenges, supports, and opportunities but also the child's expectations, aptitudes, and other characteristics. And, while part of current circumstances, such child characteristics also develop. As we describe, we attempted to measure every salient feature of developing children and their surrounding environments, age by age. Moreover, we found it necessary to study and to understand the various ways that children can be developing well at any given age, with each age defined in its own terms, as well as patterns that proved to be maladaptive.

To illustrate why we believed the study had to be done this way, we provide below the example of evaluating the role of early experience. While this was only one of the questions that inspired our work, it well illustrates the complexity of the task and the need for a comprehensive study. The same comprehensive approach is required to answer questions concerning how child characteristics and experience interact over time to produce unique outcomes, how parental care and peer experiences work together, how the impact of any experience is influenced by the point in development and previous history, and questions about processes that account for continuity and change in development.

WHY COMPREHENSIVE LONGITUDINAL RESEARCH?: THE EXAMPLE OF EARLY EXPERIENCE

Serena (SM) and Thomas (TJ) began their lives very differently. While both were born to teenage mothers, Serena was embedded in a rich network of social support. Serena's mother, Jessica, reported a history of loving relationships with her parents, and she felt unequivocally supported by them as a mother. Jessica and Serena's father decided to marry shortly after Serena was born. He had finished high school, and he worked while Jessica completed her education in a special, part-time program for teen mothers. With some financial help from Jessica's parents, they established a stable living situation. Both were dedicated to Serena and to each other. Direct observation in the home showed that Jessica was consistently responsive to Serena, providing her with appropriate stimulation and gentle care that allowed her to thrive. By the end of the first year, Serena was a confident, happy baby, who eagerly explored her surroundings, secure in her relationships with her caregivers.

In stark contrast, Thomas's mother, Veronica, had run away from an abusive home when she was 12 years old and had little further contact with her family. When Thomas was born, Veronica's mother told her that it was her problem and made it completely clear that there would be no help from her. Veronica had serious drug and alcohol problems and was mistreated by her on-again, off-again drug-dealing partner, the likely father of Thomas. Even after the baby was born, they moved from place to place, living with a parade of transient housemates. For a time, when Veronica's partner was in jail, she and Thomas lived in a shelter. At the end of Thomas's first year, they were living with Veronica's sister and her boyfriend, in another chaotic household. Direct observation showed Veronica to be notably unresponsive to Thomas, especially when she was feeling depressed, which occurred frequently. At times, she also was harshly rejecting, angrily rebuffing Thomas when he wanted contact. Not surprisingly, the relationship between Thomas and Veronica was not a good one. Thomas showed little confidence in Veronica's availability. When assessed in a standard laboratory situation involving moderate stress, Thomas explicitly would not go to Veronica for comfort. His emotions were generally flat, and his exploration superficial.

These differences in the first year of life are dramatic, even though these children are growing up in broadly the same culture and the same community. But how important are these differences? How lasting is their impact? How easily modified are they? What are the processes that govern continuity and change from the early to the later years of childhood? Most importantly, if there is a lasting influence of early experiences, how and why does this happen? What is the developmental process through which early experience has its effect on later life?

The idea that early experience plays a critical role in the development of the person is one of the oldest hypotheses in all of psychology. Freud and other early pioneers in psychology, such as James Mark Baldwin, argued that nothing is more important for the development of children than the way they are treated by their parents or others who care for them. Even before the rise of formal psychology, psychologically minded essayists and poets had espoused this idea. Alexander Pope (1731/1961, p. 149) wrote, "As the twig is bent, the tree's inclined," implying that the mature form is forecast at the very beginning. William Wordsworth (1807/1940, p. 3) captured the same idea with his famous line, "The child is father of the man." Indeed, what could be more plausible than the idea that one's expectations and beliefs about self and others should be based on past experience?

Yet this seemingly straightforward notion has proven to be deceptively complex and challenging to evaluate scientifically. At times, studies have failed to find confirming evidence. At other times, apparent confirmations have been put forward, only to be criticized on methodological grounds. The result is that many prominent psychologists have remained skeptical regarding this basic proposition (Kagan, 1984; Lewis, 1998). While recent work on how experience affects the developing brain has spurred new confidence in the validity of this hypothesis, definitive work with humans is only just emerging (Nelson, de Haan, & Thomas, in press; Schore, 2002).

Why has this task proven to be so difficult? On the one hand, failures of the hypothesis are very easy to produce. Properly measuring early experience is itself challenging. Where does one even begin? Some things, of course, like level of poverty, are easy to measure. But level of poverty often tends to be a relatively stable variable, influencing a child not just early in life but in an ongoing way. Thus, consistency in development could simply be due to continued poverty. Moreover, it is not really a measure of experience. Many parents living in poverty provide excellent care for their children. Poverty simply stands for a host of correlative challenges that some families face (Fergusson, Swain-Campbell, & Horwood, 2004).

Quality of care and other experiential measures, on the other hand, are difficult to define and measure. What is the essence of positive early experience anyway? Likewise, proper outcome measures are equally difficult to achieve. How does one know a person is developing well? Does this not change from age to age? And even if we can agree on definition, adequate measurement remains a challenge. Constructs such as high self-esteem, adequate emotional regulation, and even competence with peers are difficult to capture. With either poor early measures or poor outcome measures, the study is doomed to failure.

Just as many problems arise when a study does find that an early experience measure predicts an outcome of interest. How can we know that the early measure is not simply predictive because it is related to some other early condition (such as poverty or stress) that exerts an ongoing effect, or because the early quality itself continues to exist at the later time? Children may be doing well because of supports their parents are providing at the later age, which happen to also be reminiscent of the manner in which parents treated them in the early years. Or perhaps some inherent characteristic, or set of characteristics, of the child elicited the positive parenting in the first place and accounted for the later child outcome as well. Similarly, perhaps parents with high IQ behave in the ways identified as positive, and children with high IQ function better in terms of the outcome chosen, with parents and children sharing high IQ due to genetics. Without considering such interpretations, one cannot reach firm conclusions about the role of early experience.

The case of Thomas from our ongoing study illustrates some of these problems. As mentioned earlier, Thomas experienced clearly malevolent care in infancy. This care was characterized by both harsh treatment and chronic emotional unavailability. In light of this history, the serious inability to control his anger and other conduct problems he showed as a teenager are not surprising. However, Thomas also witnessed his father's violent suicide when he was 6 years old, his mother died of cancer when he was a teenager, and his life was completely unstable and stress filled throughout childhood and adolescence. He was also chronically rejected by peers. Might not such experiences be equally responsible for any conduct problems Thomas showed as a teenager?

Each case is, of course, even more complex than this. What if, as was true for Thomas, there were some adults who took a special interest in him, and he had an extensive period in treatment with a supportive therapist? Or what if, hypothetically, his primary caregiver had recovered from her drug dependency and other life problems, and formed a more stable social support network during the middle part of childhood? And what if, based on these changes, she then provided a more stable life situation for Thomas? We would expect child behavior to be positively influenced. What then becomes of the early negative experience? Does it still exert an influence? More to the point, in what ways or in what circumstances would we expect it to be manifest?

In light of all of this, what role do we assign to early experience? No one can doubt that the family trauma and stress of his later juvenile years would also impact Thomas's development. Developmental psychologists also are in accord in the belief that experiences with peers, as well as with parents, shape developmental outcomes. Notice that the hypothesis is not that *only* early experience is important, or even that early experience is *more* important than later experience. Rather, the hypothesis is that early experience, because of its very place in the developmental course, has some special importance for the development of the person.

An analogy of constructing a house may be helpful. We may think of early experience as the foundation for the building. The foundation cannot be more important than solid supporting beams or a sturdy roof; without these, the house will not last. But at the same time, a house cannot be stronger than its foundation, and the foundation frames or structures what the house can become, though it does not specify many details. It is in this sense that the foundation of a house has special importance.

There are, of course, limitations to the house metaphor. A developing person is not a concrete structure, but a dynamic, living system. One feature of the theoretical perspective we outline in Chapter 2 concerns the transformational nature of development. When early experience is integrated with later experience, it remains, in a sense, but in a transformed way (as suggested in our introductory quote); that is, later experience and later development can impact the influence of early experience. Development is not like building with Legos, with pieces simply added one on top of another. Development is a dynamic process wherein what evolves derives from what was there before in a logical way, while, at the same time, prior experience or prior adaptation has a fundamentally new meaning in the now more complex system.

Development is not linear; it is characterized by both continuity and change. What happens early on does not lead in a direct way to a similar-looking outcome later. There always is a complex, ongoing transaction between the person, as developed to that point, and a changing array of challenges and opportunities, stresses, and supports. What developmentalists seek to describe is the coherence of this process, the way development is organized for the individual. Thus, examining the place of early experience is just the starting point.

Such a dynamic, systemic view does not trivialize the role of early experience or early adaptation. Rather, it calls attention to the process of development, to questions about *how* early experience might exert an ongoing influence. To fully evaluate the place of early experience in development, one must go beyond simply showing a link between measures of early experience and later outcomes. A satisfactory evaluation involves also illustrating the processes and mechanisms through which any such linkages occur, including the ways in which early experience and adaptation combine with later experiences of diverse kinds.

The challenge we faced as we began our research was to evaluate issues such as the role of early experience within an emerging perspective on the organization of development, with all of the complexity of continuity and change in the trajectories of individual lives. It was a daunting task, but we believed the answer lay in conducting a comprehensive, detailed, long-term study in which the host of potential influences were considered together over time, from the very beginning of development. In the end, we did show that early experience is of profound importance in the development of a child.

OUTLINE OF THE MINNESOTA STUDY

For more than 30 years, we have pursued questions concerning the nature of individual development. The first step was a short-term longitudinal study in which children were followed from infancy to kindergarten, for the purpose of initially validating proposed early measures. In a series of studies, we showed that measures of quality of care provided by principal caregivers predicted later security of the child, as well as self-confidence, curiosity, flexible self-control, and positive functioning with peers (Arend, Gove, & Sroufe, 1979; Matas, Arend, & Sroufe, 1978; Sroufe & Waters, 1977a). These findings, which were replicated in our current sample (Egeland & Farber, 1984; Erickson, Sroufe, & Egeland, 1985; Sroufe, 1983), were the background for our ongoing, large-scale, comprehensive longitudinal study. The study is characterized by seven essential features:

- Children born into poverty
- Assessments beginning before birth
- Detailed age-by-age assessment
- Comprehensive measures across domains
- Study of normal and maladaptive development
- Considerations of developmental context
- Early assessments at the level of relationships

Each of these features is discussed in the following sections.

Children of Poverty

Deciding which children and the number of children to study were crucial decisions at the outset of this project. There are always trade-offs in deciding sample size. On the one hand, given the complexities of development and the number of questions that must be answered, a relatively large number of children is required. The need to statistically control for a sizable number of alternative explanations for any finding makes this essential. At the same time, if detailed, age-by-age measures are required, including labor-intensive direct observation of parents and children, a huge number of participants becomes impractical. Parent reports are valuable, and we used them extensively. However, relying exclusively on how parents say they treat their children and how parents (or children) say the child is now behaving is not completely adequate. Parents may say one thing and do another, have understandable biases in the way they view parenting, or simply have a different perspective than an impartial observer. We believed strongly that direct observation was essential, as were comprehensive assessments of all areas of functioning. Therefore, sample size had to be constrained. Ultimately, we followed 180 children from the last trimester of prenatal development to adulthood. We also evaluated smaller subsamples in great detail in our own preschool program and in a series of camps during middle childhood and adolescence. In part, these detailed observations allowed us to validate more global assessments made on the entire sample, as well as to examine intricate features of social behavior.

Studying children of modest poverty was both a matter of conscience and a strategic choice. In the mid-1970s, when we began this project, relatively little research, and almost no research in which children were followed over time, had been carried out with children outside of the middle class. Gathering information about the lives of these children was worthwhile in its own right. At the same time, children born into poverty in Minneapolis at this time were expected to be at risk for developmental problems, but not at such severe risk as families living in poverty for generations. Poverty was not yet entrenched in this community. Thus, factors associated with poverty—single parenthood, low education, drug and alcohol abuse—were not so consistently part of the picture as they are in some poverty samples. We would expect that while a number of these children would develop problems, many would also do well. In the end, it was the case that about half the children we studied have developed well, which is remarkable given the challenges their families sometimes faced. About half had some notable problems. Some families encountered incredible stress and difficulty, and at times, clear maltreatment of the child occurred. At other times, family circumstances stabilized and supports improved. This range of family functioning allowed us to examine the role of early experience in two ways; first, by examining the entire range of parenting differences, and, second, by looking at the results of extremely negative care. While we would never wish any children to develop with problems, from a purely statistical point of view, the variation in our sample was ideal. We have enough variation in level of competence, and in the number and type of problems to answer the important questions we set out to answer. Moreover, we believe that such a sample allows us to generalize our findings to a large number of U.S. families.

Beginning before Birth

The transactional process of mutually influencing exchanges between organism and environment begins at conception. We believed that it was important to begin our assessments in the prenatal period, both because we wanted to understand the circumstances into which the child was born, and because we wanted to study the developmental process from the beginning. This is especially important if one wants to examine the roles of parental attitudes and expectations, and any inherent child characteristics. Attitudes and expectations of parents clearly could be influenced by the behavior of the child they are rearing. Thus, we wanted to tap into such expectations before the child was born. Equally, manifest child characteristics likely are influenced by parental attitudes and expectations, and the parenting behavior they foster.

Many past studies have begun after infancy, yet have drawn conclusions concerning the role of temperament. When temperament is taken as a descriptive concept, that is, simply as a characterization of the child's style of behavior, whatever the causes, this is meaningful. Children certainly vary in terms of activity level, thresholds of responsiveness, and so forth. But when temperament is taken as an etiological concept, a reflection of endogenous child characteristics that lead to certain behavior problems or competencies, this is inappropriate. The reason is that we cannot rule out the transforming role of parental influences in the period since birth (or the role of prenatal care). We cannot infer what the child was like as a young infant from his or her behavior as a preschooler. Likewise, as valuable as it may be we cannot simply accept the report of the parent that "he was always like that" or the parents' retrospective reports about how they did and did not treat the infant. These all must be directly observed. We began our measurements of infant temperament and parental care at birth. Especially if one is interested in the early experience hypothesis, there is no choice but to start at the beginning. We also chose to study first-time mothers, so that any expectations based on a previous child would not be in effect.

Detailed Observations, Age by Age

Guided by our interest in the early-starting developmental process, we necessarily conducted very dense and detailed assessments in the early weeks, months, and years of life. As reported in Chapters 3 and 4 and in Appendix A, we carried out extensive prenatal interviews and testing of parents, and began collecting data on the infants at birth, beginning with nurses' ratings in the newborn nursery and continuing with home assessments at 7 and 10 days. We carried out 11 additional direct assessments between 3 months and 30 months, and 4 more prior to school entry. Assessments were then made almost yearly until age 13, with follow-ups at ages 16, 17½, 19, 21, 23, 26, and 28.

This pattern of assessment, with dense coverage of the early years, is important for at least two reasons. First, development is very rapid in the early months and years of life. Three-month-olds are qualitatively different than newborns. Ten-month-olds, with their capacities to recall previous experience and anticipate outcomes, are more like adults than they are like 3-month-olds. Three-year-olds, with their language and narrative memory abilities, are more like adults than they are like 10-month-olds. Dense assessments are required to track the development of individuals across these profound transitions. Second, given the rapid changes occurring, the only way to capture the transforming influence of parent on infant or infant on parent is to be there early and often. As one example, we found dramatic individual differences on the Bayley (1969) Scales of Infant Development, which we gave at both 9 and 24 months. Some children showed a 40-point decline in functioning across this age span. This change is a more important feature of development than either the starting or ending point alone. As we report in Chapter 5, this volume, such a decline was associated with a particular pattern of care.

Comprehensive Assessments

To evaluate adequately our developmental process view requires comprehensive assessment of all salient domains of experience, multiple domains of functioning, and a host of potentially mediating factors. One must, of course, measure not just parental care but influences of other family members beyond primary caregivers, as well as the influence of peers, teachers, and others outside the family. Similarly, one must measure and control for possible correlates of parenting, which themselves might be related to outcomes in question. We mentioned parent IQ and level of poverty earlier. Other personal characteristics of the parents (e.g., depression) and other aspects of the parents' circumstances, such as amount of life stress (see the section on context below), could influence parenting and through that, the child. They could also have a more direct impact on the child, for example, because of the child's direct experience of some of the same stresses. All of these features of development were assessed as part of our study.

It was also necessary to assess characteristics of the child that could be directly related to some outcomes or could influence the developmental process through their impact on the parent. Prominent here were child motor and cognitive development, IQ, and temperament. IQ was an especially important consideration with regard to certain outcomes, such as performance in school. Temperament was important to study not only as a variable to control but also in conjunction with experience. Whether experience predicts outcomes above and beyond temperament would be only one question. Other questions were as follows: Do temperament and experience together predict certain outcomes more strongly?

Do they predict better to different outcomes, or do they perhaps represent different pathways to similar outcomes? We assessed temperament at multiple times through both direct observation and parental report.

Correlated changes also had to be considered. The possibilities here are numerous, but one example will suffice, that of the child's language development. It is possible, for example, that certain parenting qualities influence both young children's sense of security and their language development. The resulting competence with peers (or success in school, in particular) may be due to the language skills of the child, and not due to the child's capacity to trust in relationships. The only way to know is to have assessed language development. Of course, if quality of care exerted its influence on development through its impact on language, or self-regulation ability, or through its support for adequate functioning with peers, then this would not really diminish its importance. But it would lead to a different understanding of the developmental process than if outcomes were mediated by early trust experiences, or by all of these. Such an understanding of the developmental process is the main goal.

Measurement of child functioning across ages also was comprehensive, capturing both positive aspects of adaptation and problem behavior. We assessed motivational, emotional, and social aspects of behavior. Thus, at various ages, we assessed exploration, curiosity, flexibility, emotional regulation and self-esteem, as well as problem-solving attitude, sense of effectiveness, and enthusiasm for new activities. We measured how well the child got along with teachers and peers, and we measured school success and failure, behavioral and emotional problems, and, ultimately, diagnosable psychopathology.

Finally, we sought to capture not just outward manifestations of the child's functioning but the child's interior world as well. If, for example, early experience is to have an enduring effect, it must somehow be internalized and carried forward. To some degree, this would involve basic patterns of emotional regulation, which we could capture through overt behavior. But it also should be reflected in children's basic expectations and beliefs about the social world and themselves in it. Bowlby (1973) argued that the child abstracts core aspects of experience, and that such mentally represented abstractions then guide subsequent expectations and behavior. Including representational measures in our study was crucial, because we were not only interested in *whether* experience influences development but also in *how* it does so. Such representations would, of course, become more sophisticated with development, so it was necessary to utilize different assessments age by age. Our measures included play, drawings, story completions, and other forms of narrative. Having these measures over time enabled us to examine the interplay between changing experience and changing representation, as well as to see whether representation "carried" prior experience forward (Carlson, Sroufe, & Egeland, 2004).

Thus, our goal was to assess all salient aspects of the child's functioning in all pertinent settings (home, school, and peer group), as well as the myriad potential influences on development. Our assessments were aimed at different levels, made use of multiple methodologies, and drew upon multiple informants. We carried out direct behavioral observation, administered formal tests, and conducted interviews with teachers, parents, counselors, and the children themselves. As often as possible, we used converging measures at the same time.

Complementary Study of Normal and Maladaptive Development

Our study is based in the discipline of developmental psychopathology. A central premise of this discipline is that the study of normative processes is informed by the study of individual differences, just as variations are informed by an understanding of normative processes (e.g., Cicchetti & Cohen, 1995). The same developmental principles govern normal and abnormal alike. Therefore, while we had a keen interest in understanding the origins of child, adolescent, and adult problems, we began at each age by examining the variety of ways that children were developing well. This set the stage for describing adaptations that were nonfunctional, in the sense that they would likely compromise later development.

In our view, all children at each age make the best adaptation possible in light of available personal resources, environmental resources, and the challenges they are facing. In some circumstances, not seeking close contact from a parent, or being highly demanding, can be the most functional thing for a child to do in an effort to meet his or her immediate needs. Sometimes, staying clear of a parent is necessary. Other times, being demanding is the only way to get any attention. But if these become the core of established patterns, they may be maladaptive in the long run because of experiences they compromise at the time and reactions they garner from others later.

Development in Context

Adequately assessing the contexts surrounding our participating families was crucial for several reasons. First, examining development in context immediately puts to rest the issue of parental blame. Yes, children develop within the context of the care their parents and other caregivers provide. But such parenting itself takes place in a broader context of challenges and support. As we report in several later chapters, we find that the stress and, conversely, the social support that parents encounter is related both to the quality of their parenting and to child outcomes. Likewise, assessments of the parents' own developmental histories, another aspect of the context of their parenting, have notable predictive power. Thus, in addition to being not at all useful, blaming parents for child problems is dramatically oversimplified and begins an infinite regress back to the earliest human couple.

Second, as alluded to earlier, the stresses and other surrounding circumstances (e.g., violent neighborhoods, substandard housing, and frequent moves) that impact on parents may also directly impact the child. As with temperament, we wanted not only to control for such variation but also to investigate how such factors, assessed age by age, combined with caregiving experience in predicting various outcomes.

Finally, our central interest was in developmental process, not simply whether some experience or some pattern of behavior at an early point was related to some later outcome. We were interested in the changing pattern of adaptation as children progressed in development, and as prior experience and adaptation interacted with current challenges and supports. We were just as interested in change as we were in continuity of individual development. In our view, as we discuss in the next chapter, such change is a lawful reflection of changing circumstances. We have found repeatedly that as family stress and social support increase and decrease, or when level of parental depression changes, child functioning likewise worsens or improves (e.g., Egeland, Kalkoske, Gottesman, & Erickson, 1990).

In the position we outline, early experience is important, but it alone does not determine child outcome. In accord with Bowlby (1973), we believe that development is always a product of the history of the child and current circumstances. Since the circumstances facing children go beyond the purview of parents alone, so then does the responsibility for the child's well-being go beyond the family to the broader society.

Early Assessments at the Level of Relationships

We felt it was essential in the first years of life to cast our assessments at the level of children's primary relationships and the contexts surrounding them. First, child behavior is notably unstable in the early weeks and months of life, and early child characteristics do not predict well to later outcomes, once context is considered (Sameroff & Chandler, 1975; Sameroff & Fiese, 2000). Second, we were seeking to predict rather complex outcomes, including the later organization of attitudes, expectations, and behavior, which is called "personality." While infant behavior is not at this level of complexity, the organized dyadic relationship is. Therefore, we thought assessments at the level of relationships would be more powerful predictors of outcome. Finally, parents are formed personalities, and parenting attitudes and expectations are established. Thus, from a purely practical statistical standpoint, it would seem that measures of parenting would have a better chance to predict child outcome. We discuss theoretical reasons for this position in Chapter 2.

These, then, are some of the practical reasons for designing our study the way we did. In part, we did it this way because there was no other way to do it properly. We wanted to provide the most comprehensive study to date of the process of individual development. Therefore, we needed to study a large number of families over time, cataloging how parents treated their children, the ups and downs of their lives, influences from outside the family, salient characteristics of the children in multiple domains of functioning, and a range of outcome arenas in the subsequent years. We knew at the outset that development was complex, and our research has only further underscored this reality.

KEY CLAIMS AND GUIDE TO THE BOOK

In this book, we claim to demonstrate important features of individual development. We conclude, among other things, (1) that nothing is more important in the development of the child than the care received, including that in the early years; (2) that individuals are always impacted by the entire history of cumulative experience, and even following periods of dramatic change, early experience is not erased; (3) that personal characteristics such as resilience and various forms of psychopathology are developmental constructions and not inherent, inborn characteristics; (4) that dichotomies such as parents *or* peers, temperament *or* experience, and past experience *or* current circumstances are almost always false; (5) that change, as well as continuity, in individual development is coherent and lawful; and (6) that ultimately, the individual person can only be understood within a model of continuing transactions between developing persons and the supports and challenges they are facing.

It is noteworthy that some of these claims are diametrically opposed to those made authoritatively by other psychologists. We need, in particular, to say a few words about genetic interpretations. We claim that parenting, not just the genes that parents provide, is an important influence on children. In a widely publicized book, Judith Rich Harris (1998) wrote that, on the contrary, peers and not parents are the major influence on development, and that any influence parents have is through the genes that they pass on, and not through anything they do. Many psychologists attribute a powerful role to genes in explaining individual behavior, although there is recently a growing understanding that genes always must be viewed in interaction with the environment (e.g., Caspi et al., 2002; Suomi, 2002). As Gottesman and Hanson (in press) have written: "Questions of nature versus nurture are meaningless, and we must return to epigenesis—the way in which biology and experience work together throughout thick and thin."

Genetic influences were not part of our study, although we did measure temperament, which many attribute to genetic influences. We did not use a twin design, and we have no DNA data. How then can we conclude anything regarding the impact of care? As one reviewer of a draft of this book asked, in response to our finding that being a single parent is a strong predictor of attention problems in children (Chapter 12), "How do we know that isn't a genetic effect? How do these mothers get to be single parents in the first place?" It was implied that our correlation was due to some shared genetic traits between mother and child that were responsible for both the mother's unwed pregnancy and attention problems of the child (e.g., low IQ, impulsivity). We argue that becoming an unmarried parent is due to complex factors and is linked to attention problems because of the ways such overtaxed parents at times stimulate and lean on their children. Can such a claim be supported?

We, of course, were not trying to prove that genes or other biological factors are unimportant. That would have been preposterous even in 1974, when we began. Indeed, much of our perspective was based in evolution and biology, especially our understanding of the kind of care children need. We were seeking merely to demonstrate that what children experience and their life circumstances *are* important. Our view of development, which is elaborated in Chapter 2, is in accord with modern biology (e.g., Goodwin, 1994). In this position, development is the result of the total "field," that is, genes, immediately surrounding context, supporting circumstances, and prior individual history.

There were many ways we were able to show that care and context are important parts of this field, parts that have been somewhat underemphasized in recent decades. We mentioned in the preceding section our finding that changes in parental depression or changes in stresses and supports that parents experience lead to changes in parenting and in child behavior. When single mothers form a stable partnership or experience declining stress, behavior problems of their children decline (e.g., Erickson et al., 1985; see Chapters 7 and 12, this volume). With such data, any genetic influences are held constant.

Furthermore, in many of our analyses of ties between experience and later behavior, we statistically controlled for variables such as IQ and aspects of temperament, which are commonly argued to have genetic bases. Also, many of the constructs we measured were at the level of relationships, not individuals, such as the child's positive expectations concerning a particular partner. When we show, for example, that at ages 8 and 11, children's positive representations of parents or peers are related to early reliability of care, controlling for IQ, the case is fairly compelling (see Chapter 8). Finally, we at times made precise, theoretically specified predictions that would require post hoc gymnastics to explain genetically; for example, that parental rejection would lead to child dependency (see Chapter 7).

Another claim we make is that early experience has lasting importance, even following changing circumstances, for example, forecasting those who recover following adversity (Chapter 11). Other psychologists have written that early experience may be of trivial importance if different experiences occur later (e.g., Kagan, 1984; Lewis, 1998). Again, the question arises, why should the reader accept our conclusions rather than those of others? Accepting our claims should be based on the degree to which you are persuaded of the soundness of our approach and the adequacy of our measurements. Our conclusions regarding the roles of parents and peers, the distinctiveness of their implications for various outcomes, and their joint, interactive, and transactive influences hinge on how adequately we measured parent and peer experiences, and carefully controlled for other major relevant factors. Likewise, the validity of our claims regarding early experience depends on the adequacy of our measures of early experience, later experience, surrounding contexts, and outcomes. Our finding that school success and failure are hugely influenced by history of care should be accepted only to the degree that we have adequately measured and taken into account IQ, socioeconomic status, and other factors known to be related to school success. We trust that the distinctiveness of this book is not the uniqueness of our claims, some of which *are* widely held, but the strength of the evidence marshaled to support them.

Therefore, in Chapters 2–4, we overview the conceptual underpinnings of our work and the methods we employed. In Part II of the book (Chapters 5–10), we describe the emergence of the person, attained patterns of adaptation, and their origins and course, age by age. We not only predict individual outcomes but also account for changes in trajectories. Part III is devoted to development and psychopathology. Chapter 11 describes the developmental process, what we have learned about the interplay of experience, representation of experience, and surrounding circumstances over time. We account for the fate of early experience following change and the development of individual constructs such as resilience. In Chapter 12, we present a developmental model of psychopathology, and provide data on the development and course of disturbed patterns of behavior, including attention/hyperactivity problems, depression and anxiety, and conduct disturbance. Implications for assessment, classification, treatment of problems, and intervention follow in Chapter 13. Then, in a final chapter, we discuss current directions of our work and present very recent data on adult disturbance, adult relationships and relationship representation, and continuity of parenting across generations, based on new studies of the children of our grown-up participants.

Some readers, perhaps because they know our project well or have an interest in a particular age, may wish to skip forward, turning back to the methods chapters as needed. But we would urge most to read the book as written, to understand both our assumptions (Chapter 2) and our methods (Chapters 3 and 4) before delving into the findings. We have tried to be concise in writing these chapters and to make them valuable reading in their own right. Some readers also may wish to skip ahead to the more clinical chapters at the end. The book is written so that this is possible. But, again, we urge most readers to read first about the normal developmental process and individual variations in adaptation. Understanding basic patterns of adaptation and maladaptation at each phase of development is crucial for all clinical work. Our view of clinical problems springs from this. The story of development is a complex tale, and to tell it completely takes time, but it is also an endlessly fascinating tale every step of the way.

CHAPTER 2

A Perspective on Development

What exists at one phase becomes transformed into
something related to, but also different than, what existed
earlier.

—BREGER (1974)

We began our longitudinal studies at a particularly interesting
time in the history of psychology. It was a time when, from one widely
held perspective, such an enterprise seemed unpromising, if not doomed
to failure. From another perspective, however, it may have been a
uniquely opportune moment.

The 1960s and early 1970s marked the demise of a certain conception of personality and at least one view of development. Social learning
theorists at the time were presenting empirical demonstrations that people behave differently in different situations, and even in similar situations at different times. As argued by Walter Mischel (1968; 1973) and
others, it was situations, not personality structures, that seemed to determine behavior. This work launched a debate about the relative importance of situations and persons that lasted for decades. For a time it also
called into question the very construct of personality itself. If people cannot be counted on to behave in a consistent way across time and situations, then is it even meaningful to talk about personality? More pertinent to our work, does it make sense to attempt to predict stable,
individual differences from earlier points in life, if such differences in
adult behavior are not meaningful in the first place?

Work specifically centered in developmental psychology at this time also was calling key constructs into question. Most noteworthy, a study that, ironically, was conducted in our own department, reported that infants' behavior with their mothers also varied from situation to situation and showed little stability across time (Masters & Wellman, 1974). Infants sometimes looked at and vocalized to their mothers a lot, or cried or hugged them a lot; at other times, or when observed on another day, they did not. Given this, was attachment a meaningful individual differences construct? Did it make any sense at all to try to predict later characteristics of children from assessments of the infant–caregiver relationship? These would seem to be two large problems for our study before we even began. We were proposing to predict individual differences in later life from experience and adaptation at earlier ages, including from relationships in infancy.

Important longitudinal studies of the time also were discouraging about the predictability of individual behavior over time. A prominent study of the era, the Fels longitudinal study (Kagan & Moss, 1962), provided only very modest evidence for the stability of characteristics such as dependency or aggressiveness. Results were especially weak predicting from the first years of life forward. Viewing a study such as ours as foolhardy, or not workable "in principle," was certainly understandable in light of these studies.

Today, we know that all of this information can be interpreted in a vastly different way. It is not personality or attachment or continuity of individual behavior that is called into question by the empirical findings presented in these studies, but rather a particular view of personality and a particular kind of developmental continuity.

Let us consider an example of infant behavior to illustrate the issues here: A mother carries her 12-month-old son into a playroom, sets him on the floor by a group of toys, and sits in a chair. The baby glances back at her, then plays quietly with the toys for 3 minutes. This ends the first episode. A stranger enters the room and also sits in a chair. The baby looks at her, then glances at his mother, then looks at her again. Then he plays again, vocalizing to his mother twice about a ball. While playing, the ball rolls by the stranger. He crawls to the ball near her feet, then looks up at the stranger. Then he turns and rapidly crawls to his mother, and stands up with one hand on her knee. From there, he turns and looks again at the stranger, who is smiling at him. He smiles back. Then he moves back to the toys and plays. In a bit, the stranger joins him in play, and he, with one glance to his mother, accepts her overtures. In the next episode, the mother leaves the room. He looks at the door and fusses briefly, but the stranger is able to attract him back to the toys. His play remains subdued, and he occasionally glances at the door. When his mother returns after 3 minutes, he scurries over to her with a toy. She picks him up and carries him to the center of the room, then sits again (the stranger leaves). He now plays facing her, looking at her twice and smiling once. His mother leaves a second time. Now he is quite upset and crying. The stranger returns and is able to settle him somewhat, but after a bit, he starts fussing again. His mother returns. He crawls rapidly to her, puts his arms up, and she picks him up. He leans in with his arms around her neck. She pats his back. His fussing stops in a few seconds, and soon he is pointing to a toy. She puts him down and takes her chair. He watches her sit, then begins playing again.

This is the kind of thing Masters and Wellman were coding for their 1974 paper, and if we examine behavior frequencies, we see the problem. First of all, many behaviors (smiling, vocalizing) are rare, so they are not likely stable. In fact, as described, the infant looks at the stranger more times than he looks at his mother in the beginning episodes, and he smiles at them equally often (once). This could suggest equal attachment to the stranger from a perspective that only frequencies of attachment behaviors matter. Second, the behaviors are not stable across the different episodes. The baby does not cry much, until the mother leaves the second time. He is in bodily contact with her only briefly early on, then a fair amount in the last episode. Clearly, these attachment behaviors are not being uniformly expressed.

On the other hand, the *patterning* of this infant's behavior is quite coherent when one considers when the baby acted, as well as what he did. That his proximity to his mother occurred precisely when he had become aroused at finding himself suddenly close to the stranger, or following stressful separations, makes sense. His looks to his mother when the stranger entered and when the stranger got down to play with him (now referred to as "social referencing"; Sorce, Emde, Campos, & Klinnert, 1985) would seem to serve as a source of reassurance. In fact, much of his behavior, including the changes in play, can be summarized as using his mother as a "secure base" for exploration. The behavior is not inconsistent; it is organized and meaningful. The behavior changes, but it does so in a coherent way in response to changes in stress. Other infants would show different, but also coherent, patterns of behavior.

In a key, early study, Everett Waters (1978) demonstrated that, in fact, such patterns of attachment behaviors were stable over a 6-month period, even though frequencies of particular discrete behaviors were not. A 20-minute observation yielded stability in patterns, whereas Waters estimated that hundreds of hours of observation would have been required for comparable stability of discrete behavior frequencies.

Thus, part of the resolution of the person–situation debate was methodological and part was conceptual. When enough data are aggregated, people in fact show some stability in their behavior, especially over time in the same situations, but even across situations. One reason for instability in individual differences, therefore, was inadequate sampling of behavior (e.g., Epstein, 1979). Even more important, however, from another conceptualization of personality, people change their behavior in characteristic ways in response to varying situational demands. (Mischel allowed for this possibility, but argued that there were no data to support it in 1968.) For the well-adapted person, there are times when constraint is called for, and other times when unrestrained exuberance is appropriate. Meaningful differences in personality concern variations in the extent to which and the way individuals adjust their behavior in terms of these demands (e.g., Block & Block, 1980). Personality is not primarily reflected in stability of behavior (in the sense of exhibiting identical behavior at all times and in all circumstances), but in the coherence of behavior, that is, the way it is organized. As with the infant behavior described earlier, individuals both vary in their behavior and show coherence in behavior across situations. Such a position is now widely accepted (e.g., Fleeson, 2001). Personality as unchanging behavior has perished, but not so for personality as the organization of attitudes, expectations, and behavior (Sroufe, 1989).

Likewise, early longitudinal studies did not discredit the continuity of functioning over time but only a view of continuity as "homotypic," that is, as frequencies of particular behavioral expressions being identical over time. Models of "heterotypic continuity"—changing forms or manifestations of an underlying construct (Kagan, 1971)—were not really tested by the early studies, nor was coherence of individual development examined. By coherence, we mean the way the organization of functioning at one age is forecast by prior organizations and leads in a logical way to later patterns of adaptation. Mischel, himself, in a later important study, showed continuity in a key self-control characteristic from ages 5 to 12 by utilizing the concept of heterotypic continuity (Mischel, Shoda, & Rodriguez, 1989).

The early studies started in a logical place, and they contributed to the field by showing that existing models of developmental continuity were not adequate. If you want to predict aggression in children, you cannot do so by looking at aggressiveness in infants, when such a construct is not yet meaningful. It turns out that aggressiveness is highly predictable from early in life, but from patterns of organization in the infant–caregiver system, not from isomorphic behaviors of infants. Likewise, characteristics such as social isolation, attention problems, and low self-esteem (or their positive counterparts) turn out to be predictable, but only within a complex model of development, emphasizing the level of organization.

The static trait views of personality and linear views of development presented earlier were consistent with the learning theories that rose to prominence in the 1950s and 1960s. These theories in their early forms attempted to explain all behavior either in terms of association and drive reduction, or as acquired bit by bit through reinforcement. These were powerful positions, and their lasting legacy is the idea that predicting actual behavior should be the final arbiter in psychological science. We are indebted to them. There is no question of the power of conditioning in the expression of behavior. However, classic learning theories lent themselves to very mechanistic views of behavior, with little room for emotions, goals, or self-organization.

If behavior is derived from the consistency with which drives are gratified, then vital individual differences in behavior should vary dimensionally, being constantly manifest with a particular frequency or intensity. Similarly, from the classic operant viewpoint, if each separate behavior is acquired separately, bit by bit through reinforcement, only frequency of reinforcement is germane, and individual differences in behavior should be similarly linear. This position quickly was fitted to (even inspired) situational specificity, because discriminatively different situations would be linked to separate reinforcement contingencies. But there could be nothing here about the individual behaving predictably differently in one situation, given his or her behavior in another; that is, no internal organizing processes were postulated.

These early learning views were not fully developmental positions. Of most note, little attention was paid to when in development something happened. Changes in the maturity of the organism or prior experiences were not considered as fundamental to the reaction to external contingencies. There was no evolving "structure" of personality that might lead to qualitatively new reactions. There was no idea of transformed meaning of prior experience based upon new development. Behavior was the simple accumulation of experience. Modern social learning views have, of course, evolved considerably, with increased roles for cognition, emotion, and self-constructs (e.g., Bandura, 1997).

CONCEPTUAL AND THEORETICAL SUPPORTS

Even as we began our study, four sets of resources were available to us. The first was a research strategy, evolved to study early disturbance and positive adaptation in a coordinated way. Second was a dynamic, nonlinear perspective on behavior. The third resource was a set of unifying principles. Finally, there were serviceably formal theories of development that could guide creation of our own theoretical perspective. We briefly review each of these resources in turn.

Risk Research

Risk research was a strategy originally formulated to shed light on the origins of schizophrenia, but it ultimately had a great range of application (e.g., Garmezy, 1975). Schizophrenia is rare, afflicting about one person out of every 100 in the general population, so studying childhood antecedents of this adult disorder prospectively would require a huge sample to net many target cases. By studying the offspring of schizophrenic mothers, one could increase the number of eventual cases (to perhaps 4 or 5 per 100 for those raised in adoptive homes), thus achieving greater statistical power. "At-risk" children could be compared to nonrisk children to seek clues to early markers of schizophrenia. Even more important, comparing at-risk children who do and do not ultimately develop the disorder, one could possible discover "protective factors," that is, resources that promote resilience in the face of risk. Ultimately, this could provide guidance for prevention and early intervention efforts.

Quickly, this strategy was applied to other outcomes and to other risk factors. Poverty, for example, was a major risk factor not only for schizophrenia but also for other problems, dwarfing maternal disorder in its general predictive power (e.g., Sameroff, 2000). Child maltreatment and even early patterns of child maladaptation also could serve to define risk groups. A risk factor is anything that increments the probability of some negative outcome. This strategy therefore led to the broad study of risk and protective factors, vulnerability and resiliency, including our own study.

Early risk research, however, was atheoretical. It provided no guidance from a developmental perspective regarding what to assess in childhood to track progress of the groups of children. At first, in fact, researchers primarily looked for similar disturbances in behavior that were ultimately shown by adults. Beyond this general strategy, we would need theoretical guidance. For example, several theorists (e.g., Erikson, 1950/1963; Havighurst, 1948/1972) had proposed the idea of development as a series of changing issues that provided foci for adaptation at different ages. Given such a changing landscape for adaptation, continuity would be reflected in qualitative similarity in the way issues were negotiated across ages, inferred from patterning of behavior. Our task was to spell out such issues age by age in a comprehensive manner, based on a coherent theoretical perspective.

The Dynamic Systems Approach

Dynamic systems perspectives provide an alternative to seeing the causes of behavior or development as simply inherent in the organism, as being stamped in by the environment, or as a linear consequence of some initial cause (Gottlieb, 1971; Gottlieb, Gilbert, & Halpern, 2002; Sameroff, 2000; Sander, 1962, 1975; Stechler & Carpenter, 1967; von Bertalanffy, 1952; Weiss, 1949). In general terms, systems imply the mutual definition and interdependence of parts and wholes. Dynamic, living systems consist of mutually influencing constituents interacting over time. Only in functioning does the whole (or a part) have meaning. Such relationships between constituents and the whole tend to be maintained even as parts (and the whole) change. In terms of human relationship systems, this is what accounts for continuity across generations (Sroufe & Fleeson, 1986). Moreover, any biological system includes not only the parts of the organism but also both organism and environment. In systems viewpoints new, nonobvious forms of increasing complexity "emerge" from the co-actions of existing parts and/or in the face of new environmental demands (Gottlieb, 1971; Gottlieb et al., 2002). Concepts such as internally generated aims or goals are needed to understand "a self-organizing, intact biological system existing and developing in constant interaction with a changing environment" (Stechler & Carpenter, 1967, p. 167).

Early experience or early adaptation is important in systems perspectives as an "initiating condition," setting the stage for subsequent transactions and providing base forms of organization. At the same time, systems theories are nonlinear in the sense that outcomes depend not only on initiating conditions but also their complex interactions with subsequent conditions. Sameroff and Chandler (1975) provided an important framework for our research, which they called a "transactional model." A key premise of this position concerns the ongoing, dynamic interchanges between person and environment. The impact of any early condition depends on the environment encountered, and responses to later conditions depend on prior history. Premature but healthy newborns go on to have problems only in impoverished environments, not in advantaged environments. The impact of particular patterns of parental socialization depend on the prior history of the caregiver–infant relationship (e.g., Belsky & Fearon, 2002; Kochanska, Aksan, Knaack, & Rhines, 2004). This has been a critical aspect of our thinking.

Again, useful as they were, systems perspectives provided no precise theoretical guidance. They pointed to neither critical initiating conditions nor to crucial aspects of the environment that must be considered. However, they did entail certain principles that would help us select the background theories for our work.

Three Guiding Principles

Our work is guided by the idea that certain principles characterize the development of all living systems, from plant life, to the human brain, to the development of the person (Edelman, 1992; Goodwin, 1994; Schore, 1994; Waldrop, 1992). The *first* such principle concerns the unity of development, the idea that the organism develops as a whole (Fogel, 1993; Thelen, 1989). As Kuo (1967) put it, "In any given response of the animal to its environment, internal or external, and at any given stage of development, the whole organism is involved" (p. 92). For us, the unit of study is the whole person. It is the person that is adapting, and the patterns of adaptation we seek to assess are at the level of the person. We may examine aspects of cognition or emotion, or social behavior, but we do this always with an eye on overall adaptation. Cognition, emotion, and social behavior develop in an integrative, mutually influential way.

The *second* principle is that development is characterized by emerging complexity or self-organization. New, more complex behavior emerges from what was present previously, and new structures show emergent properties not specified in the constituent parts.

Development of the fetus can serve as an illustration of emerging complexity and as a basic model for all development. At first, there is simple cell division, a quantitative process with an increase in number of cells but little increase in complexity. Then, there is a series of qualitative transformations "wherein an initial structuralization into layers of cells (ectoderm, mesoderm, endoderm) leads to interconnected structures and systems, which then begin to function" (Sroufe, 1996, p. 39). The changes in organized complexity are sufficiently dramatic that different names are used to label the organism at different phases (zygote, blastocyst, embryo, fetus), yet these changes are not specified in the initial cells themselves or in the early structures. Rather, it is the co-actions of the cells, and later co-actions of evolving systems, in their environment that lead to emerging complexity (Goodwin, 1994).

The developing brain provides another example (e.g., Cicchetti, 2002; Cicchetti & Cannon, 1999; Nelson, 2002; Siegel, 1999). As with the fetus, the brain does not develop by simply adding neurons one by one; rather, it entails a process of increasing organization and complexity. In the beginning, there is overproduction of neurons. Subsequent development involves both pruning and interconnecting of neurons into systems, then systems of systems. The migration of cells to their ultimate locations and their interconnections with other cells are again determined by co-actions among the constituent units.

For the fetus and the brain, and, we would argue, for the human personality as well, development is characterized by "differentiation." This is our *third* principle. At first, there is a mass of undifferentiated units (e.g., cells that are virtually all the same). Then, these form general structures. Later, these structures become more refined and specialized as they are organized into systems. It is this process of differentiation that makes early phases so important. Refinements can only operate on pre-viously existing structures. Thus, early fetal damage, or early brain dam-age, has profound effects. Massive structural damage can result. Even a relatively small insult early on can be powerful. The same principles of integration, self-organization, and differentiation govern abnormal de-velopment, as well as normal development.

Dante Cicchetti (personal communication, 2001) has described the working of these principles with regard to abnormal brain development:

> Abnormal brain development would be a self-organizing phenomenon. Perturbations that take place in the developing brain can trigger the cas-cade of growth and formation changes that could lead neural systems down a path that would deviate from that usually taken in normal neurobiological development. Abnormal perturbations at one stage of brain development could impair the construction of some new struc-tures and functions, distort the form of later emerging ones, perhaps en-able the construction of ones that would normally not emerge, and/or limit the elaboration and usage of previously emerged structures and functions. And then abnormal spontaneous or initiated neural activity could trigger the formation of a wide range of structural and functional "mis-organizations," even in sites distant from the point of the actual abnormal perturbation. Such early developmental abnormalities may lead to the development of aberrant neural circuitry and often com-pound themselves into relatively enduring forms of pathology.

We believe that these considerations that apply to the development of the body and the brain apply to the human personality. Because of emergent complexity and the phenomenon of differentiation, early dis-tortions may have profound, far-reaching implications, even though they cannot be said to specify or by themselves directly cause later forms.

Developmental Theories

A number of developmental theories available in the 1970s were either based upon developmental systems thinking or at least were congruent with it. One theory that was very influential in our thinking was that of Heinz Werner (1948). He argued that "the development of biological forms is expressed by an *increasing differentiation* and an increasing subordination or *hierarchization* of parts. Hierarchization means that for any organic structure the organization of the differentiated parts is a closed totality, an ordering and grouping of parts in terms of the whole organism" (p. 41, emphasis added). This is a structural theory, contain-ing the nonlinear idea that an acquired capacity is retained, yet changes its meaning when new capacities are acquired and organized with it into a more complex whole. In terms of personality formation, this would mean that early malevolent experience is not erased, but its meaning may change in light of subsequent development. Development is characterized by increasing complexity of organization, not simply quantitative additions. This would be central to what we would mean by a "developmental" position.

Piaget's (1952) theory, which became prominent in the United States with the publication of Flavell's book in 1963, also was important to us. Most notable were his ideas regarding the child's active role in development and the idea of qualitative change. For Piaget, the child actively engages the surround, seeking mastery and nurturing its mind through this engagement. These efforts use all the tools the child has at hand, and as the tools change, so does the child's functioning in a fundamental way. The child understands the world, and therefore experiences it, in fundamentally different ways at different ages, especially between infancy and later childhood. One reason that infancy may have special importance is because it is not subject to verbal recall and analysis. Piaget's process of "equilibration" also provided a serviceable explanation of developmental change, based upon a clash between existing structures and new goals or unassimilable demands from the environment.

Vygotsky's (1962, 1978) theory also directly influenced us. His theory represents a set of ideas about the integration of emotion and cognition, and the importance of context in development that were just beginning to become prominent in the 1970s (e.g., Bronfenbrenner, 1979). They certainly were part of our thinking from the beginning (Sroufe, Waters, & Matas, 1974). We were especially compelled by two of Vygotsky's ideas: (1) that many experiences and capacities are first mastered within social relationships and only later are capacities of the individual, and (2) that rather than the environment stamping experiences into the child, the child "appropriates" that which is provided in the surround (Rogoff, 1990). A closely related idea espoused by Louis Sander (1962, 1975) was explicitly part of our thinking. This was the notion that in the organization of the caregiver–infant system was the foundation for the organization that would become the personality. First, there is relationship; the emergent self-organization is a reflection of that prior organization.

Finally, we mention here the "genetic field theory" of René Spitz (Spitz, Emde, & Metcalf, 1970). Spitz was popular in very few circles when we began our study and has only recently achieved acclaim in light of new studies of institution-reared infants. Spitz had observed infants in orphanages in the 1940s and 1950s, concluding that their failure to thrive was due to a lack of loving care. Spitz's research was not tightly controlled, leaving open the possibility that some factor other than lack of maternal love (e.g., sensory deprivation) was the culprit, and that the rampant infections (and deaths) in these settings were not consequences of infant despondency but were causes. Recent, controlled research makes clear that he was much more right than wrong (e.g., Gunnar, 2001), and bolsters two of his concepts that strongly influenced us.

The first is the idea of "sensitive period," embraced by numerous students of animal behavior and by researchers of language development (e.g., Lenneberg, 1967). Briefly, this refers to a special openness to, or requirement for, certain kinds of experience during a particular developmental period.[1] Thus, the child may be less responsive to, or responsive in a different way to, the same stimulation occurring at another time. For example, it is difficult to acquire language unless the child is exposed to language in the first years of life. Of more interest to Spitz, if infants are deprived of responsive care, the capacity for human attachments may be compromised in a fundamental way. This notion is supported by the outpouring of information on brain development, in which neural developments have been found to be curtailed unless certain stimulation is present at particular times (Nelson, 2002; Schore, 1994; Siegel, 1999).

The second concept of Spitz that influenced us was the "developmental prototype" (Spitz et al., 1970). This is a seminal idea. A developmental prototype is a root form, the progenitor of later forms but related to them in a complex, nonlinear way. In keeping with other organization theories, such as Werner's, the later form emerges from the prototype (is inspired by it) and embodies it in its core, but it is by no means a replica. The new form is a transformation of the prototype. For example, the newborn smile is the prototype for the later social smile, but not because it is identical in form, cause, or function (Sroufe, 1996). The newborn smile involves no mouth opening, no crinkling of the eyes, nor is it based on cognitive mastery or recognition, and it is not part of a social exchange. This smile, which occurs almost solely during sleep, reflects the rising and falling of central nervous system (CNS) excitation, occurring either randomly or in response to physical stimulation. It is the prototype for the later social smile because of the arousal modulation core common to both. But arousal modulation in the 3-month-old is due to particular meanings resulting from cognitive processes, often occurring in social encounters. The latter develops from the former in a logical, describable process and embodies the initial core, but it has a fundamen-

---

1. "Sensitive period" is preferred over the term "critical period" (which Spitz used), because it does not imply the impossibility of corrective experience or a very narrow age span of influence.

tally different place in the functioning of the infant. We believe that developmental prototypes apply to broader constructs such as personality as well. We also believe they apply to individuals, as well as normatively, and that early individual adaptations are well viewed as prototypes in this sense. They will be reflected in core features of later patterns of adaptation, however much more complex these may be.

Freud's Psychoanalytic Theory

Properly situating Freudian theory in the background of our work is complicated. Freud was the original author of several hypotheses we were to test in our research, including the idea that early experience has special significance, that the emotional life of infants is of great importance, and that early primary relationships are central in the shaping of personality. Freud (1940/1964) even put forward the "prototype hypothesis" (that the early primary relationship was the prototype for all subsequent relationships). Given this, one might have expected close connections between our work and Freud's theory. On the other hand, classic Freudian theory was a drive reduction theory, with quantitative and linear predictions concerning development.

As did George Klein (1976), we distinguished between Freud's clinical observations and the drive-based explanations he evolved for them. For example, infants do develop special connections with caregivers, but not through secondary drive reduction in association with feeding. The conceptual problems of the fixed energy, hydraulic, drive reduction model were notable and thoroughly discredited (to some extent even by Freud in his later writing; Loevinger, 1976). If the master motive was to keep tension low, why would animals learn complicated behaviors simply for the reward of looking through a window (Butler, 1953), and why would children in their play, and adults in their actions, seek to reenact conflicts or repeat challenging events? If attachment to mother was based on oral gratification, why would Harlow's (1966) monkeys spend their time with the cloth surrogate that did not feed them and run to it when frightened (rather than to the wire mother equipped with a bottle)? A theory based solely on drive reduction would never be adequate.

There are, of course, other aspects of psychoanalytic theory in which mastery and meaning are emphasized rather than drive reduction (Breger, 1974; Freud, 1926). To us, it seemed entirely possible to retain certain core ideas of psychoanalytic theory while discarding the mechanistic drive concepts. We followed the lead of a long line of scholars (e.g., Erikson, 1950/1963) in (1) broadening Freud's psychosexual issues (oral, anal, etc.) to psychosocial issues (trust, autonomy, and control), (2) replacing mechanistic concepts such as fixation and regression with developmental concepts such as prototype and hierarchical organization, and (3) replacing the "pleasure" principle (keep tension low) with striving for mastery and coherence as the larger goals guiding behavior (Breger, 1974). Central roles for emotion, early experience, and vital social relationships need not be wedded to drive reduction mechanisms (Sroufe, 1996). This broader, evolved psychoanalytic theory really had not been tested and was compatible with the other developmental theories discussed earlier.

Bowlby–Ainsworth Attachment Theory

Bowlby's theory became prominent just before we began our work and was the most direct inspiration for our long-term study (e.g., Bowlby, 1969/1982). While initially rejected by many in the psychoanalytic community, Bowlby's theory is psychoanalytic in terms of the core features just described. However, rather than being couched in 19th-century physics, as were Freud's ideas, Bowlby's ideas sprang from evolutionary theory, ethology, and biological systems theory. He and Ainsworth (1969) both specifically eschewed drive reduction concepts in explaining attachment. Infants are attached to caregivers because caregivers have been interactively present in an ongoing way. That is all that is required. The disposition to organize behavior with regard to the goal of proximity to a caregiver (as well as the caregiver's inclination to be responsive to these bids) was selected through evolution. Since humans remain relatively helpless for many months, being protected by caregivers was essential for survival. Thus, infants engage in attachment-serving behaviors, because they develop the capacity to do so and are biologically disposed to do so. Just as a bird will build a nest until it is complete (or continually start over if an experimenter dissembles it), in conditions of threat, humans will direct an array of behaviors to a caregiver until proximity is achieved. No special attachment drive need be postulated.

Behavior is goal-directed, not driven, and not conditioned in a simple way. Many behaviors can serve the attachment system, and no behavior is exclusively an attachment behavior. If one behavior fails in the aim of achieving proximity (the infant calls but the caregiver does not come), another may be used (the infant raises its arms). Likewise, with development, as new behaviors become available, the infant shows increasing flexibility, readily replacing less differentiated reactions (crawling to the caregiver vs. simply crying when aroused at an earlier age). Before we began our study, Ainsworth had already shown that when mothers promptly picked up and comforted crying infants, they cried *less* by the end of the first year (Ainsworth, Bell, & Stayton, 1974). They had not been conditioned to be "cry babies." They had learned about the effectiveness of signals and could now substitute more flexible signals as they became available. In the Bowlby–Ainsworth system, the learning that takes place is a broader learning, a learning about organizing behavior with respect to the caregiver (Sroufe & Waters, 1977a).

The Bowlby–Ainsworth theory is truly developmental. In keeping with other dynamic systems positions, it has as a central premise ongoing transactions between evolving organism and surround. "The pathway chosen turns at each and every stage of the journey on an interaction between the organism as it has developed up to that moment and the environment in which it then finds itself" (Bowlby, 1973, p. 412). Since the child adapts actively, and the personality is more formed and more complex at each point, individuals are increasingly forces in their own development. This is another key developmental premise. From Waddington (1957), Bowlby borrowed the concept of "homeorhesis," the increasing tendency for "chosen pathways" to be stable as development proceeds. From Piaget, Bowlby explicitly took the idea that the child is open to different kinds of experience, and capable of different kinds of understanding, at different ages. For example, it is beyond the capacity of the young child to understand that two parental statements or a statement and an action may be contradictory (with at least one being therefore subject to explicit rejection). Explicit verbal statements ("I'm doing this for your own good") must be accepted.

Therefore, there are at least two reasons that early emotional experience has a special place in this theory. First, the initial adaptations set the direction for later development and color encounters with later experiences. Second, infants have a qualitatively different (preverbal) way of encoding experience. Early experience may be carried forward with little alteration precisely because it cannot be verbally analyzed. This is similar to Freud's idea of the "dynamic unconscious," but within a modern cognitive framework. Research during the last two decades has made it clear that there is not only an early emerging "procedural memory" system, but that this system also has a different neural base than the later emerging verbal ("semantic") memory system (e.g., Nelson, 2000).

The child is not viewed as "fixated" at an early stage, but as "guided" in subsequent encounters by what Bowlby (1973) refers to as "working models." These are abstractions of direct experiences with caregivers, and they guide future expectations the way all generalizations do, although early models are outside of verbal awareness. Unlike fantasies emphasized by some other psychoanalytic theorists, these models are viewed as "tolerably accurate reflections of the experiences those individuals have actually had" (p. 407). If caregivers have been consistently responsive, then infants evolve expectations that caregivers (and, by generalization, others) will be so in the future. At the same time, in a complementary way, the infant evolves a model of the self as worthy of care and as effective in eliciting it. Such preverbally established expectations (or their converse) have a powerful influence on later social encounters. "[A]n unwanted child is likely not only to feel unwanted by his parents but to believe he is essentially unwantable, namely unwanted by anyone" (p. 238). Again, these ideas are well supported by contemporary research on "scripts," narrative construction, affective memory, and other advances in cognitive science (Belsky, Spritz, & Crnic, 1996; Bretherton & Munholland, 1999; Nelson, 1999; Nelson & Gruendel, 1979; Waters, Rodrigues, & Ridgeway, 1998).

As a structural dynamic theory of successive adaptations, the Bowlby–Ainsworth theory is developmental in the sense of making important nonlinear, nonobvious predictions. One clear example concerns the growth of self-reliance or independence in the preschool years. In contrast to all other theories of the time, infants who were effectively *dependent*, that is, who directly signaled their caregivers when threatened, and who elicited consistent responsiveness, were predicted to be more self-reliant as preschoolers. This is because, in having their security needs met through responsive care, they acquired a sense of themselves as effective and capable. Infants who do not experience responsiveness, including those pushed toward precocious independence, will later show dependency problems. As presented later, we obtained complete confirmation of this hypothesis in our work.

Finally, Bowlby's theory is a suitable framework for developmental psychopathology research such as ours. As were we, Bowlby was interested in explaining both normal and disturbed development. In contrast to Freud, however, and more in keeping with the now established principles of developmental psychopathology (Cicchetti & Cohen, 1995; Rutter & Sroufe, 2000; Sroufe, 1986; Sroufe & Rutter, 1984), Bowlby began by seeking an understanding of normal development. Beginning with the study of normal development led Bowlby to a very different view of emotions than that of Freud. Emotions such as fear, anxiety, and anger are normal reactions to naturally occurring circumstances and can guide individuals in maintaining vital relationships. Disturbance, therefore, is seen both when such reactions are chronic, misdirected, or inappropriately triggered, *and* when they fail to happen when needed. For example, failure to grieve following a significant loss is pathogenic. In general, much disturbance is the result of failures by significant adults to respond appropriately to the young child's normal needs for closeness to caregivers and fears of separation in threatening situations, or by direct or implicit threats of abandonment made by caregivers. Most forms of psychopathology entail either problems of emotional dysregulation or distorted personal relationships (Cole, Michel, & O'Connell-Teti, 1994;

Sroufe, Duggal, Weinfield, & Carlson, 2000). According to Bowlby, the root of such problems is often caregivers' failure to help the young child regulate normal emotional reactions (or even to contribute to their dysregulation) and being untrustworthy as the child's primary relational partner.

SYNTHESIS: AN ORGANIZATIONAL PERSPECTIVE ON DEVELOPMENT

We have integrated the various conceptual and theoretical ideas discussed earlier into what we refer to as an "organizational perspective" on development (Sroufe, 1979; Sroufe & Waters, 1977a; Sroufe et al., 1974). This was the guiding framework for our research. The first premise of this perspective is that *the fundamental feature of behavior is organization.* Recall from our example of the infant in the playroom (p. 24) that it is the patterning of behavior that was critical. It is not the mere occurrence of a behavior alone, or even its intensity, that reveals its meaning, but its organization—with other behaviors, with regard to social partners, and with other aspects of context.

Consider another example. A 12-month-old is playing with toys in an unfamiliar playroom, with her mother seated behind her several feet away. After examining several items in succession, she comes upon a toy elephant. She briefly puts it aside, then looks at it again with rapt attention. Then, with widened eyes, she picks it up and, in a smooth movement, turns and shows it to her mother, smiling broadly and vocalizing. Were this remarkable reaction described merely as "child smiles" or "child shows toy to mother," the richness and meaning present would be missed. The integration of the show, the broad smile, and the vocalization has vastly different meaning than any of the behaviors individually. Infants virtually never show such organized "affective sharing" with a stranger, though they do frequently look at them, smile at them, *or* show them toys (Waters, Wippman, & Sroufe, 1979). The organized sequence of behavior also reveals the emotional meaning. The child "recognizes" the object (imbues it with meaning), then directly, automatically shares her delight. Clearly, her caregiver is tied together with such experiences of joy. This is distinct from affiliative gestures to strangers, which are not organized in the same way with respect to exploration of the object world.

A second premise of the organizational perspective is that *organization is revealed in the interplay of emotion, cognition, and social behavior.* Consider, for example, a preschooler, AK, running with companions down to a sand-filled play area. On spotting a wooden structure in the center of the area, AK, shouts gleefully, "Hey, it's a boat," and flops onto the sand and "swims" over to the structure. The others follow, with laughter and shouting all around. Notice what is involved here. There are cognitive features, as in seeing the analogy between a boat in water and the wooden structure (which was not literally boat-like) in the middle of the sand. There are affective elements, as in AK's delight and enthusiasm. And there is the communication and other aspects of social sharing. But what is most revealing is how they all work together. The others follow not only because AK asks them to but also because of the cleverness of the idea and the contagious emotion. AK's competence is revealed by this organization, and our assessments were based on this proposition.

A third premise is the key proposition. *Development is defined by changes in organization of behavior over time* (Sroufe, 1996). Consider a comparison of a 6-month-old and a 10-month-old playing the "cloth-in-mouth" game with their fathers. The parent puts the cloth in his mouth, then moves it back and forth by shaking his head. This will capture the 6-month-old's attention. She stops, stares, then methodically reaches for the cloth, pulling it free. She likely will then put it in her own mouth. At 10 months, reaction to this situation is dramatically different. The infant stops, looks, perhaps glances back and forth between cloth and father's face, then, smiling broadly, tugs the cloth free. Then, commonly laughing uproariously, she tries to stuff it back into her father's mouth. The dramatic development revealed in comparing these two reactions is not best seen by considering individual capacities. Indeed, the 6-month-old has many of the capacities of the 10-month-old. She can recognize her father as distinct from other people; she will laugh in many situations (such as when being tickled); and she has the motor skill to put the cloth back into her father's mouth. To be sure, the 10-month-old has advanced capacities, especially in the realm of memory, and those advances make possible the new levels of organization. But qualitative change in development is revealed primarily by the new level of organization—recognizing the simultaneous existence of father-without-cloth and father-with-cloth, acting to reverse the visual transformation of the father, and laughing *in anticipation* of recreating the incongruity again— all as an integrated behavioral–emotional sequence. It is this integration that defines the game; there was no game at all for the 6-month-old.

Our fourth premise is that *organization of behavior is central to defining individual differences*. Not frequencies of behaviors, but how behaviors are organized with other behaviors and with regard to context reveals meaningful individual differences. As one example, two preschool children may both be highly active, but one is curious, sociable, empathic, and rule abiding, while the other is unfocused, uncooperative, aggressive, and noncompliant. The high level of activity has completely different meaning within these patterns of organization. It likely is a positive aspect of adaptation in the first child (perhaps contributing to peer leadership), whereas it is a problem for the second child (see also Suomi, 2002, for a contemporary discussion).

Defining individual patterns of organization is complicated, and increasingly so with development. As capacities expand, perhaps especially representational and memory capacities, so too does the complexity of the organization of cognition, affect, and social behavior. Likewise, since organization is always with respect to context, complexity is increased as contexts expand with age. In the end, there is enormous complexity in patterns of personality organization, both those that are functional and those that are maladaptive. Still, we describe a general strategy that holds: First, describe normative patterns of organization with regard to the issues and contexts of the age, then define meaningful deviations from these patterns.

This brings us to the fifth and final premise of our organizational perspective, derived from the work of Bowlby (1973), Ainsworth (Ainsworth, Blehar, Waters, & Wall, 1978) and, especially, Louis Sander (1962, 1975): *Central aspects of individual organization originate in the organization of early primary relationships.* This represents our solution to the problem of predicting complex adaptational outcomes from early in life, when the organization of infant behavior alone is so relatively simple. There is in infancy an organization of attitudes, expectations, and behavior that is at a high order of complexity. This organization, however, is not at the level of the individual infant, but at the level of the infant and the caregiving system (Sroufe, 1989). While, at first, it is best thought of as an organization in which the infant is simply nested, increasingly, during the first year, the active role of the infant as a participant in the organization expands. In time, it is truly a dyadic organization of varying pattern or quality, and from this an individual organization of the self emerges (e.g., Kochanska et al., 2004).

IMPLICATIONS FOR ASSESSMENT

The purpose of this lengthy discussion of developmental concepts and theories is to provide the background for explaining why we did our study the way we did it. We only briefly sketch the rationale for our assessment strategy here and lay out in more detail the study plan and how we carried it out in Chapters 3 and 4.

Adapting Organism and Surround

Based in a systems perspective, at every age we carried out assessments of both the organism and the surround, since emerging complexity is always a product of both. This included frequent assessments of caregiving and the broader caregiving context. Development always occurs in context. Thus, while caregiving provides a crucial near-in context, and received ample attention in our study, caregiving too occurs in a context of supports and stresses. These concentric rings of context (cf. Bronfenbrenner, 1979) were as important to us as prior adaptational history, which also is part of the current context of adaptation.

In time, we further assessed the dynamic child–environment transaction by examining the predictability of environmental "response" from earlier child adaptation in numerous ways. For example, a subset of participants participated in a nursery school that we controlled. Since teachers were constant, and were blind to history, their attitudes, expectations, and behaviors toward the various children could be examined in light of the children's early adaptations. We found that, indeed, the general way teachers treated different children, the standards they held up for them, and their varied reactions to failures of compliance, were distinctly predictable from each child's early history of experience and adaptation (see Chapter 7).

Patterns of Organization versus Developmental Milestones

In addition to assessing broad, comprehensive domains of functioning, our behavioral assessments especially were aimed at the integration of affect, cognition, and behavior. Assessments of child functioning were designed to be age-appropriate challenges to the child's adaptive capacities, taxing the child's ability to remain organized. Either some problem or a series of problems was posed that was certain to arouse affect, or we took advantage of naturally occurring challenges (e.g., peer group interaction, transition to school) that were affectively arousing. In this way, we could see how the child drew upon personal and environmental resources in order to meet challenge and therefore promote further development.

Our interest was in processes versus achievements. We were not primarily concerned about ages at which children reached milestones, or ages when behaviors were first manifest. Rather, we were interested in variations in organization or adaptive response at ages when all children had reached the developmental milestone in question. For example, we were not primarily concerned with whether a child first had an enduring close friendship at age 6 or 7, or at age 8 or 9. Rather, we were concerned about the degree of smooth organization the child achieved in the middle childhood social world. Yes, they should develop the capacity to form close friendships, but they also must be able to function effectively in the peer group. Most important, they must be able to coordinate the competing demands of individual friendships and group functioning; that is, maintain the special tie to a friend even while also engaging others (see Chapter 8). In brief, the objective was to assess how well the adaptation that had evolved, as reflected in the organization of behavior, was serving the child's development.

Focus on Salient Developmental Issues

When the focus is organization of behavior, one must ask the question, organized with respect to what? Our answer to this question is: issues salient for the particular developmental period. We describe the series of issues that guided us in Chapters 3 and 4. Here we just make the general case regarding selection of issues for targeting assessments.

First, each age can be described in terms of the central challenges for development, the central capacities that must be acquired to promote subsequent development, the dominant concerns of the child, and the central venues of environmental engagement. For the latter part of the first year, for example, formation of an effective attachment relationship is clearly a salient developmental issue. A central challenge for the infant is emotional regulation, and attachment *is* the "dyadic regulation of emotion" (Sroufe, 1996). The infant must learn to draw effectively upon external resources in the service of emotional regulation and mastery of the object world. Attachment, supporting exploration, is critical in this regard. Object play, and encounters with novel objects and people, are principal venues. Effective attachment enables the infant to remain organized in the face of novel experiences. Moreover, attachment is an integrative construct: It lies at the intersection of all of the cognitive, emotional, and social development occurring in the first year. One must discriminate attachment figures, understand them as independent sources of action, and form expectations regarding their likely reactions. Moreover, in seeking caregiver assistance, one is guided by serviceable emotional reactions. When an effectively organized attachment is achieved, subsequent development is clearly served. The object mastery skills, the entrained capacity for emotional regulation, and the positive expectations regarding self-in-relationships together provide a platform for later autonomy and effective relationships with peers.

Attachment formation represents a prototypical salient issue given its clear centrality to infant functioning and its promotion of subsequent development. As is described later, salient issues for other ages may be defined using the same criteria. Not surprisingly, given the developmental principles we have been discussing, the task becomes more complex with each age. As venues of environmental engagement expand, and as the complexity of developmental challenges being faced increases, it becomes increasingly difficult to define a singular issue. The number of salient issues expands, and assessments must expand in a commensurate way. In the preschool period, for example, salient issues include self-management and entering the world of peers, as well as continuing to draw effectively upon parents. Each of these entails considerate complexity. Peer relationships, for example, are very complex and become more so at each developmental period. Still, the same rules apply for assessment. Tap the organization of affect, cognition, and social behavior, and focus on the way the adaptation likely would serve or compromise later development. For example, is the child able to regulate emotion and engage others in ways that will allow him or her to elicit return engagement from them and sustain interactions, so that skills for reciprocal sharing and conflict resolution can be developed and carried forward?

It should be clear that these developmental issues are not viewed as tasks to be passed or failed; rather, they are reference points for looking at behavioral organization. Every child, whether doing well or not, negotiates every issue and moves forward. However, the way the issues are negotiated—the organized adaptation evolved—sets the stage for negotiating subsequent issues. For example, self-isolated preschoolers will find close friendships in middle childhood more challenging, with their demand for sustained emotional investment even in the face of inevitable conflicts.

Normal First, Then Disturbances

In keeping with the central premises of developmental psychopathology (Cicchetti & Cohen, 1995; Sroufe, 1997), we begin always with questions about how most children organize behavior with regard to the issue of the age and how they are able to do so. Then, we ask how the process can go awry. To understand, for example, why some children have a set of problems that leads to a diagnosis of attention-deficit/hyperactivity disorder (ADHD), we would ask first why most children do not (see Chapter 12). How do children typically develop the capacities to regulate arousal, to reorganize following disruptions, and to focus attention? What are the phases in these developments? How does the emergence of these capacities proceed, age by age? What prior organizations are the foundations for functionally organized arousal, attention, and behavior in the school years? What are the supports needed at each age?

There is not a single pattern of organization that "works" at a given age. There always are variations in organization that have in common allowing the child to meet challenges adequately, while garnering the necessary experiential resources to promote subsequent adaptation. Understanding what needs to "work" and describing various serviceable organizations is prerequisite to defining maladaptive organizations. In our view, the problems most children have are best seen in terms of variations in organization. For the most part, children who are functioning well and children who are troubled are not qualitatively different.

Ainsworth's attachment work can again provide an example. She described not one, but four patterns of effective (secure) attachment organizations. On the surface, these were quite distinctive. Some infants, for example, become quite distressed during brief separations from the caregiver. Upon reunion, they approach directly, actively seek contact, hug, and cling until settled. Others are not acutely distressed by separation (but perhaps simply subdued) and seek no physical contact upon reunion. Instead, they broadly smile, show toys, and otherwise reengage the caregiver through interaction. What these two distinctive organizations have in common is active initiation of reconnection with the caregiver that, in each case, promotes a subsequent return to active play and exploration. Disturbed organizations, while also varied, in one way or another compromise emotional regulation and exploration.

At each age, then, we ask questions about what challenges the child is facing and describe the various patterns of organization that enable children to rise to the challenges and utilize the opportunities available. Then we ask: How can this go wrong? What ways of functioning can cause the child to struggle unduly with the challenges or fail to take advantage of the available opportunities? In the early years, the patterns we examined were in the caregiving relationship. At later ages, we examined the child in other relationships, as well as the organization of the child's expectations and behavior.

Progressive Validation

There is an inherent and troublesome circularity in much competence research, wherein competence and doing well are mutually defining. The problem can be illustrated with the concept of "resilience." For example, why do some children do well in the face of adversity? Because they are resilient. How do we know they are resilient? Because they are doing well in the face of adversity. It can be seen that resilience treated in this way is simply a name for doing well in the face of adversity, not an explanation. Within a developmental approach, however, there is a solution to this problem. There is a way of progressively validating constructs, of becoming incrementally confident in the constructs, assessments, and underlying theory.

When we determine that a pattern of organization is adaptive, or functional, or effective, how can we know we are correct? If we have selected the proper series of issues, and properly defined the range of normative and nonfunctional patterns of organization, these should forecast effective and nonfunctional patterns at the next age. If predictions fail, this may mean, of course, that we selected the wrong issues, that our assessments of the patterns of organization are weak, that the underlying theory is wanting, or all of these. If, however, patterns of behavioral organization show cross-time coherence (despite changing issues, assessment contexts, and measures), we gain a bit of confidence in the framework and both sets of assessments. The second pattern, of course, should not only relate to the first but also to organization in the next developmental phase, and so on. In the end, one can have considerable confidence in the validity of the constructs and the approach, though perhaps not based on a single study. It is a self-correcting research strategy.

CONCLUSION

We had a number of important conceptual supports available to us as we began our project. There were theories that informed us about the nature of development. There were systems perspectives that provided a framework for dealing with the complexities of normative and individual growth. And perhaps most important of all, there was an emerging perspective regarding the interplay of child and surroundings. Known as the transactional or ecological model, this was a critical influence as we initiated this study. In 1973, Arnold Sameroff visited our department and shared with us a draft of his classic paper on this model (Sameroff & Chandler, 1975). This paper confirmed our own preconceptions about the interaction of developmental risk factors and environmental supports and inspired us in the early phases of the project.

As we began our study of individual adaptation, it was clear what was needed. We needed to select the right set of salient developmental issues; we needed to measure organized patterns of adaptation properly with regard to them at each age; we needed to simultaneously carry out ongoing assessments of relevant context factors; and we needed to employ a sufficiently complex model of continuity and change. Our goal was to track the changing organization of behavior that resulted from the interplay of a variety of forces at different levels of context acting over time. This is what we set out to do.

CHAPTER 3

Inception

> ... competence implies a competent mother–infant pair—an
> infant who is competent in his pre-adapted function ... and
> a mother who is competent in the reciprocal role to which
> the infant's behavior is pre-adapted.
> —AINSWORTH AND BELL (1974)

An idealized study of individual development would involve
measuring virtually everything at every time period on a very large number of people. One would wish to tap all meaningful experiences, all features of the child, all relevant aspects of context, and all possible outcomes. In practice, of course, no study, however well funded, and no
consortium of studies, however large, could really carry out such a project. It is not possible to measure everything and still measure it well. Developmental research must be strategic; choices must be made. Here and
in Chapter 4, we will discuss the research strategy and assessment principles that guided our study and describe the measurements that we carried out age by age. We begin with infancy.

The principles that guided our approach to assessment are well illustrated by the infant period. These included (1) a focus on salient developmental issues; (2) an ecological approach, entailing measures of individual adaptation, surrounding care, and broader context (Belsky,
1980; Bronfenbrenner, 1979; Sameroff, 1983); (3) use of multiple methods and multiple sources of information; (4) use of previously validated
measures; and (5) emphasis on measures at the level of organization.

The critical issues of adaptation in infancy that were central for us

46

were *initial state regulation* (0–3 months), *reciprocal exchange* (4–6 months), and *formation of an effective attachment* (7–12 months). Initial state regulation refers to establishing regular sleep–wake cycles, the capacity to modulate reactivity to stimulation, and developing the capacity to focus attention and to follow changing stimulation. Reciprocal exchange refers to the capacity to coordinate and sustain interactions between infant and caregiver (e.g., Stern, 1985). Such coordinated exchanges are a crucial training ground for expansion of the infant's capacity to remain organized in the face of arousal (Sroufe, 1996). They are "opportunities for the infant to learn how to contain *himself*, how to control motor responses, and how to attend for longer and longer periods" (Brazelton, Kowslowski, & Main, 1974, p. 70). Formation of an effective attachment, a competent infant–caregiver pair, has already been discussed as the pivotal issue in all of infancy (see Chapter 2). Our assessments were comprehensive with regard to each of these issues.

In addition to measuring diverse aspects of infant behavior, we carried out comprehensive measures of caregiver behavior and caregiver life circumstances from the first days of life onward. Parental care represents the innermost ring of influences surrounding the infant in the Bronfenbrenner (1979) model. In this model of reciprocal influences, however, parenting itself is influenced by the broader context surrounding the family. We sampled this context of care extensively, including not only current supports, stresses, and economic challenges but also the parents' own developmental history. In the end, we had captured the effectiveness of the entire infant and caregiving system.

Multiple methods of assessment and multiple independent sources of data were utilized throughout the infancy period. Prenatally, most of the data came from interviewing and testing parents, but some data were based on objective records (e.g., regularity of prenatal physician visits). Following the infant's birth, interviews, formal testing, and direct observation by multiple persons all were utilized. For example, with regard to early infant characteristics, nurses made daily ratings in the newborn nursery, trained project staff administered a neonatal neurological status examination on two occasions, and detailed observations were carried out in the home at 3 and 6 months. Thus, in addition to parent questionnaire measures of temperament, which are standard in the field, we had numerous converging observational measures, each independent of the others.

Our practice in the infant period and throughout the study was to emphasize measures that had been validated by previous research. At times, this meant conducting short-term studies of our own in advance of this work (e.g., Arend et al., 1979; Matas et al., 1978), and sometimes it meant drawing upon the work of others (J. Sroufe, 1991). In a longitudinal, process-oriented study, each measure is crucial, and there is no going back. If, for example, we want to know whether an uncovered link between infant attachment and certain qualities of adult romantic relationships is mediated by peer competence in middle childhood, then measures of peer competence, as well as the other two measures, must be sound. If we find that we used inadequate procedures in middle childhood, for example, we cannot go back and do them over in adolescence.

Attachment assessment can again serve as an example. We used Ainsworth's Strange Situation procedure, which had been well validated, and we used it *exactly* the way she did, so that we could draw upon her norms and her validation data. Just as in giving a standard IQ test, one cannot "modify" the procedure and still reference the norms. Moreover, our primary coders established reliability with Ainsworth, and we had previously shown with another sample that our attachment classifications had the same home correlates as in Ainsworth's work. Subsequently, we again demonstrated the relations with the current sample (e.g., Egeland & Farber, 1984).

We conducted the Strange Situation at both 12 and 18 months. This was important for several reasons. First, combining the assessments would yield a more powerful predictor. Second, the 18-month assessment could provide additional validation of our 12-month measure (i.e., the stability of the classifications made by independent coders). Third, the two assessments would allow us to document and explain change in adaptation. With a middle-class sample, trained coders demonstrated strong stability in classifications across this period (Waters, 1978). This was critical, because we anticipated considerable change in our new sample given the greater instability in life circumstances. Use of a previously validated measure let us know that changing classification likely meant changing adaptation, not simply an inherently unstable measure. Indeed, while we found significant stability, there was considerable change as well, and we were able to demonstrate that this change was lawful (see Chapter 5).

Finally, the last principle that has guided us throughout the study was an emphasis on measures at the level of organization. Ratings of "caregiver sensitivity" and "caregiver intrusiveness" (Sroufe & Sampson, 2000) are such measures. As we describe, these are ratings that take into account not only what caregivers do and how frequently they do things, but when and in what sequence. Thus, playing pat-a-cake with a 6-month-old is a perfectly reasonable thing to do. But it is not sensitive and responsive *if* the child is already overaroused and fussing (perhaps because she is hungry), and especially not if this is a child easily pushed to overarousal and disorganization. Thus, sensitivity reflects how the caregiver organizes his or her own behavior with regard to the infant's nature, mood, immediate state, and the particular circumstances. It was at this level that we made our ratings. We did supplement these with detailed behavioral codings, but we found repeatedly that integrative ratings of child, parent, and social relationships were the most powerful measures.

These, then, are the principles that guided us in our assessments during infancy and at all other age periods. Before presenting in more detail the array of prenatal and postnatal measures, we first describe how and why the study was initiated, and the nature of the sample of participants we recruited.

INITIATION OF THE STUDY

We originally recruited the participants in our long-term study with somewhat more modest goals in mind than those laid out in the previous chapters. The study was begun by Byron Egeland, along with Amos Deinard, a pediatrician and outstanding advocate for children and families. Egeland and Deinard believed that if more could be understood about what led parents to sometimes mistreat their children, much more could be done to help families. It was only when these children were approximately 18 months old that the goal became to follow children through development in order to explore the consequences of variations in early care and later circumstances. By that time, we knew there was great variation of parenting in this sample, and we knew from the results of our short-term longitudinal study of middle-class families that infant experience was related to outcomes in the preschool years (Arend et al., 1979; Matas et al., 1978).

The decision to study the origins of child maltreatment in a comprehensive way was important for two reasons. First, a great deal indeed was learned about the complex factors that lay behind child maltreatment, as we present in Chapter 5. Second, the question posed by Egeland and Deinard led them to carry out one of the most comprehensive and detailed investigations of very early development ever conducted. As we detail later, there were comprehensive assessments of parents' prenatal care, child-rearing beliefs, expectations, personality characteristics, and caregiving behavior. Likewise, very detailed assessments of all aspects of infant functioning were made beginning at birth. Finally, what Jay Belsky (1980) referred to as the "ecology of child maltreatment," or the context surrounding parenting, received extensive study. All of this would prove to be critical for our later study of the unfolding of individual development.

The situation in the child abuse field as the study began was in many ways similar to that in developmental psychology as a whole. Researchers were having a difficult time predicting which parents would abuse or neglect their children. Simple linear models were found to be inadequate, and no single factor could be isolated as an infallible risk indicator (Egeland & Brunnquell, 1979; Pianta, Egeland, & Erickson, 1989). For example, early investigators hypothesized that psychosis or gross psychopathology of parents was the cause of maltreatment, but subsequent investigations showed that such disturbance only accounted for a very small number of child maltreatment cases (Gelles, 1973). While poverty did prove to be a risk factor, child maltreatment clearly crossed all social class boundaries and, as we discussed in Chapter 1, poverty itself likely was predictive because it stood for a host of other factors (e.g., high stress, family instability, domestic violence). Even history of abuse experienced by the parents, which is a dependable predictor (Egeland, Jacobvitz, & Papatola, 1987), was not an infallible predictor (Kaufman & Zigler, 1987). Many parents "break the cycle" (Egeland, Jacobvitz, & Sroufe, 1988), and one wants to understand why some carry forward the abuse history into the next generation and others do not.

Likewise, no child factors had proven to be strong predictors of maltreatment (Egeland & Vaughn, 1981). Premature birth and difficult temperament were once thought to be determinants of maltreatment. But such conclusions were based on retrospective interview studies. Parents who mistreated their children frequently reported that their children had been premature or had always been difficult. But these studies suffer from what Garmezy (1971) referred to as "etiological error": Looking backward in time always provides a cause, but the inferred linearity is misleading. Moreover, factors such as prematurity are confounded with other variables, such as poverty. There were no studies prior to the mid-1970s following children forward from birth to ask, for example, what proportion of premature children, objectively assessed, in fact are mistreated compared to full-term children, especially those from the same socioeconomic status (SES). This is what Egeland and Deinard did.

At one point, the "child factors" interpretation went so far as to assign blame for mistreatment almost totally to children. The low point of this era was marked by a publication called "Bringing Up Mother" (Segal & Yahres, 1978). The article was published in *Psychology Today*, which at the time was a prestigious journal published by the American Psychological Association. Segal and Yahres argued, based on a classic paper by Richard Bell (1968), that children influence their parents, as well as being influenced by them. Such an idea of "bidirectional" or, as we prefer, "transactional" effects is reasonable, especially placed in a comprehensive developmental model. Indeed, parents must be influenced by children if they are to provide the care children need. But Segal and Yahres went further to argue that extreme parental behavior would be *caused* by extreme child characteristics. Some children, they argued, by their inborn nature elicited abuse. Beyond this rationale, the "proof" they put forward for this assertion was the fact that abused children often are reabused by foster parents following out-of-home placement. Again, we see an argument from outcome to cause, as well as a lack of developmental thinking. There is no understanding that children internalize experience, turning it into expectations for self and others. Children with histories of maltreatment may indeed behave in challenging ways and elicit exasperation and anger from adults. But this likely is due to the dysregulating sequelae of abuse. At the least, such a claim as made by Segal and Yahres should not be put forward in the absence of prospective, longitudinal data. One would need very early, direct observation of child characteristics to make such a case. Egeland and Deinard were to provide just such data. As we discuss later, it turns out that neither prematurity nor perinatal infant difficulties, nor early measures of temperament, play much of a role in child maltreatment (Egeland & Vaughn, 1981; see also Gottfried, 1973), yet maltreatment is predictable (see Chapter 5).

At the time we began our study, researchers also were having a difficult time demonstrating the consequences of maltreatment. Shortly after our study began, Elizabeth Elmer (1977) published a book entitled, *Fragile Families, Troubled Children*, in which she concluded that abuse had no harmful impact on development over and above that associated with lower SES. Future research on child abuse was threatened, because Elmer was such a major figure in the field. But the study underlying this conclusion was not strong. Groups were quite small, and it is quite possible that the poverty control group contained cases of neglect and other forms of maltreatment. Both groups showed serious impairment. The large-scale study launched by Egeland and Deinard would control for level of poverty (largely by looking at variations within a poverty sample). It would also entail comprehensive, well-validated assessments. In the end, it demonstrated profound consequences of maltreatment (e.g., see Chapter 12) and spurred continued research. The impact of abuse and neglect has now been widely demonstrated (e.g., Cicchetti & Toth, 2000).

Recruitment of Participants

The participants in this study were recruited through the Minneapolis Department of Public Health and the Hennepin County General Hospital. Pregnant women entering the third trimester of pregnancy were recruited. Only two selection criteria were used: (1) It was a first pregnancy and (2) the mother qualified for public assistance for prenatal care and delivery (i.e., income below the official poverty line).

First births were studied because we wanted to rule out variations in expectations and parenting experience based on raising a previous child. Ultimately, we did also study the first 75 second-born children in a short-term study. Among other things, this allowed us to investigate sibling relationships (see Chapter 8).

The poverty requirement was to create a sample at higher risk for parenting difficulties than the general population. Poverty, with its attendant stress and instability, certainly makes parenting more challenging. However, despite all falling below the poverty line, there was great variation in the circumstances of our participants. Some, for example, were only temporarily poor (e.g., students). Some had excellent support networks, including grandparents, and other relatives and friends. Some had little support, and some, like Veronica, described in Chapter 1, faced numerous adversities.

More specifically, 61% of the mothers were not married when the child was born and about 50% were teenagers, with an age range from 12 to 34 years. Only 59% had completed high school. In keeping with the demographics of Minneapolis at that time, 80% of the mothers were European Americans, with about equal numbers of African Americans and Native Americans, and a very small percentage of Latin Americans.

In addition to these demographic aspects of risk, these mothers as a group also showed elevated medical risk during pregnancy, including serious infections (15%) and venereal disease, use of hard drugs, or excessive weight gain (5% each). Clinic staff judged 37% to have inadequate nutrition, 33% to be unprepared for the birth of the baby (e.g., no sleeping arrangements), and 21% to be generally "at risk." Independent of our study, public health nurses or social workers were assigned to these latter cases.

A high proportion of the infants were considered to be at risk for medical reasons. Medical data were available on 214 infants (118 males and 96 females). Some of the reported anomalies and clinical difficulties included the following: 18 had elevated bilirubin (severely jaundiced); 9 had instances of intrauterine growth retardation—dysmaturity; 3 had severe tremors; and cases of Potters syndrome, Holt–Oram syndrome, cleft palate, and respiratory distress syndrome were reported. In addition, 27 infants were born prematurely, as defined by birthweight of less than 2,500 grams.

In the first phases of the study, we made no attempt to pursue families that moved out of the state. There also were 5 infant deaths, and we could not locate 15 participants after birth. This left us with 240 participants of an original 267 we had recruited. By participant age 24 months, we had 212 participants, and 85% of these were still in the study 20 years later. We do know that those lost between age 1 and 2 years were some of the most high-stress, unstable families. More will be said about participant "attrition" where it is appropriate in the book.

The Character of Our Participants

Two questions often come up when we present talks based on our study: (1) Aren't you blaming mothers (because we find that quality of care is a robust predictor)? and (2) Isn't this study pretty pessimistic (because we predict far-reaching negative outcomes from the early years)? We answer "no" on both counts.

As pointed out earlier, when one studies the circumstances surrounding parents, one quickly abandons any tendency to assign blame. The parents in this study virtually without exception wanted the best for their children, and they wanted to do their best for them. Sometimes the difficulties of their circumstances simply were beyond their resources. We could provide many anecdotes regarding how much they cared for their children, but one will suffice. As part of the study, we were able to provide one term of a high-quality preschool program for a subset of our participants (described in Chapter 4). When we were seeking funding for this program, reviewers asked if we could be certain that parents of the selected children would allow them to participate. In fact, each and every one agreed, and the typical response was one of overwhelming gratefulness that someone would provide such an experience for their child.

For similar reasons the study did not lead us to pessimism. In fact, we were impressed by how well these parents and their children did given the challenges of their lives. Some did very well indeed, even given difficult beginnings. Many more of the parents could have given more to their children, and their children could have fared better, had the families had more support. The study did not make us pessimistic about the character of parents living in poverty, but it did make us at times question the priorities of our society.

Finally, we comment on the generosity of our participants. They have given much to our study and to the field of developmental psychology. There are several reasons why they joined the study and stayed with it over the years. One reason, at the beginning, was their respect for and confidence in Dr. Deinard. We hope another reason is that all of us on the project have at every point treated them with respect. We have had great stability in core staff members, yielding continuity in contacts. These staff members care about the individual participants. But at least one reason our participants have stayed with us is their belief in what we are doing. They hope that what we find out will be of use to families, and that other children will benefit.

ASSESSMENTS IN THE INFANCY PERIOD

A list of the measures used in our study can be found in the Appendices at the end of the book. Here, we provide an overview of the key measures, describing them in narrative form.

Prenatal Assessments

At approximately 36 weeks of pregnancy, a battery of tests was given that assessed personality characteristics—aggression, defendence, impulsivity, succorance, dependency, depression (Jackson, 1974), anxiety (Cattell & Scheier, 1963), locus of control (Egeland, Hunt, & Hardt, 1970; Rotter, 1966), and parents' feelings and expectations regarding pregnancy, delivery, and their expected child (Cohler, Weiss, & Grunebaum, 1970; Schaefer & Manheimer, 1960). Specifically, these latter tests measure characteristics such as fear for self and baby, lack of desire for pregnancy, appropriate versus inappropriate ideas about control of a child's aggression, valuing of reciprocity, and feelings of competence in meeting a baby's needs. Some of the measures were from Cohler's Maternal Attitude Scale (Cohler et al., 1970), and they tapped the parent's understanding of the psychological complexity of the child, that is, that the baby is a separate person from them, and at the same time needs a lot from them. In addition, Broussard and Hartner's Neonatal Perception Inventory (1971) was used to assess parental expectations of what an "average" baby is like and what their own baby would be like in areas such as amount of crying and trouble with feeding and sleeping. Finally, the parents were given an expectation measure that assessed knowledge of a child's development; for example, when a child typically crawls, feeds itself, and talks, and the age at which a child can be expected to obey commands, be toilet trained, and so forth (Egeland, Deinard, & Brunnquell, 1975). The battery of tests given to the parents prenatally was administered again, when the infant was 3 months old.

Focusing on assessment of parental beliefs, feelings, and expectations regarding the infant, and on understanding the development and functioning of the baby, our measures were distinctive from measures of general attitudes. The popular measures of child-rearing attitudes, such as the Parent Attitude Research Inventory, had generally not been shown to relate to actual parental behavior or to the later development of the child (cf. Becker & Krug, 1965). On the other hand, measures of parents' expectations about and understanding of their children were known to relate to later development (Broussard, 1976).

Separate factor analyses of the parental measures given prenatally and at 3 months yielded six factors that were similar across the two testing periods (Brunnquell, Crichton, & Egeland, 1981). The factors included self-assurance, rejection of the baby and anxiety regarding pregnancy, expectations about the infant, and sensitivity and psychological awareness of baby's complexity.

Groups of mothers with similar characteristics and profiles were formed using multidimensional classification procedures (Brunnquell et al., 1981). The three groups that emerged were differentiated along the lines of positive and negative feelings, perceptions and expectations of the child, and certain constellations of personality characteristics. While two of the groups had many positive characteristics, the other group of mothers was characterized as being highly dependent, suspicious, and feeling unable to act or behave in a way that would affect their lives; in addition, they were frightened of their hostile impulses and unable to express them in an acceptable fashion. Broussards's expectation measure and Cohler's measure of the understanding of psychological complexity formed one of the dimensions along which the groups of mothers clustered.

In summary, some mothers had many conflicted feelings, were still struggling with problems of growing up, and somehow felt that the baby was going to make things better by being a companion or "somebody to love me." They hoped the baby would meet their needs, rather than understanding that the infant was an autonomous being who would be needing a great deal of care from them. This seemed like a blueprint for parent–child difficulties, especially in the unsupportive contexts in which many of these mothers would be operating. As we report in Chapter 5, it proved to be so.

Postnatal Assessment

The Infant

It was critical to begin assessment of the infant in the first weeks of life. "Temperament" is generally defined as relatively enduring, inborn characteristics of the child (Goldsmith et al., 1987). At the same time, most contemporary temperament researchers believe that temperament may be modified by the environment (e.g., Bates, 1989). This means that, increasingly with development, temperament is a blend of constitutional and experiential factors. For some purposes, this does not matter. If the goal is simply describing the developmental process, how child characteristics interact with circumstances, it is not so important whether these characteristics are inborn or not. It is certainly the case that even later emerging child characteristics can be demonstrated to have some degree of heritability (O'Connor & Plomin, 2000). But to examine etiological claims about temperament per se causing later outcomes or influencing the quality of parenting, one must start early. We began at birth.

We used four different approaches to the young infant's temperament. First, nurses made ratings in the newborn nursery at the end of each shift for the 4 days during which infants and mothers stayed in the hospital (routine practice during the mid-1970s). The nurses rated characteristics such as irritability, activity level, and soothability. Second, we conducted direct assessments of the neonate at ages 7 and 10 days using the Brazelton Neonatal Assessment Scale (Brazelton, 1973), designed to capture the infant's neurological integrity and early capacity to organize states. For most infants, the 7-day assessment would mark the adjustment to the transition to home. We also observed infants in interaction with their mothers on three occasions in the first 6 months. (These observational settings are described in the following section). Finally, at both 3 months and 6 months, mothers completed the Carey Infant Temperament Questionnaire (Carey, 1970), designed to capture the nine temperament dimensions put forward by Thomas, Chess, and Birch (1968). While there are better questionnaires today, this was state of the art at the time. We used another questionnaire measure at age 2½ years, designed by Buss and Plomin (1975), and we used a measure of minor physical anomalies developed by Waldrop, Pedersen, and Bell (1968). (While we obtained this latter measure at age 8 years, we assumed that such indices would be unchanging measures of neurological intactness.)

A detailed analysis of the three major infant measures of temperament (Taraldson, Brunnquell, Deinard, & Egeland 1977) showed that interrater reliabilities for the Nurse's Rating Scale and the Brazelton were very good. However, the stability of the baby's behavior across the 4 days in the newborn nursery was moderate, and the correlations of Brazelton scores from day 7 to day 10 were quite low. In order to improve reliability, Brazelton scores from day 7 to day 10 were combined. Stability of Carey scores from 3 to 6 months showed moderate correlations on 7 of 9 scales (.44 to .58); the canonical correlation across the 3-month period was .78. However, the Carey scores did not relate to the observation-based temperament measures. Thus, there was a problem of limited stability of the very early measures and, while more stable, the questionnaire measure may actually have been tapping stability of parental point of view rather than stability of infant behavior.

These early infant measures highlight an issue that runs throughout the study, namely, the large number of variables. (In the study as a whole, there are well more than 10,000; we stopped counting long ago). Here, there are numerous nurses' ratings (done 12 times); numerous Brazelton scales and scale combinations, assessed twice; and dozens of infant home-observation variables, obtained on three occasions. Add to these the measures of prematurity and other birth difficulties, and it is a large number indeed. Even combining a number of individual scales, in one paper we created an infant risk index based on 42 variables (Aguilar, Sroufe, Egeland, & Carlson, 2000). Clearly, if one looks at these one at a time with regard to some outcome, many spurious, chance findings would result. There is a need to reduce this number of variables through some form of combination.

Throughout the study, we used various methods for combining measures and "reducing" data. Sometimes we used rational methods, for example, combining measures based on a priori theoretical concerns, or making an overall global rating of functioning. Sometimes we simply averaged measures after standardizing them. And sometimes we used formal empirical techniques, such as factor analysis (which groups variables) or cluster analysis (which groups individuals on the set of variables). The resulting number of factors or groups was generally much smaller than the original number of variables.

For example, factor analyses yielded six factors for the Brazelton scales (irritability, orientation, physiological maturity, consolability, direct arm control, and habituation) and four factors in the Nurse's Rating Scale (Activity–Alertness, Mother Interest, Fussiness–Soothability, and Ease of Care) (Vaughn, Taraldson, Crichton, & Egeland, 1980). A factor analysis of the Carey items resulted in 25 factors that were obviously impossible to interpret. A cluster analysis of the temperament data yielded groups similar to the "easy" and "difficult to care for babies" described by Thomas and colleagues (1968); in addition, two groups formed along the dimensions of orientation, consolability, and activity. In Chapter 5, we present the results of these efforts, in terms of how well various infant factors or cluster groupings predicted parenting or later infant development.

Caregiving Assessments in Early Infancy

We also began our assessments of parental care at birth.[1] The hospital nurses rated mothers, as well as infants, a key variable being "the mother's interest in the baby." This measure proved to be remarkably

---

1. "Parental" here means maternal care. Only one-third of the infants' fathers were still involved with the child by age 18 months.

powerful. Then, there were systematic observations of mother–infant feeding during a 1-hour home visit at 3 months, and two visits to assess feeding and play interactions at 6 months. Some of the variables observed were quality of verbalizations, quality of physical contact, expressiveness, responsiveness to infant interactive bids, positive and negative affect, and facility of caretaking.

Home visitors also made ratings on two of Ainsworth's 9-point caregiving sensitivity scales, Sensitivity to Infant Signals and Cooperation–Interference. These were critical variables in our study. Ainsworth (1970) has provided on overall description of sensitive care, which guided her development of these measures:

> The sensitive caregiver responds socially to his attempts to initiate social interaction, playfully to his attempts to initiate play. She picks him up when he seems to wish it, and puts him down when he wants to explore. When he is distressed, she knows what kinds and degree of soothing he requires to comfort him—and she knows that sometimes a few words or a distraction will be all that is needed. On the other hand, the mother who responds inappropriately tries to socialize with the baby when he is hungry, play with him when he is tired, or feed him when he is trying to initiate social interaction. (p. 3)

More specifically, sensitivity to infant communications requires being aware of the infant's signals, interpreting them accurately, and responding both appropriately and promptly. Sensitive care also is reflected in responses that are "well rounded" and "completed." For example, when the baby wants to be held, the mother holds him long enough that he is truly comforted, so that when he is put down, he does not want to be picked up again immediately.

The Cooperation–Interference Scale is centered on the degree to which the caregivers' ministrations and other actions fit smoothly with the infant's mood, state, or current interests, or interrupt, break into, or cut across the baby's ongoing activity. Cooperative caregivers guide rather than control their infants. Interfering or intrusive caregivers behave in ways the infant is not, or even cannot be, prepared for and are thus very dysregulating. Cooperative caregivers are engaged "with" the infant rather than always being "at" the infant.

These scales were most pertinent to our predictions of later organization given how integrative they are—how much they encompass regarding the organization of infant and caregiver behavior. As complex as they are, given ample observational opportunity, our observers were able to rate them reliably (Egeland & Farber, 1984).

Later Infancy Assessments

Infant Cognitive and Motor Development

At 9 months (and again at 24 months), we administered the Bayley Scales of Infant Development (Bayley, 1969). These scales yield a motor index, a verbal index, and a profile of scores regarding the infant's handling of the test. While not well related to later IQ, these scales nonetheless tap the infant's current developmental status and are useful control variables. Also, change between 9 and 24 months is a useful measure of developmental trajectory.

At 12 months, we administered the Uzgiris–Hunt Assessment in Infancy Scales (Uzgiris & Hunt, 1975). These scales are based in Piaget's theory and measure the infant's development with regard to object concept, means–ends relationships, and causality.

Attachment Classifications

The Ainsworth and Wittig (1969) Strange Situation procedure was administered at 12 and at 18 months. This procedure involved a series of separations and reunions, following a period of play, and the introduction of a stranger in an unfamiliar room (see Chapter 2, pp. 24–25). The relationship is classified as secure, anxious–avoidant, or anxious–resistant based upon the overall patterning of infant behavior, but with special emphasis on the reunions. "Significant individual differences lie not so much in the relative quantities of attachment and exploratory behavior as in the quality of each and the smoothness of the transition from one to another" (Ainsworth & Bell, 1974, p. 116). Scales of proximity seeking, contact maintenance, avoidance, and resistance guide classification. Reunions are critical theoretically; since the connection has been threatened by the brief separations, infants are expected to be both *active* and *effective* in reestablishing contact. For relationships that are classified as secure, infants either pursue direct and thorough physical contact (expected with distressed infants) or immediately initiate interaction with the caregiver (nondistressed infants). In either case, such activity promotes a return to exploration. Based on such active behavior, and in consideration of the patterning of the four scales of interactive behavior across the two reunions, four subtypes of secure attachment are identified (Ainsworth et al., 1978; Sroufe & Waters, 1977b).

The first anxious attachment group, anxious–resistant attachment, comprised 22% of our sample at 12 months. Infants in this relationship group become very distressed by the procedure (as do some secure cases) and desire contact upon reunion (as do some secure cases), but they are

ective in using the caregiver to become comforted. Either
ntact seeking with squirming to be put down, angry rejection
,iver, and/or general petulance (thus the term "resistance"), or
assive and weak in their efforts to achieve contact despite be-
ssed. In both cases, they show poor exploration throughout, in
stark contrast to the secure groups.

Those classed as anxious–avoidant (20%) explore at least superfi-
cially prior to separation and are not upset when left with the stranger
(and perhaps not when left alone). But this also is true of some secure
cases. What distinguishes these cases is the infant's active avoidance of
the caregiver upon reunion. One subgroup may give no greeting or acknowledgment whatsoever; or infants may greet then markedly turn
away (and perhaps stay unresponsive despite the efforts of the caregiver). Another subgroup may begin to approach and then markedly
turn away from the caregiver. Strikingly, both groups show greater
avoidance following the second separation, belying the idea that they
simply were not interested. Also, concurrent heart rate recordings show
that the heart rates of this group remain elevated during reunion, in contrast to secure cases (Sroufe & Waters, 1977b). They are indeed aroused,
but do not use contact with the caregiver to alleviate that arousal, and
quality of exploration is compromised.

A final category, "disorganized/disoriented" attachment (Main &
Hesse, 1990; Main & Solomon, 1990), was not available when we
started our study. By the time it was available, only 157 assessments
were available to code due to deterioration of old-style videotapes.
These 157 cases were coded in the early 1990s. We describe this pattern
in later chapters, when it is especially germane to the discussion.

We view these attachment classifications as relationship assessments, even though they are based on examining infant behavior. The
many reasons for this have been widely discussed (e.g., Sroufe, 1985).
They include the fact that the infant may well be classified differently
when seen with a different parent; that is, they reflect expectations built
up over weeks of interaction with the particular parent. Also, they are
linked to earlier parental treatment and the classification predicts later
maternal behavior (e.g., Chapter 6). Moreover, they predict attachment
relationships for siblings and the caregiver. Finally, as we report in Chapter 5, security of attachment is not predicted by infant temperament (for
relevant reviews, see also Thompson, 1998; Vaughn & Bost, 1999).

Maltreatment Caregiving Groups

By the end of the infancy period, 44 cases had been identified as providing care that was sufficiently inadequate to be designated as maltreat-

ment. Maltreatment judgments were based on a variety of sources of information, including statements made by the parent during interviews, and observer ratings and judgments made during the various observational assessments (Child Care Rating Scale; Egeland & Brunnquell, 1979).

Four patterns of maltreatment were identified: physical abuse, physical neglect, psychological unavailability, and verbal abuse. (At later periods we identified a pattern of seductive behavior and, ultimately, experiences of sexual abuse, though generally not at the hands of the mother.) "Physical abuse" refers to inflicting actual physical harm to the child through hitting, beating, burning, or some other means. "Physical neglect" entailed failure to provide adequate care for the child in terms of food, shelter, clothing, or supervision. "Psychological unavailability" was an especially important pattern. It involves a complete lack of emotional engagement or emotional responsiveness to the child. The mother is either affectively flat or simply does not resonate with the child's emotional expressions. It is the psychological counterpart of physical neglect (Egeland & Erickson, 1987; Egeland & Sroufe, 1981). Finally, "verbal abuse" involved chronic verbal expression of hostility and derision directed at the child, or chronic yelling and verbal threats. We were conservative in all these judgments. Placement in these groups required extremely negative parental behavior. Generally, when we made such a decision, the family already had been called to the attention of Child Protection or had been assigned a social work caseworker, separate from our study.

The Context of Infant Care

During the infant period, we obtained extensive information regarding the context in which each caregiver was operating. We relied on four approaches: (1) a self-report life stress scale completed at 3 months, 12 months, and 18 months; (2) information from social work files available for each family; (3) an extensive interview regarding demographics, living arrangements, social support (e.g., who they turn to for advice), and problems in raising their baby; and (4) the mother's own experience of care, including any history of abuse.

SES was derived from scores on the Duncan Socioeconomic Index (Stevens & Featherman, 1981). This score is based on equations using percentages of occupation holders in the population who have achieved given levels of income and education.

To measure the stress being experienced by our families, we initially used an adaptation of the Cochrane and Robertson (1973) Life Events Inventory. In this procedure, parents answer questions about whether a large number of events has occurred during the given time period (e.g., illnesses, moves, job changes). Ample research had shown a powerful impact of experiencing a large number of such life changes. However, it became apparent that this instrument was not fully applicable for our sample. It contained items that were not pertinent (e.g., trouble with investments) and lacked items tapping salient matters (e.g., trouble with the landlord). Moreover, it provided no information on the degree of disruptiveness caused by the particular event.

Therefore, we adapted the instrument by adding and subtracting items (see Appendix B) and by weighting each item in terms of its severity (Egeland, Breitenbucher, & Rosenberg, 1980). For example, a life-threatening illness of someone a person is dependent upon is more stressful (rated 3) than a routine virus (rated 1). In the early years of the project, we used a total life stress score, cumulating these weighted items. In later years, as we describe, we sometimes also examined different subcategories of stressors (e.g., personal stress and instrumental stress; Pianta & Egeland, 1990).

In infancy, at ages 3, 6, 9, and 12 months, and throughout the study, we interviewed the mothers regarding the general circumstances in their lives, how it was going with their parenting, and the social support that was available to them. We asked them about problems they were having and things they enjoyed about being a parent. We asked about their living arrangements, about partners (whether living in or not), and about who they talked to when they needed someone and, in general, who was there for them. (A sample interview format for age 12 months can be found in Appendix C.) From these interviews we were able to make ratings of the quality of adult partnerships (e.g., "relationship tension") and the quality of social support available to each of our participants.

Finally, every participant was given a brief life history interview, including questions about maltreatment and alternative sources of support (e.g., adults other than parents who cared for the child, therapy experience). For a subset of participants, a much more detailed clinical interview was given (Morris, 1980). For these participants, it was possible to gather information about childhood exploitation and sexual abuse that did not surface in the brief interview. Such detailed analyses of subsamples established a pattern we followed throughout the study.

CONCLUSION

This is how we began our study. Data collection was very intensive in the earliest phases of life. The infants were observed by nurses on each of the first 3–5 days infants were in the hospital, were tested by us at days 7 and 10, were observed with their mothers at 3 months and twice at 6 months of age, were evaluated in terms of motor and cognitive development at 9 and 12 months, and were seen in the Strange Situation at 12 and 18 months. Thus, by the end of the first year, infant assessments of some kind had been made 11 times on over 200 participants. Mothers, likewise, were seen on numerous occasions. They filled out questionnaires and were interviewed extensively throughout the prenatal and postnatal periods. We probed not only their expectations and viewpoints but also personal characteristics and ways of interacting with the infant. But, in addition, we obtained detailed information about the array of circumstances in which their parenting was taking place.

This extensive information allowed us to understand the similarities and differences in the early development of children like Serena and Thomas, discussed in Chapter 1. We knew, for example, that both were robust newborns. Neither was born prematurely or showed signs of compromised neurophysiological development. Both reached early developmental milestones on time. Neither was temperamentally difficult. We also knew that the maltreatment and lack of emotional responsiveness experienced by Thomas began early, that his family life was chaotic, that his mother faced chronic stress, and that she suffered from depression and other personal problems. Finally, we knew that while both mothers were poor at the time of their child's birth, the economic situation of Serena's mother, Jessica, improved dramatically. Moreover, she formed a stable relationship with a partner, and all four grandparents were involved in supporting this family.

Thus, we came to understand a great deal about how our child participants began their lives. In Chapter 4, we describe, age by age, all of the ways we followed them through time.

CHAPTER 4

The Follow-Up Strategy

> Development turns at each and every stage of the journey on
> an interaction between the organism as it has developed up to
> that moment and the environment in which it then finds
> itself.
>
> —BOWLBY (1973)

A central premise of our hierarchical, organizational view of development is that each preceding phase of development provides the foundation for subsequent phases. Thus, caregiver regulation of infant arousal in the first months of life sets the stage for the quality of attachment later in infancy, with its attendant expectations regarding self and other. These two issues, then, set the stage for the more autonomous functioning of the toddler. The cumulative negotiation of these issues is then the foundation for the growth of self-management and the other salient issues to be negotiated during the preschool years, and so on, through the years of development.

Our major assessments at each age concerned the central adaptational issues of the time. Likewise, our first analyses concerned the continuity between variations in negotiating these issues and variations in negotiating past and subsequent issues. However, since coherence of development rather than stability is the target, we measured changing circumstances and specific aspects of individual growth that might mediate or reflect change. Thus, in addition to general measures of adaptation, in the toddler and preschool years, we assessed, for example, language development and other aspects of cognitive functioning; in the school years, we measured intelligence and achievement, and so forth. Routinely, we assessed problems as well as strengths. We also routinely assessed characteristics of the principal caregiver, especially those such as depression, which may fluctuate over time. Finally, at each age, we measured the stresses and supports presented by the current family environment.

This was an unusually comprehensive study, and thousands of pages would be required to fully describe it. Assessments were very extensive at each age. Listing all measures, age by age, would make for tedious reading and a ponderous book. At the same time, we do wish to convey fully the rationale for our assessments of adaptation and the meaning of the various codings and ratings we made. Therefore, we focus on our assessments of quality of care and of the adaptation of child, teenager, and young adult, providing most detail regarding our behavioral assessments. We do this age by age. Then, we provide a very brief overview of the assessments of caregiver characteristics and the measures of context across ages. For readers who wish a complete listing of everything we measured at any given age, see Appendix A.

SALIENT ISSUES OF ADAPTATION

Here, we briefly overview the key issues for adaptation at each age. These receive some elaboration in later chapters when we present our findings with regard to them. We organize the issues into three broad domains: individual development, relationships with parents, and functioning in the broader social world. Note also that there are recurrent issues in each of these domains that run throughout development. For example, as we elaborate below, self-regulation is such an issue on the individual level. At each age, there are different, culturally based expectations with regard to this capacity, and quality of adaptation is judged, in part, with reference to these expectations. At the level of the parent–child relationship a recurrent issue is "autonomy with connectedness," the degree to which the child is increasingly independent of parents, yet remains connected with them. Finally, with regard to peers, one continuing issue may be labeled "deepening and expansion of relationships." With age, the child has a more complex network and also deeper friendships. In keeping with our organizational perspective, at each age, we are tapping into the same issues, yet they are transformed by the developmental level of the child. The array of issues is outlined below and summarized in Table 4.1. Since infancy assessments were presented in Chapter 3, we begin here with the toddler period.

Numerous theorists have described the challenges that come with

TABLE 4.1. Salient Issues of Development

Toddler period

Major issue: "Guided self-regulation"
Subsidiary issues
　Increased autonomy
　Increased awareness of self and others
　Awareness of standards for behavior
　Self-conscious emotions

Preschool period

Major issue: "Self-regulation"
Subsidiary issues
　Self-reliance with support (agency)
　Self-management
　Expanding social world
　Internalization of rules and values

School years

Major issue: "Competence"
Subsidiary issues
　Personal effectance
　Self-integration
　Competence with peers
　　Place in group
　　Functioning in group
　　Loyal friendships
　Competence in school

Adolescence

Major issue: "Individuation"
Subsidiary issues
　Autonomy with connectedness
　Identity
　Peer network competence
　　Place in network
　　Functioning in network
　　Intimate relationships
　Coordinating school, work, and social life

Transition to adulthood

Major issue: "Emancipation"
Subsidiary issues
　Launching a life course
　Financial responsibility
　Adult social competence
　　Coordinating partnerships and friendships
　　Coordinating colleagues, partners, and friends
　　Stable partnerships
　Coordinating work, training, career, social life

the toddler's emerging autonomy (e.g., Mahler, Pine, & Bergman, 1975). On the one hand, it is vital for the toddler to express strivings and desires, because this is the bedrock for agency and purposefulness. The enthusiasm of toddlers for exercising new capacities and tackling new experiences is often noteworthy. On the other hand, such exploration must occur within a field of containment, so that overwhelming arousal is not repeatedly experienced. We therefore label the major issue of this phase "guided self-regulation," because, paradoxically, the toddler shows notable advances in doing for him- or herself and in self-regulation, but only within the framework of caregiving relationships; that is, a toddler can inhibit a response, modify an action, or comply with a request to do something he or she does not want to do, but all of this is heavily dependent on adult presence and guidance.

The toddler period is also the age of the emergence of self-awareness (and a parallel increasing awareness of others), as is shown by the classic mirror self-recognition studies (Lewis & Brooks, 1978; Mans, Cicchetti, & Sroufe, 1978). With this awareness comes the beginning sense of standards for behavior, which is the cradle of morality (e.g., Kochanska, 1997). The toddler understands that some things ought not be done. This is one reason that compliance with adult requests is to be expected in most circumstances. Congruent with all of this is the beginning of self-conscious emotions (Lewis, 1992). Just as toddlers can feel ebullient, they also have the capacity for shame, feeling intensely bad about the self—shriveled, defeated, and unworthy. It is a vulnerable period, as well as an expansive period. For this reason, we conducted a major assessment during this developmental period.

Preschoolers are capable of self-direction and self-management, and we expect it of them. They need supervision, of course, but we expect them to follow rules, without constant enforcement, and to refrain from certain actions, such as hitting someone, even when adults are out of arms reach. In brief, we expect them to have internalized the rules and values of caregivers. This internalization makes possible not only feelings of pride when a standard is met but also feelings of guilt when it is not. Entrée into the world of peers also is a hallmark of this period. While toddlers certainly have playmates, preschoolers more actively select partners and sustain interactions with them, and they participate in groups. These are critical training opportunities for later peer competence. All of these experiences are crucial for consolidating the sense of self or personality. Some children emerge from this period with positive self-esteem; others do not. Our assessments at this age tapped into all of these issues.

Competence is the central issue for middle childhood, competence in every domain. This is not the competence of imagination and play of the preschooler, but competence in the real world. It is manifest in school, in the peer group, and in the development of special talents and skills. Whereas the preschooler has a sense of agency, of doing things on his or her own, the elementary school child has a sense of effectance, of doing things well and to completion. Children at this time also forge a more integrated and realistic sense of themselves. Elementary-age children are more autonomous *vis-à-vis* parents; at the same time, they are generally aligned with them, accepting their rules and their authority. Parenting now is more a matter of supervising and monitoring, as opposed to direct guidance. But perhaps the major manifestation of growing competence is seen in the world of peers. Elementary schoolers have not just play partners, but important, deep, and loyal friendships. They not only sustain interactions but also maintain relationships, despite the attendant conflicts. Highly organized peer groups emerge. Moreover, elementary-age children coordinate group functioning with maintaining friendships (see Table 4.2).

The adolescent brings the process of self-development to a new level, developing the sense of being a unique, differentiated person, connected with the past and projecting into the future. "Identity" and "individuation" are two of the terms used to describe this issue. More recently, however, it has been recognized that this new autonomy is not at the expense of continued closeness with parents (and now with others as well). The connection now is more between equals; adolescents recognize shortcomings of parents and their parenting. But individuation generally does not mean separateness. The individual now has greater responsibility for decisions, and to some degree, they must self-monitor. But parents retain the vital role of monitoring the teen's monitoring. Adolescent life is qualitatively more complex than life in middle childhood. Teens generally must coordinate school with work and/or extracurricular activities, as well as with a complicated social life. Teens function in a social network, often including same- and other-gender friends, same- and mixed-gender groups, and intimate partnerships. All of this must be coordinated.

Emancipation really is an issue for adulthood rather than the teenage years for most people in Western society. The young adult must set a life course, as well as begin assuming financial self-responsibility. If not, in fact, living separately, the young adult in some way functions as a more independent unit. The coordination tasks of the teen years are expanded. Now training and/or advanced education must be coordinated with work, activities, and a social life. On the personal front, the individual must evolve a sense of direction and an attitude of reflection, that is, the capacity to examine one's own trajectory, to appraise it, and to al-

TABLE 4.2. Changing Issues in Childhood Peer Relationships

Preschool: "Positive engagement of peers"

1. Selecting specific partners
2. Sustaining interactive bouts
   a. Negotiating conflicts in interaction
   b. Maintaining organization in the face of arousal
   c. Finding pleasure in the interactive process
3. Participation in groups

Middle childhood: "Investment in the peer world"

1. Forming loyal friendships
2. Sustaining relationships
   a. Negotiating relationship conflicts
   b. Tolerating a range of emotional experiences
   c. Enhancement of self in relationships
3. Functioning in stable, organized groups
   a. Adhering to group norms
   b. Maintaining gender boundaries
4. Coordinating friendships and group functioning

Adolescence: "Integrating self and peer relationships"

1. Forming intimate relationships
   a. Self-disclosing same-gender relationships
   b. Cross-gender relationships
   c. Sexual relationships
2. Commitment in relationships
   a. Negotiating self-relevant conflicts
   b. Emotional vulnerability
   c. Self-disclosure and self-identity
3. Functioning in a relationship network
   a. Mastering multiple rule systems
   b. Establishing flexible boundaries
4. Coordinating multiple relationships
   a. Same-gender and cross-gender
   b. Intimate relationships and group functioning

ter the course if necessary. No one else can do this for the person. The social world, too, increases in complexity. Stable partnerships occur and colleagues join the social network. Integrating these relationships with the already complex social network is the challenge.

This, then, was the set of developmental issues that guided our key assessments. Our goal was to examine the adaptation of individual children over time with regard to this series of developmental issues, rather than asking, for example, whether quality of attachment per se remained stable. Each issue we have defined persists, though they may not be most salient for defining later ages and may not be so readily assessed at those times. During the toddler and preschool years, for example, normally developing attachment relationships remain integral in the child's world. However, tapping the underlying attachment organization becomes more difficult due to the extensive behavioral repertoire and expanding cognitive capacities of the child (Solomon & George, 1999). Fewer situations are seen as threatening, and mere knowledge of the parents' accessibility is effective in terminating attachment behavior (rather than physical proximity). Children may use eye contact, nonverbal expressions of affect, and conversations about feelings and activities to organize interactions with attachment figures. Therefore, brief observational measures are less sensitive. At the same time, representational assessment is not yet very reliable due to variability in language and symbolic capacities (Cicchetti, Cummings, Greenberg, & Marvin, 1990). For these reasons, we did not directly assess attachment during these ages.

THE ASSESSMENTS

The Toddler Period

The key assessment in the toddler period was a videotaped laboratory session including 10 minutes of free play, a cleanup session, and a series of four problems, solved with the caregiver's assistance. The play segment was relatively stress free for most pairs; it allowed us to see the child's capacity for symbolic play and enthusiasm for play. The cleanup session taxed the caregiver, because the child was not likely to want to stop playing with the attractive toys provided. We could assess the caregiver's ability to structure the task, and to set and maintain limits, as well as negative behaviors, such as hostility, coerciveness, or seductive manipulation. Finally, the tool problems taxed both partners and their relationship. The first two problems were relatively easy, involving getting rewards from a slot and from a tube using sticks. The third problem was a bit more difficult, because two short sticks had to be put together to obtain the reward. The fourth problem was very difficult. Here, the child had to weight down a long board with a wooden block, so that candy would be raised through a hole in the top of a large box (see Matas et al., 1978). The problem had to be solved at a distance, using a tool that was not obvious. It was expected that all children would reach a point where their capacities were exceeded. Caregivers (almost always mothers) were told the following: "See what she can do with it first on her own; then, give her any help you think she needs."

We viewed this procedure as ideal for tapping into the salient issues of this age (i.e., emergence of autonomy, beginnings of standards and guided control). We could assess the child's enthusiasm, compliance, persistence, positive and negative affect, anger, and frustration. We also gave the child an overall rating with regard to these variables, taking into account support she got from her mother; for example, persistence in the absence of support is more impressive than when the caregiver is very helpful. For the caregiver, key ratings were of Supportive Presence and Quality of Assistance. Supportive Presence refers to the emotional aspects of her support; for example, encouraging the child's efforts, drawing closer to the child when needed, sharing the joy of problem solution, anticipating frustration, and taking action to deal with it. Quality of Assistance referred to the timing, clarity, and appropriateness of clues; that is, did the caregiver give clues such that the child could do everything he could, while not being asked to do too much, and were the clues such that the child actually came to understand the solutions to problems. These two 7-point caregiver scales are found in Appendix D. We also rated caregivers on hostility, derision, and boundary violations. These kinds of ratings had been shown in our previous research to be related both to earlier attachment assessments and to outcomes in kindergarten (Arend et al., 1979; Matas et al., 1978), and they would prove to be useful again.

Finally, we used a global rating of the child's "Experience in the Session." At the positive end of this scale, the child was viewed as having a positive, growth-enhancing experience. She was receiving the help she needed to be both enthusiastically invested in the problems, yet contained when arousal and frustration made this necessary. If this were a microcosm of the child's daily life, this was a child who later would have a high sense of self-esteem, a belief in her own competence, and in the support of others. At the negative end of the scale, the child had a profoundly deflating experience, likely to leave him with less confidence in himself and in the availability of his caregiver: Specifically, "in the end, the child is feeling abandoned or outside of the support of the mother, and impotent in the face of the tasks and his feelings" (from scale point 1). Such experiences would lead to profound feelings of self-doubt. This was the key measure for this age period (see Appendix D).

During this same time, we also carried out a series of measures on facets of the child's development and another measure of parenting. For example, at 24 months, we administered the Bayley Scales of Infant Development (Bayley, 1969), which had been given previously at 9 months. The EASI (Emotionality, Activity, Sociability, and Impulsivity) Temperament Survey (Buss & Plomin, 1975) was given at 30 months. Finally, the Caldwell HOME Inventory (Caldwell, 1979) was used to measure the quality of social, emotional, and cognitive stimulation provided to the child in the home at age 30 months.

The Preschool Period

We conducted major videotaped, observational assessments during the preschool period at ages 42 and 54 months. At 42 months, we saw the child *with* the caregiver, doing a series of teaching tasks, and *without* the caregiver present, facing an unsolvable problem. The Teaching Tasks (building block towers, naming things that have wheels, tracing a maze, and completing a multidimensional form board) were adapted from the Berkeley Longitudinal Study (Block & Block, 1980). They were primarily used to assess caregiver behavior, although we did assess child behaviors such as enthusiasm, positive and negative affect, and compliance as well. Both child and parent ratings were similar to those used at age 2, with some additions (e.g., caregiver's respect for the child's autonomy; caregiver's confidence in his or her ability to deal with the child). The situation was indeed taxing, because the tasks were difficult. For example, children cannot do two-dimensional classification tasks, much less the three-dimensional size, shape, and color-sorting task that we used, and children at this age do not like tasks in which they simply must talk to their mothers. Likewise, it is more fun to play with the Etch-A-Sketch or with the blocks than follow a prescribed route on the maze, or build a specific model tower repeatedly. Noncompliance and efforts to quit the tasks early were frequent. The caregiver's flexibility and continued patient support of the child were key features.

In the barrier box situation, when the caregiver was not present, the child's interest was first aroused by a set of attractive toys. He or she was then told that to play with the toys a locked box must be opened. This was virtually impossible for a child to do and provided an excellent vantage point for evaluating the child's sense of agency (strength of efforts), flexibility, frustration tolerance, and self-regulation. For example, could he or she modulate arousal by taking breaks, trying other strategies, and so forth? In addition to rating these variables, we also rated self-esteem. This was an integrative scale that captured the projected self-confidence, enthusiasm for working on the problems, persistence, and capacity to have fun. (After the children worked on this problem for 10 minutes, we did open the box so that they could enjoy the toys!)

At 54 months, we observed the child in a series of engaging tasks utilized by Block and Block (1980) to assess a control dimension (from impulsiveness at one end, to inhibition at the other) and a flexibility dimension (the degree to which the child could loosen or tighten self-control as appropriate). The procedures included the Lowenfeld Mosaic Test (Block & Block, 1973), in which the child used a set of plastic tiles to make potentially elaborate designs; tasks that required divided attention; a delay of gratification measure, in which the child got a larger reward if he or she was able to wait, or a small reward immediately; a Curiosity Box (Banta, 1970, described in Chapter 7); and the Shure and Spivak (1974) Interpersonal Problem-Solving Test (PIPS). Various indices were composited to capture flexibility and control (Troy, 1988). The PIPS, which involved asking the child to describe various ways a set of interpersonal problems could be solved, also yielded an early measure of attachment representation; that is, from the child's responses, one could determine his or her internalized expectations regarding parental availability and support (see Carlson et al., 2004).

Additional measures we obtained during this period included a role-taking measure (Borke, 1971) and a language-development assessment (Zimmerman, Steiner, & Pond, 1979) at 42 months, and assessments of both self-help and language skills at 48 months. At 64 months, we administered the Wechsler Preschool and Primary Scale of Intelligence (WIPPSI; Wechsler, 1967) and the Slaby and Frey (1975) Gender Constancy Test.

In addition to these assessments that were conducted with all participants, 98 children were observed in nursery school, including 40 children seen in classrooms that we controlled. In selecting the children for our nursery school, a history of anxious attachment was overrepresented, such that in one class (n = 16), half of the children had clearly anxious histories, and in our second class, two-thirds had anxious histories (i.e., there were 8 secure, 8 avoidant, and 8 resistant children). Such a distribution allowed us to make the comparisons we wished to make. Half were males, and half were females; otherwise, children were selected at random (see Sroufe, 1983).

All 98 of the nursery school children were assessed with the Behar and Stringfield Preschool Behavior Questionnaire (1974) measure of behavior problems and strengths and were rated by teachers on agency, self-confidence, social skills, positive and negative affect, and compliance. For the subsample of 40 children, there also were detailed observations of social behavior, dependence, self-regulation, and emotion; for example, what proportion of contacts with another child were initiated with positive affect (Sroufe, Schork, Motti, Lawroski, & LaFreniere, 1984)? Ratings and Q-sorts were made by multiple teachers and staff (Sroufe, 1983). The 100-item California Child Q-Sort allows researchers to generate scores on flexibility, control, self-esteem, and dependence, among other things. Typical items included "impulsive, acts without thinking," "empathic, shows concern for others," "curious, likes to explore," "is physically cautious," "is admired and sought out by others," and "falls to pieces under stress." Items were placed by the rater into nine categories along a dimension from least characteristic of the child to most characteristic.

An advantage of the Q-sort approach is that one can create new "mega-items" or scales at a later time. For example, by treating placement of items pertaining to empathy (e.g., "is considerate and thoughtful") as scores and adding them together (with negative items reversed), one obtains a variable value for each child. Even constructs not being studied by the field when the project began (e.g., childhood depression) can later be studied.

Children also were extensively videotaped, and these recordings were used to derive a variety of measures, including empathic behavior of children and treatment of individual children by teachers. We provide more details on these measures when we present results from the nursery school study in Chapter 7.

Finally, we obtained rankings of children's popularity, neglect, and rejection, using a sociometric technique and a procedure for tapping the classroom attention structure. In addition to asking children to nominate three children that they "especially liked to play with" and three that they did "not especially like to play with," we carried out paired comparisons with photos, asking them in each case which child they preferred as a playmate. The attention-structure procedure involves observing all children in a cyclical fashion, noting each time the target of each child's looking (Vaughn & Waters, 1981). A structure (and ranking) emerges, with some children receiving many looks. This measure of popularity and the sociometric measure were highly correlated, and both agreed with teacher ratings and rankings (LaFreniere & Sroufe, 1985).

As can be seen, this subsample study allowed great strength in measurement. As one example, dependence was measured in four ways: (1) the Q-sort dependency index, (2) composited teacher ratings of dependence, (3) observed time with teacher, and (4) "circle time" contact. Each day for 15 weeks, during the three circle times, for example, a record was made of where each child sat and whether the child touched the teacher or sat on her lap. There was great convergence among the four dependence measures, and they were powerfully related to earlier attachment and later dependence measures (see Chapter 7).

In all, our preschool assessments allowed us to capture individual variations in self-management, self-regulation, and independence; the growth of initiative and agency; and immersion into the world of peers. Some children, like Selena, did well on all of these. Others, like Thomas, did poorly on all. Still others showed various combinations of strengths and problems. At the same time, we monitored variations in the continued support by parents.

Middle Childhood

During the elementary school years, the assessment strategy changed to fit the development and changing circumstances of the child. Many assessments were carried out at school. And the children were directly tested, interviewed, and asked to engage in a variety of expressive procedures. So teachers, parents, and now children themselves were informants. Direct observation of social behavior was carried out with all of the participants during kindergarten, and a majority of them were also observed at school. A smaller subsample was observed intensively in a series of summer camps.

School functioning is a critical arena, and we obtained comprehensive school assessments in kindergarten and grades 1–3 and 6. These included teacher rankings of Emotional Health–Self-Esteem and Peer Competence. Teachers were given paragraphs describing these constructs prior to ranking each child in their class, including our participant. The peer competence description included the characteristics of close friendship and successful group functioning presented in our discussion of peer competence earlier, and the emotional health/self-esteem description captured the child's integrated emotional functioning and sense of well-being (see Appendix E). Teachers, as well as parents, also made ratings of behavior problems and deportment, using the Teacher's Report Form of the Child Behavior Checklist (Achenbach & Edelbrock, 1986) and the Devereaux Preschool Behavior Rating Scale (Spivak & Swift, 1982). In addition, teachers were interviewed regarding the child's academic performance and other aspects of school functioning, and information from school files on attendance and other matters was obtained. We also conducted our own assessments of reading and math achievement using the Peabody Individual Achievement Test in grades 1–3 and grade 6 (Dunn & Markwardt, 1970). The Harter Perceived Competence and Acceptance Scale for Young Children was obtained from the teacher at school and from the child at home in grades 1 and 2 (Harter, 1979).

In other assessments, we measured the child's impulsivity using Porteus Maze Performance (Porteus, 1965) in grade 1, depression (Children's Depression Rating Scale [CDRS]; Poznanski, Cook, & Carroll, 1979) in grades 2 and 3, and intelligence using four subscales of the Wechsler Intelligence Scales for Children—Revised (WISC-R; Wechsler, 1974) in grade 3. We obtained drawings of a person in preschool and in grade 1, and family drawings in grade 3. The family drawings were scored for attachment representation, using a system first developed by Nancy Kaplan and Mary Main (e.g., Main, Kaplan, & Cassidy, 1985) and expanded by us (see Fury, Carlson, & Sroufe, 1997). In grade 6, we gave a battery of projective tests to probe the child's representations of self and others. These included Thematic Apperception Test stories (Cohen & Weil, 1971; Murray, 1938/1943), a Sentence Completion Test, a moral fable (Johnston, 1988), and the Seligman Explanatory Style Questionnaire (Homan, 1990; Seligman et al., 1984). We gave the child an extensive friendship interview that was used both as a measure of representation (the child's expectations regarding relationships) and as a basis for some factual information regarding friends.

Sometime between grades 3 and 5, observers went to the schools of 108 children on three separate occasions and observed them in a variety of settings. Following these observations, both the observers and the children's teachers completed the Block Q-sort (see p. 73).

At age 10 years, 48 children (39 from our nursery school study, plus additional randomly selected children with secure attachment histories) were seen in a series of 4-week summer camps (16 children in each). Half of the children had anxious attachment histories and half had secure histories, and boys and girls were equally represented (see Elicker, Englund, & Sroufe, 1992). As we did in the preschool, multiple counselors completed rankings or ratings of social competence, dependence, self-confidence, agency, and other scales, as well as completing a Q-sort. Observers made detailed records of the social behavior of the children (e.g., isolation, contact with adults, frequency of participation in groups, contact with particular children). We obtained sociometrics from the children themselves. Thus, there were comprehensive assessments of social competence and the organization of peer behavior. Special strengths of these data were the density of observation and the possibility of using convergent measures. As one example, friendships were scored in three ways. First, based upon hundreds of observations of each child in turn, we could determine the density of contacts with a particular partner. This ratio of contacts was a "friend" score. Second, counselors nominated pairs of children that they viewed as forming clear friendships. Finally, if the children themselves reciprocally nominated each other as friends, they were viewed as friends. These three measures showed strong convergence and yielded powerful links to earlier measures of adaptation and to later outcomes.

The children were extensively videotaped at the camps, and these tapes were used to derive a variety of important measures after the fact. As one example, we were able to make reliable ratings of the degree to which children maintained or violated age-typical gender boundaries (see Chapter 8). All observers and counselors were blind to the histories of the children.

Information on parenting when the child was in elementary school came from observations and interviews in the home. At age 6, the

Caldwell HOME scales (Caldwell, 1979), administered at age 2½, were repeated to assess quality of cognitive, social, and emotional stimulation. In addition, following lengthy interviews of the mothers in grades 1–3 and 6, interviewers made global ratings of quality of child care, which, among other things, allowed detection of child maltreatment. From the interviews, more specific ratings of monitoring of the child, parental involvement at school, and involvement and support from men in the child's life were also made.

Adolescence

Three major direct assessments were carried out during the junior and senior high school years, one at age 13, one at age 16, and one at age 17½. In addition, teachers were interviewed, and school records were obtained at age 16 and also at the end of high school to monitor dropping out and other school problems.

Early adolescence is a critical time for families, since every member is taxed by the child's newly expanding autonomy (Collins, 1995). Family conflict is at its height (Collins & Laursen, 2004; Steinberg & Morris, 2001), in contrast to the later teen years. For some families, it is difficult to let the child assume more autonomy and a more egalitarian role in the transformed relationship. In light of this, we carried out a key assessment of parent–child relationships at age 13. This was the last time we observed parents and children together in our laboratory. We were able to recruit 175 mothers and 44 fathers or father substitutes. When fathers were present, the child was seen with each parent separately; then the three family members were seen together.

The procedures, many of them adapted from the Berkeley Longitudinal Study (Block & Block, 1980), were specifically designed to probe issues surrounding the adolescent's emergence from childhood and changing role in the family (see J. Sroufe, 1991, for a description). For example, the pair was asked to plan an antismoking campaign designed to appeal to teenagers (mothers) or an antishoplifting campaign (fathers). In each case, the young person had a clear expertise. Could the parents acknowledge this? Could the child step up to a leadership role? In a task we created (Wiens & Collins, 1983), the parent was asked to assemble objects from the Wechsler Intelligence Scales (the apple, the person) while blindfolded, with the teenager giving directions. Again, it is a transfer-of-power problem, and this task yielded remarkable variation. Other tasks involved discussing imaginary happenings, for example, "What would happen if scientists discovered a tasty, inexpensive pill that would meet all needs for nutrition?" We considered whether the pair could talk together and collaborate. They also completed a Q-sort of an "ideal person." This last task inevitably produced disagreements; for example, exactly how important is "independence" compared to "follows the rules"? Young teens often have different opinions from their parents on such matters. How these conflicts were resolved was of great interest. Two tasks were used only with triads. One was a revealed differences task, using a case scenario in which the child arrives home 2 hours late on a school night. The members first considered separately what they thought should be done in such a situation; then, the three of them had to agree on a joint solution. In the other task, they planned a vacation together.

Engagement, several emotional scales (positive affect, negative affect, anger, and hostility), conflict and conflict resolution, certain relationship structure scales, and overall quality of functioning scales were coded (following J. Sroufe, 1991). An important distinction was made between anger and hostility when we used these ratings here and in later observations of couples. With anger, the emotion is directly expressed, and behavior shown is congruent with underlying feelings. The goal of anger is changing the partner's behavior, and there is some expectation that this might happen. With hostility, in contrast, there is indirectness and lack of congruence (as when a parent smiles and says in a sarcastic tone, "Oh, you're being so helpful," implying that the child never has been and never will be helpful). Hostility and cynicism imply a lack of hope.

The relationship structure scales concerned maintenance or breakdown of roles (child-like parent, adult-like child, seductiveness, boundary violations, triangulation). Despite encouraging autonomy, the parent must still remain the more adult person, and parents must meet emotional and sensual needs with their partner, not with their child.

Overall functioning was assessed using three scales tapping "balance" in the relationship systems. First, there must be balance among the persons, with each person having a safe place in the relationship. This is manifested primarily by spontaneity and being able to retain a position despite disagreement. The second balance scale concerned balance between the relationship and the individuals. The relationship must serve each person's development; for example, does the parent support the child's emerging autonomy? Can the child engage in the tasks versus having to take care of the parents or put all of his or her energy into fighting with them? The third balance scale concerned balance between the relationship and the outside world. Could the partners marshal resources to address the tasks at hand and work as a team? Two coders rated a subsample of 129 dyadic assessments with good reliability (kappa for these scales averaged .78).

At age 16, we conducted major interviews with the teen concerning school, identity, friendship, and dating. In addition to factual information, the friendship interview was again used as a measure of representation. Participants were asked to share what they liked and disliked about the friendship, how their friend treated them, and to describe several positive and negative emotional experiences in the friendship. They also were asked to describe the biggest fight they had ever had with the friend, including the topic, circumstances of the argument, reactions of both individuals, and resolutions. Coders rated audiotapes of these interviews on several 7-point scales. The intraclass correlations between two coders' scores ranged from .74 to .84. A composite variable labeled "friendship quality" was formed by summing ratings of security, presence of conflict (reverse-coded), conflict resolution, disclosure, and closeness. This scale had high internal reliability (alpha = .88).

We also administered the Adolescent Health Survey (Blum, Resnick, & Bergeisen, 1989), with wide-ranging coverage of physical and mental health, including drug use and suicidal ideation. We obtained behavior problem checklist data from parents, teachers, and the young person, and we administered the Harter Self-Perception Profile (competence, appearance, global self-worth; Harter, 1979). Reading and math achievement were assessed using the Woodcock–Johnson Psychoeducational Battery—Revised. Finally, we obtained the youth's report of family functioning, conflict, and life stress using the Adolescent Perceived Events Scale (Compas, Davis, Forsythe, & Wagner, 1987).

A major clinical interview was carried out at age 17½: the Schedule for Affective Disorders and Schizophrenia for School-Age Children (Puig-Antich & Chambers, 1978). This 3-hour interview allows one to assign symptom scores and diagnoses for all of the major categories of the fourth edition of the *Diagnostic and Statistical Manual of Mental Disorders* (DSM IV-R; American Psychiatric Association, 1994). In addition, we interviewed the young person extensively about school, work, dating, living situation, and so forth.

The procedures described were carried out on all project participants. Moreover, 41 of the 48 young people previously seen in summer camp were brought to a series of weekend, overnight reunions at age 15. The teens were seen in a variety of settings—large-group outward bound–type activities, small-group problem-solving tasks, meals, free time, planned recreational activities, and a party. Observations were again made of isolation and other aspects of social behavior. Interviews were conducted to obtain the young people's judgments about the other campers. Multiple counselors made ratings of social competence and other pertinent dimensions. One scale of particular interest at this age was Capacity for Vulnerability, that is, the young person's willingness to participate in the range of activities, including those in which some vulnerability is involved (see Appendix F). This proved to be a powerful outcome measure. In all, we felt that we were able to capture the complexity of adolescent functioning at these camp reunions.

Young Adulthood

At age 19, we made a very comprehensive assessment of participants' adjustment. This included administering the Adult Attachment Interview (George, Kaplan, & Main, 1985), a procedure designed to assess the person's "state of mind" regarding attachment. Based on the way they characterize their earlier relationships with parents, and the nature and coherence of the evidence they use to support such characterizations, individuals are classified into one of three major categories. In the first category, individuals are classed as "autonomous." These persons are open to examining their attachment experiences, and whether they describe their history in positive or negative terms, their characterization is done in a coherent and balanced way. If the experience is described as negative, there is evidence that this experience has been integrated and that some understanding has been achieved. If experience is described in generally positive terms, specific examples are provided, making it clear that it was indeed positive. In the second category, individuals are described as "dismissing." Either they disown the importance of attachment experiences, claim lack of memory for them, or fail to acknowledge that negative experiences had any effect on them. Most positive descriptions of history are idealizations, without support from, or contradicted by, specific examples. For example, having claimed to have had very loving parents, the individual may provide as an example being locked outside barefoot in the snow as punishment "because it showed they wanted me to be a better person." In some way, they keep a distance from their attachment feelings. Members of the third category are referred to as "preoccupied." These individuals talk about their feelings but tend to be entangled with the past, at times revealing an ongoing anger. Often there is a lack of precision and conciseness in their discourse, and they are unable to present an integrated view of their experience. Finally, independent of the three major categories, some individuals are judged to be unresolved–disoriented regarding past trauma or losses. Such an unresolved state is also revealed in discourse, for example, speaking about a deceased person in the present tense, as though he or she were still alive.

We also carried out another extensive interview at ages 19 and 23, covering work, education, religion, politics, living arrangements, and interpersonal relationships, including both friendships and romantic partnerships. We again administered the Adolescent Perceived Events Scale (Compas et al., 1987), and also administered two clinical instruments:

the Adult Health Survey (Blum et al., 1989), which included information on drug use, and the Dissociative Experiences Scale (E. B. Carlson & Putnam, 1993). We gave the participants a sentence-completion task to assess inner models of self and other. From the extensive interviews, we were able to make an integrative rating of the emerging adults' overall quality of functioning. To receive the highest rating on this scale participants had to be working and/or in school or training full time, have a viable social support network that included at least some experience with serious relationships, and they had to have acquired a reflective attitude. This meant that they had to be examining their life course and have some plan for moving forward. If a participant's situation was unsatisfactory, he or she must be taking steps to change it.

For those participants involved in a romantic relationship of at least 4 months' duration, we carried out an extensive assessment at age 20 or 21 ($n = 74$). First, we observed couples in two challenging procedures: In one procedure, they reviewed together a series of problems typically faced by couples, talking about the degree to which each applied to them and subsequently selected a major problem for discussion. This was then discussed for 10 minutes, or until they felt they had reached a joint resolution. In the other procedure, they worked together to complete a Q-sort of the ideal couple. Both procedures were emotionally engaging. Rating scales coded were parallel to those used at age 13 (engagement, four emotional scales, conflict and conflict resolution, and the three balance scales; see page 78).

These couples also completed a relationship interview and an extensive battery of relationship questionnaires. The Current Relationships Interview (Crowell & Owens, 1996) is parallel in administration and scoring to the Adult Attachment Interview discussed earlier, focusing on the couple's relationship qualities. The questionnaires focused on the couple's perceptions of their relationship (e.g., closeness), their problems and conflicts, and their tactics for resolving conflicts (see Appendix A).

Our study is ongoing. At this writing, we are carrying out assessments of participants at age 28. In the final chapter of this book, we outline our assessments for ages 26 and 28, overview some key findings, and point toward the future.

ASSESSMENTS OF CAREGIVERS AND CAREGIVING CONTEXT

In Chapter 3, we described measures of caregiver personality, expectations, and attributions, as well as measures of context, obtained during the prenatal and postnatal periods. Comparable measures were obtained at numerous times in childhood and adolescence, with some changes, of course, due to the age of the child. For example, instead of expectations about how easy it will be to care for the baby, in middle childhood, we assessed expectations regarding educational attainment. Again, a listing of these measures may be found in Appendix A. Here, we provide a brief overview.

Various measures of parental mood, anxiety, alcohol use, and personality were administered during the preschool years. The parental tendency toward dissociation was assessed twice at a later point in time. Finally, depression was assessed five times across the study. This was critical, because it enabled us to demonstrate the impact of changing caregiver depression on the child's behavior problems. We also measured caregiver intelligence using the Wechsler Adult Intelligence Scale (Wechsler, 1955).

We continually probed caregivers' expectations and understanding regarding children and child development. In the early years, this involved primarily the parents' knowledge of child care, their developmental expectations, and their sources of information. Later, perceptions of the school and their child at school, their views on parenting and discipline, and their feelings of autonomy and influence on the child were assessed.

The caregiving context was assessed intensively and extensively. We administered our life stress interview, described in Chapter 3, and interviewed the parents in detail about their life circumstances on 11 occasions over the course of childhood and adolescence. The interviews were the basis for some of the information regarding expectations. They also allowed us to gather information on parents' social support and partnerships, which were at times probed in great detail. We assessed both changes in partnerships and the quality of partnerships. These interviews allowed us to gauge not only support for the mother but also the role of men in the lives of the children, which turned out to be important even after taking into account the quality of parenting by mothers, whether single or married. The interviews further allowed us to assess all other aspects of the caregivers' life circumstances, including their fluctuating economic situations. All of these proved to be powerful sources of information.

We have stated several times that these assessments of fluctuating life circumstances were important, because they placed issues of parenting and parental care into perspective. The tendency to blame parents is greatly reduced when one sees the challenges parents are facing. At the same time, by monitoring the supports and stresses of families at multiple points in time, we were able to account for change in adaptation, as well as in continuity. Finally, this is one way we address the concern of some researchers and clinicians that all of our findings on the impact of experience on child adaptation may be reduced to shared genes between parents and children. Fluctuations in parental depression, life stress, quality of partnerships, or general social support account for changing child competence or behavior problems, and this does not lend itself readily to a genetic interpretation. There are other ways that we draw upon the comprehensiveness of our assessments to address this issue. For example, we, as well as others (e.g., Patterson & Dishion, 1988), find that direct measures of what parents do with their children are better predictors of child outcome than measures of parent personality. Measures of parent aggressiveness as a trait do not predict later child conduct problems nearly as well as do those of observed parental rejection, hostility, and abuse of the child (Egeland, 1997). Similarly, inconsistent, chaotic care (and the anxious–resistant attachment to which it leads) predicts later anxiety problems in the teenager far better than do general measures of mothers' anxiety (Warren, Huston, Egeland, & Sroufe, 1997).

OVERVIEW

Several important features characterized our assessments. First is the use of multiple informants, including trained observers, parents, teachers, counselors, peers, and the children themselves. This is critical both for validation and in order to be comprehensive. While there is some concordance across informants, each also sometimes adds a valuable perspective. The teacher sees the child in the formal school setting, and only the caregiver sees the child at home. Peers at times are the clear experts (e.g., in determining how well a child is liked). For some characteristics, such as adolescent depression, the young person's own vantage point is critical.

The second feature is the use of multiple methods. These include formal tests, expressive procedures (e.g., drawings, stories), questionnaires, interviews, and direct observations. Given our interest in all aspects of functioning, including the inner world of the child, as well as overt behavior, this was a necessity. We put much energy into direct observation, because we believe it holds a pivotal place in developmental research, but our questions could not have been answered without all of the supplemental measures.

Finally, many of the same or similar constructs were measured at multiple points in time. For example, behavior problems and psychopathology were assessed in preschool, kindergarten, grades 1–3 and 6, and at ages 16 and 17½. With the exception of age 17½, peer competence was assessed at all of these same points in time and at age 19. Representation of self and others was assessed in preschool, in grades 3 and 6, and at ages 16, 19, and 26. Parent–child relationships were assessed using direct observation in infancy, the toddler and preschool periods, in early elementary school, and at age 13, and, via interviews, at ages 16 and 19. Context was assessed at every age. We continue to assess each of these constructs at this time. Such cross-time assessments are critical for tracking individual trajectories of development and for carrying out studies of continuity and change in adaptation. These are the tasks we take up in Part II of this book.

A NOTE ON ETHICS

At some point, if not already, a question may enter the reader's mind regarding the ethics of following children over time and tracking the development of problems for many of them. How can one simply observe, while problems in children like Thomas unfold, age by age? It is an issue that we struggled with and continually discussed over the course of this study. There are several reasons why, in fact, we did not directly intervene in the lives of these participants. First, of course, we really had no right to do so. Our participants did not sign up to be part of an intervention study. Second, our predictions about development may have been wrong. What if, for example, those showing patterns of avoidant attachment were actually robust and precociously independent infants, as many psychologists at the time suggested? What business would we have trying to alter parenting patterns in such families? In general, as sound as we might have thought our theories and predictions were, they had only the status of hypotheses. We believe that intervention should only be based on solid evidence. Third, one thing we wanted to study was the response of current institutions to the problems of children and families. Who received special education services? Who got psychiatric care? These questions could only be studied by documenting problems and recording what interventions occurred. We were reporters, not service providers.

Still, it was difficult to embrace the ideas we were pursuing and not take action, especially as early results became available. Ultimately, our solution was to, in fact, conduct an intervention project—not with these participants, but with another large group of families with even greater levels of stress. This project, Steps Toward Effective Empowered Parenting (STEEP), began in the 1980s and has subsequently inspired a number of intervention efforts (e.g., Egeland & Erickson, 2004). It was based upon what we learned in the first 5 years of our study about the need for multipronged supports for families.

PART II

Development and Adaptation

CHAPTER 5

Adaptation in Infancy

> She holds the infant with her hands, with her eyes, with her
> voice and smile, and with changes from one modality to
> another as he habituates to one or another. All of these
> holding experiences are opportunities for the infant to learn
> how to contain himself. . . . They amount to a kind of learning
> about the organization of behavior in order to attend.
> —BRAZELTON, KOWSLOWSKI, AND MAIN (1974)

As we discussed in Chapter 3, critical developmental issues for
the infant concern regulation in the service of engaging the surrounding
world. At first, this involves establishing state and arousal regulation.
These support periods of being awake, alert, and attentive, so that physical and social stimuli can be processed. Progressively, with development,
the infant becomes capable of more sustained engagement, wider fluctuations in arousal, or what we have called "tension modulation" (Sroufe,
1996), and a range of early emotions. Tension and emotion regulation
are critical, because they are inevitable by-products of exploration, and
exploration provides *aliment* for cognitive and social development.
Therefore, early regulation is the platform upon which individual adaptation is constructed.

Yet, at first, such regulation is not an individual matter. As numerous scholars have suggested, and as research has confirmed, effective
regulation of the infant is only possible within a supportive caregiving
system (Ainsworth & Bell, 1974; Fogel, 1993; Sroufe, 1996; Stern,
1985). By providing appropriate and changing stimulation in response
to perceptions of infant state, moods, and interests, caregivers not only

87

help keep arousal within manageable bounds, but they also entrain the infant's own capacities for regulation (see opening quotation). Moreover, additional entrainment of the infant's nervous system occurs when caregivers "repair" breaches in tolerable arousal (Tronick, 1989); that is, assisting the infant to recover and settle following overarousal and brief periods of disorganization promotes a more flexible and resilient nervous system (e.g., Schore, 1994). As freestanding entities, infants have notable limitations in their capacities to do all of this on their own, but with sensitive and responsive caregivers, they can be very well regulated and adaptive. Their inborn reflexes and their emerging capacities for attention and engagement prepare them exquisitely for being part of a smoothly functioning system. They do the things, such as attend, vocalize, smile, and fret, that encourage caregivers to provide the regulatory help they need, and, typically, they respond quickly to caregiver ministrations (Sroufe, 1996). So much is this a dyadic process that D. W. Winnicott (1965, p. 39) once wrote that there is "no such thing as an infant," by which he meant that the human infant can be emotionally functional only within a caregiving context.

These considerations led us to see our major task in the first phases of our study as twofold: (1) to understand in a comprehensive way how caregivers support and respond to initial state and arousal variations in their infants in the first months of life, and (2) to assess variations in achieved effectiveness of regulation within the attachment relationship at ages 12 and 18 months. It was Bowlby's (1969/1982) explicit hypothesis that variations in the quality and effectiveness of infants' attachments would be in important ways outcomes of the responsiveness of the earlier care they received. As we discussed earlier, evaluating this seemingly straightforward hypothesis required comprehensive, broad-ranging assessments of caregiver, infant, and the surrounding context. While our primary interest was in infant outcome, our focus on the role of early care required that we also understand the origins of variations in care, which clearly are governed by multiple influences.

One central premise of the organizational transactional model that guides our work (Sameroff & Chandler, 1975; Sroufe, 1996) is that the environment and the organism are mutually influencing from conception forward. Quality of care may predict infant functioning, but newborn characteristics also may impact quality of care. Newborn characteristics themselves, of course, may be influenced by prenatal experience. Maternal anxiety and amount of stress during pregnancy predict newborn functioning (Molitor, Jaffe, Barglow, Benveniste, & Vaughn, 1984; Schneider & Moore, 2000). To take the circle back to the beginning, adult anxiety is predicted by early experience (see Chapter 12).

Infant adaptation or maladaptation depends upon environmental support, while infant characteristics, in part, may determine the nature of the environment. The relative role of the infant or caregiver may vary for different dyads, with some caregiver characteristics (e.g., depression) and some infant characteristics (e.g., irritability) being especially important. In either case, individual factors do not operate in a vacuum. Each individual infant is born into a unique set of circumstances. We share with others the idea that infant characteristics are important, but we also maintain that such characteristics develop in interaction with the environment.

The same infant characteristic may have a different meaning in a different set of caregiving circumstances. Suomi (2002) has illustrated this dramatically in his studies of cross-fostering in rhesus monkeys. Some of the animals studied had a genetic variation, often associated with impulsiveness. However, when these animals as infants were experimentally assigned to foster mothers with established records of being highly nurturing, the infants did not grow up to be impulsive, hyperactive, and distractible. In fact, they were likely to become leaders of the troop. Thus, the potential negative characteristic was transformed in the context of nurturing care. Some human studies are equally revealing. For example, Mangelsdorf and colleagues found that infant proneness to distress by itself did not predict later attachment problems, nor did maternal personality characteristics (Mangelsdorf, Gunnar, Kestenbaum, Land, & Andreas, 1990). However, when infants who were prone to distress had caregivers with high needs for control, this combination was associated with increased anxious attachment; that is, there was a statistical interaction between the infant variable and the personality variable. This is an illustration of what has been referred to as the "match–mismatch" hypothesis—that some caregivers will have special problems with some infants.

In our work, we began with the notion that infant characteristics would have their impact primarily in interaction with caregiving and other aspects of surrounding context. Since so many of our parents were living in conditions of high stress, this could also lead to some small direct effects of early infant difficulties, but interaction effects should nonetheless be more substantial. We also hypothesized that there would be considerable predictive power in measures of caregiver sensitivity and responsiveness in the first 6 months of life. Conceptually, this is because such measures already take into account the caregivers' capacity to be attuned to the particular signals, needs, and moods of their individual infants. This is what responsiveness means (see Chapter 3). Empirically, Ainsworth (e.g., Ainsworth et al., 1978) had demonstrated such a connection, as had we in our previous sample (Sroufe & Waters, 1977a). We also were interested in the origins of extreme variations in caregiving, especially the negative patterns of care that are properly described as child maltreatment. In all of this, we expected there to be an important role for context. Context was expected not only to forecast variations in parenting and initial infant adaptation but also to underlie changes in adaptation.

To address these issues, we assessed caregiver personality and expectations, beliefs, and understandings regarding the infant, the organization of neonatal behavior and infant temperament, caregiver responsiveness to infant signals during the first year, general treatment of the infant, and the ultimate dyadic organization of the attachment relationship. Finally, we assessed the broader environmental context of life challenges and supports for care. Given the rapid growth and transformations occurring during infancy, assessments were made early and often. Our plan at each phase of infant development was to investigate how factors individually and in combination predicted subsequent outcomes. These assessments were reviewed in Chapter 3.

Our overall strategy here and in subsequent chapters is to proceed chronologically. We begin by describing the origins of variations in caregiving quality (including maltreatment) in the first year, then describe our findings on attachment outcomes at the end of the first year, examining in detail combinations of caregiving history and our assessments of infant factors. Finally, we describe factors involved in changing attachment between 12 and 18 months.

In this and in other chapters in Part II of this book, we try to strike a balance between narrative flow and necessary statistical detail. Especially where published papers are available, we use statistics mainly to convey the strength and nature of the findings, with only infrequent use of more complex examples to illustrate the kinds of approaches we took. In the text, we make considerable use of correlations and regressions, since these are most widely understood. At times, we present actual correlations. We also use a consistent terminology to describe the obtained associations. When we refer to a correlation as "very modest," that means that it is significant, but only in the teens. "Modest" means in the .20s, and "moderate," in the .30s. With the kinds of things we were trying to measure and the developmental spans we often traversed, correlations beyond .40 are fairly impressive, and these are referred to as being "strong." We also keep the reader apprised of the sample sizes in the analyses, especially whether we are discussing the entire sample of 170–180 cases in various analyses or smaller subsamples that participated in parts of the project. Both correlations and sample size are required to understand "effect size," that is, the robustness of the finding.

THE FOUNDATIONS OF CAREGIVING QUALITY

Our first general question concerned the influence of maternal, infant, and environmental features on caregiving quality during the first year (e.g., Egeland & Farber, 1984). A key measure of caregiving was a composite of the Ainsworth ratings of sensitivity and cooperation, made in the middle of the first year (see Chapter 3). We found that one of the strongest predictors of this measure of quality of care was the caregiver's psychological understanding of the infant (the "psychological complexity" variable described in Chapter 3), which was correlated in the moderate range ($r = .35$). Recall that this refers to the caregiver's understanding of the infant as an autonomous being, separate but also very much in need of care. Caregivers who scored low on this dimension did not understand why young infants were so needy, perhaps having the misapprehension that the baby was there to meet their needs. It is not surprising, then, that they were unable to perceive properly the infant's signals and moods, and respond to them in a prompt and sensitive fashion. This variable proved to be potent in all of our analyses of quality of care in infancy.

Related contextual variables, including low socioeconomic status, single status at time of birth, and emotional support available to the mother, were significant, with correlations ranging from very modest to moderate (see Table 5.1). When these measures and the psychological understanding measure were combined in a multiple correlation, a strong relation was obtained ($r = .49$).

The mother's interest in the baby, as rated by nurses in the newborn nursery, her expectations regarding the caregiving relationship, and her reaction to pregnancy all were significant predictors, in descending order of strength (again, see Table 5.1). We also found that a few composite measures of infant temperament gathered between birth and age 3 months showed very modest to modest correlations with caregiver sensitivity at 6 months (Susman-Stillman, Kalkoske, Egeland, & Waldman, 1996). For example, when we standardized and combined irritability measures from hospital nurses' ratings, our observations in a home feeding, and caregiver questionnaire responses, the resulting correlation was significant but very modest (.14). A similar composite for "sociability" yielded a somewhat larger but still modest correlation (.25).

Thus, the responsiveness and sensitivity of care in infancy, which for us became a major predictor of adaptation from the early infancy period on, was itself forecast by earlier factors. It is the nature of the developmental process that any predictor that can be defined is itself an outcome as well. Most notably, a caregiver who failed to grasp the autonomous and needy status of her newborn infant (which we suspect was a

TABLE 5.1. Correlations between Maternal Characteristics/Experience and Caregiving Quality (6 Months)

Variable	Caregiving quality		
	Cooperation	Sensitivity	Composite
1. Socioeconomic status (prenatal)	.33*** (221)	.35** (221)	.36*** (221)
2. Single-parent status (birth)	.15* (221)	.17* (221)	.17* (221)
3. Maternal psychological understanding (prenatal)	.35*** (217)	.32*** (217)	.35*** (217)
4. Nurses' observation of maternal interest (birth)	.24** (136)	.31*** (136)	.28*** (136)
5. Maternal reaction to pregnancy and birth (3 months)	.16* (217)	.14* (217)	.16* (217)
6. Maternal expectations of baby (3 months)	.26*** (217)	.22*** (217)	.25*** (217)
7. Maternal anxiety/impulsiveness (3 months)	−.22*** (217)	−.18** (217)	−.21** (217)
8. Maternal emotional support (birth–12 months)	.24***	.22**	.24***

* $p < .05$; ** $p < .01$; *** $p < .001$.

product of her personal needs and history), and who was notably poor and unmarried at the time of her child's birth, and herself had little emotional support, was at risk for providing insensitive care. Measurable qualities of her infant in the early months were predictive to a lesser degree.

Predicting Maltreatment

Maltreatment of the child was to become another predictor from infancy on in our study. It, too, was first treated as an outcome. During the infancy period, we sought to define a distinctive group of caregivers who were providing clearly inadequate care and to compare them with contrasting groups of mothers in terms of antecedents (Brunnquell et al., 1981). Group assignment was based on home observations and completion of the Child Care Rating Scale (Egeland & Brunnquell, 1979) at 3, 6, 9, and 12 months (see Chapter 3). The inadequate care group of mothers ($n = 32$) showed some clear evidence of abuse or neglect of the child in physical or emotional areas. The second group, the adequate/excellent care group of mothers ($n = 33$), met the physical and emotional needs of the child well, showed sensitive and cooperative handling of interactive situations, and encouraged child growth and development. Another comparison group (n = 32) included mothers matched to the inadequate care group in terms of age, education, and marital status, but with no history of abuse or neglect. A final comparison, labeled the random group (n = 31), included other mothers selected randomly from the total sample, excluding the inadequate care group.

Maternal personality and mother–infant interactive variables, factors, and constructs were all examined with respect to their ability to discriminate the adequate and inadequate groups (Brunnquell et al., 1981; Egeland & Brunnquell, 1979). We found that the adequate and inadequate groups were best discriminated by broadly defined factors, again related to the caregiver's understanding of the psychological complexity of the infant, and by her positive reactions to pregnancy, measured in the prenatal period. Adding high hostility–suspicion scores from personality tests and a global measure of poor personality integration increased the risk for inadequate care. Even when age and education were controlled, maternal hostility–suspiciousness, among all of the personality factors, best discriminated groups.

In another analysis, we explored the relative predictive power of maternal factors and infant variables to distinguish between our parenting groups. We first examined which variables from each set predicted quality of mother–infant feeding interactions at 3 months, using the entire sample. In addition to the caregiving variables cited earlier, some infant indicators also predicted feeding interactions, including Brazelton factors of orientation and irritability, and nurses' ratings of newborn activity and alertness. Based on these findings, we conducted a discriminant function analysis, a procedure designed to determine the relative strength of different predictors, as well as their combined strength. In this analysis, we included maternal psychological characteristics, infant characteristics, and mother–infant interaction variables. In combination, the variables distinguished between adequate and inadequate care with 85% correct classification (Egeland & Brunnquell, 1979). The most highly predictive measures of quality of care were the ratings of caregiving sensitivity and cooperation, comprehensive measures of the caregiver's understanding of the psychological complexity of the infant, and the caregiver's understanding of the nature of the child care task.

In keeping with our interest in the broader context of care, we examined the influence of environmental stress on quality of care, both independently and in combination with other factors. We found that even though, overall, caregivers in the inadequate caregiving group experienced more stressful events than controls, many maltreating families experienced relatively small numbers of stressful events, and many families providing adequate care experienced stressful events (Egeland et al., 1980). It was not the number or type of stressors that distinguished the groups; rather, the interaction of psychological characteristics of the caregivers (e.g., high levels of anxiety, aggression, dependence, and defensiveness) and environmental stress best predicted inadequate caregiving.

Finally, we examined environmental stress in combination with maternal characteristics, infant temperament, and qualities of mother–infant interaction to distinguish between adequate and inadequate caregiving groups (Pianta, Egeland, et al., 1989). The groups did *not* differ with respect to infant gender, prematurity, infant abnormalities, Apgar scores, gestational age, or type of delivery. There were modest differences in pregnancy and delivery complications. Pregnancy complications were reported for 45% of the adequate caregiving group and 58% of the inadequate caregiving group, and delivery complications occurred for 45% and 68% of the groups, respectively. More dramatic in distinguishing the groups were contextual factors, such as the mother's emotional support, age, education, preparation for the infant (e.g., childbirth class, planned pregnancy, informal preparation rated by nurses), her understanding of the psychological complexity of the infant, and her relationship with the infant. These findings both highlight the importance of environmental factors, such as emotional support and preparation for child rearing, and call into question the view that child characteristics cause maltreatment (see Chapter 3, this volume; Sameroff & Chandler, 1975; Werner, Bierman, & French, 1971).

Summary

During the infancy period, across the total sample and with group comparisons, analyses employing individual variables, factors, and rationally derived constructs reflect the complex nature of the development of variations in caregiving. The results emphasize the importance of the caregiver's understanding of the complexity of both the infant and the caregiving relationship, and the ability to integrate life experiences as bases for adequate caregiving.

Factors and processes contributing to caregiving quality are complex. However, our data suggest that maltreatment or grossly inadequate caregiving evolves from the interaction of psychological characteristics of vulnerable, at-risk mothers in the context of environmental stress and lack of support. Isolation in the midst of challenging life events, as well as a history of unresolved, harsh caregiving experiences may all contribute to feelings of powerlessness, suspicion and fear, and the inability to control hostile impulses that influence caregiving ability. In a separate study (Egeland, 1988), we found that comprehensive intervention was effective in helping young mothers develop greater parental awareness and in improving their capacity to keep their own feelings from interfering with taking the infant's perspective.

CONTINUITY AND CHANGE IN MALTREATMENT: BREAKING THE CYCLE OF ABUSE

Although a history of maltreatment in childhood is an established risk for quality of parenting in the next generation, there is clear evidence that intergenerational continuity is not complete. Many children who have experienced maltreatment do not grow up to mistreat their own children. To better understand the intergenerational continuity of maltreatment in the longitudinal study, we analyzed child care practices of our participants who had been abused as children (Egeland et al., 1988). In this study, 40% of parents who were identified independently as having experienced childhood abuse were observed to maltreat their infants, and 30% provided borderline care (e.g., suspected maltreatment) for their own children. In contrast, all but one of the mothers with a clear history of supportive and loving parental care provided adequate care for their children. Of course, this degree of continuity may be especially high due to the high level of stress that characterizes our sample.

Even though the findings support the notion of intergenerational continuity, 30% of the parents who had been abused themselves provided clearly adequate care for their own children in the next generation. In subsequent studies, we sought to identify experiences that distinguished mothers who broke the cycle of abuse from those who were abused as children and mistreated their own children (Egeland & Susman-Stillman, 1996; Egeland et al., 1988). We wanted to understand external influences and internal processes that enabled some caregivers to provide adequate care for their children despite harsh caregiving histories. Based on maternal interviews and questionnaires completed over a 64-month period, measures of the mothers' past and current relationship experiences, stressful life events, personality characteristics, and associated symptomatology were obtained.

Three factors stood out in protecting these women from perpetuating the cycle of abuse (Egeland et al., 1988). First, we found that abused mothers who provided adequate care were significantly more likely to have received emotional support from an alternative, nonabusive adult during childhood, and/or, second, to have participated in a therapy experience of at least 6 months' duration during some period of their lives. In each case, such a circumstance applied to approximately 50% of the group, whereas it was the case for virtually none of those who perpetuated the cycle of abuse. Third, those who broke the cycle had an emotionally supportive and satisfying relationship with a mate as adults. This was true for almost all of the cases in which the pattern was broken. We were struck by the fact that each of these change-promoting factors was a relationship experience.

In addition, we found that mothers who broke the cycle of abuse were more likely to be able to integrate past abusive experiences into a coherent sense of self, compared to mothers who repeated the cycle (Egeland & Susman-Stillman, 1996). In contrast, abused mothers who reenacted their maltreatment with their own children had experienced significantly more life stress and were more likely to be anxious, depressed, dependent, and immature. These mothers received higher scores on the Dissociative Experiences Scale (see Chapter 4), and in early interviews were more likely to recall childhood experiences in a fragmented, idealized, or unintegrated fashion (even controlling for IQ). Recent adult attachment work suggests similar relations between the ability to integrate early caregiving experiences and perspectives, and positive parenting quality and, conversely, between denial, or the inability to integrate experience, and the reenactment of harsh experience (for review, see Hesse, 1999).

ATTACHMENT QUALITY

For the infant, the central challenge is to engage the novel world of objects and people, yet maintain a degree of emotional regulation. Arousal in the face of novelty is inevitable, yet novelty must be engaged if the infant's world is to expand. Therefore, the infant must not only learn to use its own capacities for regulation but also draw effectively upon external resources to regulate emotion. Primary attachment relationships are critical in this regard. When this relationship is effective, the infant is able to balance exploration with proximity and interaction with the caregiver, exploring when arousal is manageable, and monitoring caregiver availability or seeking reassurance or contact when threatened. Attachment draws upon and integrates all development in the first year, tapping the infant's organization of affect, cognition, and social behavior in a way that may serve later development.

In our longitudinal study, attachment assessments were conducted at 12 and 18 months using Ainsworth's Strange Situation procedure (Ainsworth et al., 1978), designed to assess the organization of attachment and exploratory behavior around the caregiver (see Chapter 3). At 12 months, the distribution of attachment classifications was 55% secure,

22% avoidant, and 23% resistant (n = 212). At 18 months, it was 61% secure, 22% avoidant, and 17% resistant (n = 189). Of the 189 dyads assessed at both time periods, 74% of secure infants remained secure, 45% of avoidant infants remained avoidant, and 37% of the resistant infants remained stable (Egeland & Farber, 1984). This is not only significant stability but also substantial change, as we discuss in a later section. In keeping with our goal of understanding how caregiving supports infant development, we attempted to distinguish the caregiving histories associated with different attachment classifications. In the next section, we examine the relations between attachment organization and measures of earlier maternal and infant characteristics, caregiving interactions, maltreatment, stressful life events, and maternal social support.

Secure, Avoidant, and Resistant Attachment

Overall, our longitudinal data affirmed Bowlby's (1969/1982) hypothesis that differences in quality of care lead to differences in quality of attachment, as well as Ainsworth's findings (e.g., Ainsworth et al., 1978) that attachment relationship quality is related to caregiver responsivity at various points in the first year (see also Thompson, 1998, for an extensive review of the broader literature). Mothers of securely attached infants were consistently found to be more cooperative and sensitive with their infants in feeding and play situations than were mothers of anxiously attached infants (Egeland & Farber, 1984). These mothers were more responsive to their infants' cries, more sensitive in pacing and timing of care (e.g., beginning and terminating feeding), and they tended to hold their infants in an affectionate fashion. These relations between attachment security and insecurity in the laboratory and caregiver sensitivity at home have now been widely demonstrated (e.g., K. Grossmann, Grossmann, Spangler, Suess, & Unzer, 1985; National Institute of Child Health and Human Development [NICHD] Early Child Care Research Network, 1997; Stovall-McClough & Dozier, 2004), especially by research that approximates Ainsworth's methodology (including extensive observation, adequate measures, and comparable infant age; e.g., Pederson, Gleason, Moran, & Bento, 1998; Posada et al., 1999).

As described in Chapter 3, those infants classified as having anxious–resistant attachment relationships cannot be easily settled by their caregivers during reunions that follow the brief separations in the Ainsworth procedure. They may be explicitly angry, squirm, push away after seeking to be held, and bat away toys, or they may simply fuss and cry, and not be consoled. In contrast, in the anxious–avoidant pattern, infants fail to seek out or reestablish contact with the caregiver during reunions. They may simply ignore caregivers or actively turn or move away from them. Caregiver sensitivity was comparably low for these two groups earlier in the first year, yet there were some distinctive aspects of their histories as well. Mothers of infants who later showed resistant attachment were the least psychologically aware group of mothers. The infants themselves tended to lag behind their counterparts developmentally and were less likely to solicit responsive caretaking (Egeland & Farber, 1984; Waters, Vaughn, & Egeland, 1980). At 9 months, anxious–resistant infants scored lower on Bayley mental and motor indices than did infants classified as secure and avoidant.

In contrast, those who later had anxious–avoidant relationships, although robust, were more likely to have mothers who had negative feelings about motherhood, were tense and irritable, and engaged in caregiving in a perfunctory manner. Feeding interactions were not adapted to the pace of the infant. In addition, mothers of avoidant infants were less responsive and effective in responding to infant crying and appeared at times to avoid physical contact. This is reminiscent of one of the key findings in Ainsworth's research (Ainsworth et al., 1978), replicated by Isabella (1993). Ainsworth found that mothers of those infants who became avoidant held their babies as much as other mothers, *except* when infants signaled explicitly that they wanted to be picked up; then, they turned them away. Maltreatment in the form of lack of emotional responsiveness and psychological unavailability was also highly related to avoidant patterns of attachment; at 18 months, every infant experiencing this pattern of maltreatment was avoidant (Egeland & Sroufe, 1981).

Thus, in general, caregiving difficulties related to maternal lack of knowledge and understanding, and low functioning in newborns were related to resistant attachment, whereas maternal physical rejection, lack of affection, and lack of interest appeared to be related to avoidant attachment. The findings reflect Ainsworth's characterizations of resistant caregiving patterns as unreliably responsive, and avoidant patterns as chronically rejecting.

Disorganized Attachment

Mary Main, Judith Solomon, and Erik Hesse introduced the concept of disorganized/disoriented attachment when our project was more than a decade old (e.g., Main & Hesse, 1990; Main & Solomon, 1990), but we were able to recode 157 videotapes for this category (Carlson, 1998). This category (type D), which, as it turns out, is the most clinically significant, is distinctive from both the avoidant (A) and resistant (C) patterns. As ineffective or maladaptive as A and C patterns may be in the long run, they are nonetheless "organized"; that is, they encompass coherent patterns that can be described in terms of expectable behaviors and functions.

In Main's terms, both A and C represent "strategies" for enhancing opportunities for care in the face of particular patterns of caregiving. In the face of chronic rebuff when their tender needs are expressed, the avoidant infants learn to *minimize* expression of attachment behaviors. While this may not be effective for ensuring regulation, it does not alienate further a rejecting caregiver and, by keeping mother and infant in some kind of proximity, leaves open the possibility that the caregiver will be available for the infant in dire circumstances. In contrast, in the face of inconsistent care, the C's must *maximize* expression of attachment behaviors in an effort to compensate for the caregiver's lack of dependability. By being constantly vigilant and expressing needs with intensity in the face of the slightest threat, they may be in proximity to their mothers when the threat is serious. The intense and almost chronic arousal, however, makes it difficult for them to be settled, and their preoccupation with seeking care interferes with exploration. Nonetheless, all of their behavior makes sense in light of this "strategy." (The word "strategy" should not be taken to mean that these infants have a thought-out plan; it is simply a summary term, borrowed from ethology, for their emotionally guided behavior.)

What kind of strategy can the infant adopt, however, if the caregiver's behavior is incoherent, or if the caregiver is a source of threat? Humans are motivated to flee *from* a source of threat and also, when threatened, to flee *to* the caregiver (who can protect or carry the infant to safety). This is a key part of human adaptation and survival. However, if the caregiver *is* the source of threat, the infant is placed in an irresolvable paradox. It is not possible to flee toward and away from the same locus simultaneously, or to maximize and minimize expression of attachment behavior at the same time. What one would expect to see in the Ainsworth procedure in such circumstances are contradictory behaviors, unfocused or anomalous behavior, a collapse in organized functioning, and other signs of behavioral conflict. This is exactly what Main and Solomon (1990) described and what we also coded with our sample. Such a pattern was hypothesized to reflect a seriously compromised attachment relationship.

We reasoned that both our measure of cooperation–interference (intrusiveness) and our measures of maltreatment would predict disorganized attachment. Intrusiveness, which entails doing things for which the infant is unprepared, likely would be confusing, while physical abuse would be frightening. Chronic emotional unavailability (another form of maltreatment) might seriously compromise the infant's capacity to organize behavior around the caregiver in the first place.

In accord with accumulating attachment research (Carlson, Cic-chetti, Barnett, & Braunwald, 1989; Cicchetti & Toth, 2000; Lyons-Ruth & Jacobvitz, 1999), infants with high ratings of disorganization in our study were indeed more likely to have experienced generally insensi-tive/intrusive caregiving and also some form of maltreatment during the first year (Carlson, 1998). Both correlations were in the moderate (.30s) range. In this sample, attachment disorganization also was associated with other environmental risks, including single parenthood and nurses' ratings of general caregiving risk, but it was not associated with endoge-nous (inborn) infant risk factors. Disorganization was not related to ma-ternal history of serious medical problems, pregnancy or delivery com-plications, infant anomalies, nonoptimal neurological status at birth (NBAS; Brazelton, 1973), infant temperament (ITQ; Carey, 1970), or in-fant behavior ratings at 3 months. This is important for discriminant va-lidity. It is difficult to distinguish disorganized attachment behavior from anomalous or stereotypical behavior shown by some disabled infants (Barnett et al., 1999). Therefore, our demonstration that the behavior we scored was not related to early infant difficulties was critical. If disor-ganized attachment is a reflection of a particular relationship history, it should not be strongly related to endogenous variables.

Our work is supported by studies specifically confirming a link between disorganized attachment and frightening or confusing parental behavior (Jacobvitz, Hazen, & Riggs, 1997; Lyons-Ruth, Bronfman, & Parsons, 1999; Schuengel, Bakermans-Kranenburg, van IJzendoorn, & Blom, 1999) and with parental experiences of loss and depression (there-fore, presumably unfathomable parental behavior due to state fluctua-tions) (Lyons-Ruth, Repacholi, McLeod, & Silva, 1991; Main & Hesse, 1990; O'Connor, Sigman, & Brill, 1987; Radke-Yarrow, Cummings, Kuczynski, & Chapman, 1985; Rodning, Beckwith, & Howard, 1991). Because of these findings, we expected that disorganization would be re-lated to later pathology (see Chapter 12).

INFANT CHARACTERISTICS AND ATTACHMENT

Conceptualizing the place of infant characteristics in the creation of at-tachment variations is necessarily complex. A simple, direct tie, for ex-ample, between infant temperament and attachment security, is unlikely due to the nature of the attachment construct. Attachment security is a relationship construct. It refers to the degree of confidence the infant has in the responsiveness of the particular caregiver, as reflected in the in-fant's comfort in exploration and ease of settling with *that* caregiver. In-fants of quite different temperaments could be confident about their caregivers or not. Moreover, the quality of attachment with two care-givers often may be different, with the infant being stably secure with one and anxious with the other (Fox, Kimmerly, & Schafer, 1991; Main & Weston, 1981; Sroufe, 1985). As we discuss in the next section, at-tachment patterns also may predictably change over a period of a few months. These and other observations make it clear that temperament variations cannot be causes of attachment variations in any simple way.

Research has consistently failed to demonstrate a direct link be-tween early infant temperament and attachment quality (see Vaughn & Bost, 1999). This may at first seem somewhat surprising given the role of distress and other aspects of emotional response in the Ainsworth as-sessments. Indeed, measures of temperament do predict certain aspects of *behavior* in the Strange Situation. For example, proneness to distress and cortisol reactivity at age 9 months predict crying during separations in the Strange Situation (Gunnar, Mangelsdorf, Larson, & Hertsgaard, 1989; Spangler & Grossmann, 1993). However, the amount of crying during the separation episodes is not a criterion for attachment security. Amount of distress during separation does not predict *organization* of attachment behavior or ease of gaining comfort in the presence of the caregiver, the hallmark of security. Other studies also show that temper-amental variations predict crying during separation, but not during re-unions with the caregiver (Vaughn & Bost, 1999).

Still, even though temperament cannot explain differences in attach-ment security, numerous possible roles for temperament and other infant characteristics are possible, and we explored a number of these in our re-search. As has been true of the field in general, we investigated both early anomalies and newborn neurological status and observational and parent report measures of infant temperament in the early months. In each case, we believe our data show that the place of infant characteris-tics (whatever their origins) may best be seen when considered with other aspects of context.

We were the first to report that an infant measure, nonoptimal neu-rological status on our 7- and 10-day Brazelton NBAS assessments (see Chapter 3), predicted anxious attachment, specifically, the resistant pat-tern (Waters et al., 1980). It is noteworthy, however, that Crockenberg (1981), in a completely parallel study with *middle-class* families, found no such relation. The two studies together suggest that in the context of highly stressful lives, such as in our poverty sample, nonoptimal status may be an additional risk factor. On the other hand, in conditions where support is adequate, nonoptimal newborn status is overridden by quality of care. Crockenberg found that, indeed, when she looked at only the subgroup in her study that had low social and emotional support, infant status was predictive of anxious attachment.

An intervention study by Dymph van den Boom (1989) also supported the notion that, under conditions of support, care can override infant difficulties. In the Netherlands, in contrast to the United States, newborn irritability is related to avoidant attachment, likely because of the difference in cultural context. Nonetheless, when van den Boom gave parents of irritable infants support and training to enhance sensitivity, a substantial majority of these infants were secure at 12 months, dramatically more so than her control group.

Our analyses of the role of temperament at 3 and 6 months were guided by two hypotheses: (1) that temperament might interact with responsiveness of care in some way, such that certain combinations of temperament and caregiver sensitivity might best predict attachment security; and (2) that temperament might be related to subtype of attachment rather than to attachment security, since subtypes are manifest in particular behaviors, while security versus nonsecurity reflects confidence in care (e.g., Sroufe, 1985). Confidence or lack of confidence in the caregiver can be shown in a variety of ways.

We focused on the dimensions of irritability and sociability, and combined our observational and parent report data to obtain more robust measures. While neither temperament dimension independently predicted attachment security, we did find that at 3 months, maternal sensitivity and infant irritability interacted in a particular way in predicting security (Susman-Stillman et al., 1996). Specifically, we found that when infant irritability was low, there was a stronger effect for sensitive care (i.e., a "moderator" effect). Put another way, high irritability muted the effect of sensitive care. Moreover, while at 6 months, irritability was not directly related to attachment security, it was related to 6-month sensitivity and through that, indirectly to attachment security; that is, its impact on security was "mediated" by caregiver sensitivity. Sensitivity remained a significant predictor even with both infant temperament measures taken into account. The findings support the influence of sensitive and responsive caregiving in aiding infants in modulating affective expression and arousal (Sroufe, 1996). Our general finding that infant characteristics have their impact in interaction with caregiving is consistent with the broader literature (e.g., Thompson, 1998).

In addition, we found some relation between temperament and type of anxious attachment. For example, while at 3 months, sociability did not distinguish secure from nonsecure infants, sociability scores were higher for those who were later avoidant than for those who were later resistant. An opposite trend was found for irritability at 6 months, with the resistant group having higher mean scores than the avoidant group. In general, the resistant cases and the subgroups of secure infants with high crying scores (B3 and B4) had significantly higher irritability as 6-

month-olds than the avoidant cases and the secure subgroups having low crying scores (B1 and B2). Again, as hypothesized, this confirms that irritability predicts crying in the Strange Situation, especially during separations, but not settling and returning to play during reunions. Thus, maternal sensitivity distinguished secure and insecure infants, and temperament predicted type of insecurity and subcategory placement.

CHANGING ATTACHMENT

In our view, attachment security derives from experience. Infants are confident regarding the availability of their caregivers and have positive expectations about their responsiveness precisely because, in their experience, their caregivers have been reliably responsive. This is what our data show. Therefore, because attachment security with a caregiver is a reflection of interactive history, attachment category should be subject to change. It may change from secure to anxious when parents become more overwhelmed and therefore provide less responsive care, or it may change from anxious to secure with the same parent when circumstances improve.

   In a first analysis, we were able to test directly a part of this hypothesis by examining changing life stress between 12 and 18 months for those cases in which attachment changed compared to those in which it stayed the same. In our sample, 62% of the participants in the study were assigned to the same attachment classification at both 12 and 18 months, and 38% changed. We found that, in general, anxious attachment was associated with less stable caregiving environments than was secure attachment. In addition, parents of those who changed from anxious to secure attachment reported a greater reduction in stressful life events than those who were anxious at both ages (Vaughn, Waters, Egeland, & Sroufe, 1979).

   In a subsequent analysis, we examined stability and change in attachment organization in relation to maternal and infant characteristics and environmental context (Egeland & Farber, 1984). The data suggested that specific maternal and infant characteristics that are important for the formation of attachment may not be the same characteristics that account for change. Mothers of infants securely attached at 12 months but insecure at 18 months demonstrated similar caregiving skills in infancy but differed in affective and personality characteristics compared to mothers of stably secure infants. Both groups were observed to accommodate to newborn cues and needs; however, declining security was related to low ratings of maternal joy, pleasure, and gratification, as measured in feeding interactions at 6 months. Thus, whereas specific caregiving skills, such as pacing and timing, may contribute to the formation of attachment, affective behavior appeared to be influential in maintaining adaptive relationships. The prominent role of affect may reflect changing child capacities and needs for interaction in the second year (Sroufe, 1989). In contrast, change from insecure to secure attachment from 12 to 18 months was characterized by maternal and infant growth and development. Mothers in these relationships had often been young and relatively immature, and initially responded negatively to pregnancy. Over the course of the first year, maternal negative attitudes became more positive, and mothers became more skillful at caregiving. Such changes in the caregiving environment were reflected in infant development. Infants who were once rated as less cuddly and responsive at 3 months were rated as fairly robust according to Bayley Scales of Infant Development scores at 9 months. Thus, as their mothers matured and took to the caregiving task, the infants began to thrive.

Gender differences were also noted in this study. For boys, 12- to 18-month change was related to changes in mother–child interaction, the mother's relationship status, and life stress. For girls, personality characteristics of the mother were more predictive of change (Egeland & Farber, 1984). This was the kind of finding with regard to gender that was to appear repeatedly in our study.

CONCLUSION

During the infancy period, we focused on the determinants of caregiving quality (including maltreatment), the links between caregiving and quality of infant–parent attachment relationships, and contextual influences on development. The findings from early analyses illustrated the multiple levels of influence and the transactional nature of early development. Overall, global factors and constructs (e.g., psychological complexity) rather than individual variables (e.g., personality characteristics) best accounted for differences in caregiver sensitivity. In turn, caregiver sensitivity and responsiveness predicted the quality of the attachment relationship, the most integrative measure of adaptation in infancy, summarizing all of the developmental achievements of the first months of life. Furthermore, differences in caregiving interaction and infant–caregiver relationship quality were best distinguished by combinations of caregiver and infant strengths and vulnerabilities in the broader context of environmental stress and support. We were to obtain such a pattern of findings repeatedly as our study progressed.

Harsh or neglectful treatment of infants was, not surprisingly, related to general insensitivity of care and to the psychological complexity variable that preceded it. Moreover, for some mothers, such difficulties understanding their infants and their own feelings, in combination with stressful, unsupportive living situations, a history of abuse in their own childhoods, and personality characteristics of hostility and suspiciousness, all converged to predict abusive care.

CHAPTER 6

Adaptation in the Toddler Period
Guided Self-Regulation

> A positive, reciprocal interpersonal set between parent and
> child, which renders the child ready, receptive, and positively
> motivated to respond to parental socialization . . . and to
> internalize parental standards and values may be the result of
> a long-term positive relationship.
> —KOCHANSKA (1993)

For each of us, self-regulation is a dual task, involving both expression and containment of impulses, desires, and feelings. For toddlers, this task is extraordinarily challenging, and the consequences of success or failure are profound. Regulation is such a difficult problem for toddlers, in part, because of emergent capacities for goal directedness, persistence, and expressiveness. Not only do impulses feel imperative, toddlers *will* to carry them out. While their capacities to modulate arousal and inhibit responses are dramatically greater than those of infants, such capacities still are no match for the strength of toddlers' impulses in many cases. To express the range of emerging impulses and feelings, both joyous and rageful, yet be able to contain them adequately, is not possible for the toddler alone. But it is possible for the toddler within a supportive caregiving system.

The exuberance and strength of toddlers' desires are important human characteristics. With caregiving assistance, they can become the cornerstones of later creativity and agency. Without appropriate help, however, toddlers are not able to sufficiently contain and direct impulses. Their options are to become chronically undercontrolled or unduly inhibited (to restrain unremittingly). For this reason, Erikson (1950/1963) described the salient issue for this era in terms of a polarity between a burgeoning sense of autonomy and profound feelings of shame and doubt. It is a critical time for parents and children.

Thus, the adaptation of the toddler remains fundamentally a dyadic adaptation. The dyadic "training program" in emotional regulation continues. As was true for infants, toddlers require responsive and consistent involvement by caregivers to remain regulated. Caregivers provide scaffolding for regulation and a protective envelope (Mahler et al., 1975) within which the toddler can freely explore new capacities and desires. Toddler development and the caregiver–child relationship builds on foundations laid down in infancy and, at the same time, consolidates what was established before (Kochanska et al., 2004). When willful challenges to the caregiving relationship are met with firm limits and emotional support, trust is deepened and regulatory systems emerging in infancy are strengthened and elaborated.

Toddlers contribute a great deal to this dyadic regulation. Not only can they contain themselves to a much greater degree than infants, they can be much more explicit in expressing needs, and their receptive language skills allow them to be reassured and directed at a distance. They are not capable of self-regulation, but within a supportive relationship, they are capable of "guided self-regulation."

The expanding language capacities, motor skills, and self-awareness of toddlers are both a boon and a bane for parents. On the one hand, toddlers can do more for themselves, and it is easier to communicate with them than it was with infants. On the other hand, they can and do get into things. They can engender anger by explicitly going against parental wishes that parents know they understand, and they can be persistently willful. Toddlers do not, however, simply oppose their parents' wishes; they retain equally a motivation to maintain a harmonious relationship. The child's bids are "not all in a direction away from or contrary to the mother but are balanced by bids for reciprocation with her" (Sander, 1975, p. 140). Or, as psychoanalyst George Klein (1976) put it: "Two components of selfhood must be recognized: a centrifugal assertion of autonomy, and a centripetal requirement for being an integrated and needed part of a larger, more encompassing entity or social unit" (p. 33). The parental task at this time is challenging, because parents must recognize these dual tendencies, allowing the child enough room to explore, while also recognizing the child's need for continued closeness and guidance. Overall, in our work, we observed some decline in the number of children showing a positive adaptation during this period, as parents struggled with issues of limits and control. Nonetheless, there was great variation in parenting and in toddler functioning.

For some dyads, coordinated functioning continued to evolve, with things perhaps going even better than they had in infancy. Many toddlers were cooperative with their parents in joint activities, and this ability to use the caregiver as a resource led to an enthusiasm for problem solving on the tool tasks (see Chapter 4). Our thesis was that such a readiness for collaboration was based upon the relationship established in infancy (for independent confirmation of this idea, see Kochanska et al., 2004; Main & Weston, 1981). In the "cleanup" situation, they may have at times been noncompliant, for example, when they wanted to play with toys and their parents wanted them to stop. However, when their caregivers followed through and were firm, the toddlers went along. When the limits were clear, toddlers were pleased enough to adhere to them (see Waters, Kondo-Ikemura, & Richters, 1990, for a theoretical discussion of this issue).

Other toddlers, however, seemed entrenched in their noncompliance with caregivers who were themselves inconsistent in setting or maintaining limits. These toddlers quickly became frustrated in working on the tool problems, and were fussy and angry instead of enthusiastic. Caregivers lost patience with them, and the two became locked in a struggle, with the tool problems fading into the background. In other cases, there was a notable emotional distance between caregivers and toddlers. These toddlers were in trouble when the problems became difficult. They did not tend to seek help from their caregivers, and their caregivers gave them less help as the problems got harder.

Our task in this chapter is to describe further and explain the origins of these and other variations in parenting and in toddler adaptation, in light of the assessments available from our study. We examine predictors of both the measures of toddler functioning and measures of the quality of care. Some consequences of observed parenting variations are also presented here, but these are discussed in detail in later chapters, as we continue to trace patterns of adaptation from childhood to adulthood.

PREDICTING TODDLER ADAPTATION

Security of Attachment and Overall Quality of Toddler Adaptation

Our approach to research dictates that, in predicting to each age, we first select the single most representative measure of earlier adaptation as a predictor and a comparable single measure as an outcome. The most integrative measure of adaptation in infancy is the quality of the attachment relationship. Moreover, as we presented in Chapter 5, security of attachment was predicted by earlier measures of sensitive care, thus attaining validity from our theoretical perspective. The comparable molar measure of dyadic adaptation in the toddler era is the child's "Experience in the Session" from the 2-year laboratory assessment (see pp. 70–71 in Chapter 4). This scale, which is aimed at capturing the overall quality of the toddler–parent *relationship*, tapped the degree to which guided self-regulation was being achieved. Progress in this regard was revealed in the child's enthusiasm in engaging the problems, persistent effort in the face of difficulty, and effective utilization of help available from the caregiver. A high score on this scale meant that the child was able to manage the attendant challenges and frustrations in the situation using the caregiver as a resource and, in the end, have a rewarding experience of being supported and of prevailing in the face of difficulty. Relating attachment security to this variable is therefore the most appropriate starting place for our developmental analysis. It is a single statistical test that takes into account all of the information in our integrative assessments and allows examination of continuity in adaptation at the level of organization in a direct way. Subsequently, we also sought to examine links at the level of child and caregiver behavior.

In infancy we measured attachment at both 12 and 18 months, and we first examined continuity to age 2 for those toddlers whose attachment status was stable. Even though change in attachment security between 12 and 18 months was to some degree predictable (see Chapter 5), it is nonetheless the case that using stable cases reduces error of measurement. Therefore, this was the basis for our first test of continuity of adaptation from infancy to toddlerhood. We found that, indeed, those with stable secure attachments received dramatically and significantly higher scores on the toddler Experience Scale at age 24 months than did those with stable anxious attachments (equivalent to a strong correlation of .46). While such a finding indicates that continuity is by no means complete, we are impressed with its magnitude for several reasons. First, the behavioral constructs in question are very difficult to measure. Here, we are traversing an important developmental transition, carrying out challenging behavioral observations, and using very different, completely independent procedures at each age. It is also the case that predictions of toddler adaptation are improved by combining attachment with other measures of early care (see below). Finally, genuine lawful change is taking place, as we discuss later. The demonstrated continuity is occurring within the context of this change.

While correlations were more modest, other analyses of continuity also yielded significant results. The next most representative attachment measure utilized all 180 participants and combined the 12- and 18-month assessments by giving each child a 0, 1, or 2 for the number of times they were secure. This resulted in a correlation with the Experience Scale of .31 (again significant beyond the .001 level of confidence). In addition, both 12- and 18-month attachment security assessments separately yielded significant but somewhat more modest correlations.

Attachment security in infancy was also found to be significantly related to ratings of child functioning at age 2, although these correlations at the level of the child were more modest in every case than those at the level of the relationship (i.e., the Experience in the Session Scale). For example, the correlation between the stable attachment security variable and the Overall Child Rating (in which we rated the quality of the child's behavior and not how well the pair functioned; see Chapter 4) was .33. For more specific variables (enthusiasm, positive affect, etc.), correlations were generally lower, although differences in compliance were notably distinguished for secure versus insecure attachment groups. This finding is consistent with the position later developed further by Kochanska (1993), as described in the introductory quotation for this chapter. Our interpretation of the total array of findings is that continuity at this age is still primarily at the level of the relationship; that is, the quality of the parent–child relationship is more stable than is child functioning.

Continuity of Individual Patterns of Adaptation

Beyond the question of whether there is some kind of general continuity in quality of functioning, we are keenly interested in whether there is continuity in particular patterns of behavioral organization. Given the problem of transformation in development, and the fact that the child remains so tightly nested in the caregiving relationship, this is a challenging task; nonetheless, we believed we could define profiles of expectable behavior for the three primary attachment groups in the toddler tool problem situation at age 2. If the attachment classifications do reflect *patterns* of dyadic organization, these should be reflected in later patterns of behavioral organization. For example, those with secure histories should engage the problems with enthusiasm and at least some degree of positive affect. They should at first attempt to tackle the problems on their own, rather than immediately seeking help. Still, when their personal resources are exhausted, they should readily turn to the caregiver for help, clearly expecting a positive response, and they should effectively use this help. That is the nature of their relationship. Thus, they should not wind up frustrated or angry, and in the end, they should manifest the sense that *they* solved each problem. This is the legacy of their history of responsive care and the confident exploration it promoted.

In contrast, those with histories of avoidant attachment would be expected to show some investment in the problems and some persistence (because of their acquired object-oriented style). But they should not readily seek help from their caregivers, who had previously proven to be unavailable in times of need. They should fail to seek more help as the problems get harder. They would not directly express their frustration toward their caregivers, though they might express it through indirect anger or by seeking help from the experimenter. On many variables in this setting, their scores would be moderate.

For toddlers with histories of anxious–resistant attachment, this should be a very difficult situation. They have not been supported in the development of emotional regulation, and they are easily stressed, over-taxed, and frustrated. We expected them to show increasing negative affect, and low and declining enthusiasm and positive affect. They would seek a great deal of interaction with the caregiver, but they would be unable to use the inconsistent help that was offered. The toddler and caregiver would become embroiled in a struggle. In contrast to the avoidant group, a great deal of anger and frustration would be clearly directed at the caregiver.

Can such hypothesized patterns be predicted from infant attachment variations? In this case, we used the stable attachment groups, since no obvious prediction could be made for those who changed classification. The first step was establishing prototype scale score patterns for the three attachment groups (Gove, 1983). For example, the secure prototype was assigned high scores on positive affect, enthusiasm, and compliance; low scores on negative affect, frustration, and time off-task; and changing (increasing) scores on help seeking across the problems. Each child's observed scores were then checked for degree of correspondence with this prototype and with comparable prototypes for the avoidant and resistant patterns (using simple correlations). If the highest correlation was, for example, with the secure prototype, the child was judged to fit that pattern, and so forth. We were able to predict whether children fit the secure pattern or not with 70% accuracy, and for exact matches for the three groups, there was 62% accuracy. Both of these are significant predictions, although they are not strong.

A second approach yielded identical results. Here, experienced attachment researchers, blind, of course, to the child's history, classified each toddler based on the profile of scores, noting especially whether help seeking, if present, increased across tasks, and whether anger and frustration, if present, were expressed directly to the caregiver. The secure group was distinguishable from the avoidant group by increased help seeking, and from the resistant group by lower ratings on negative affect and frustration. Avoidant and resistant groups were distinguished by directness of negative expression and by help seeking, which were expected to be greater in the resistant group. A later detailed analysis showed that those with resistant histories showed more dependent entanglements with their mothers, yet a poorer quality of help seeking than those in the other two groups (Hatem, 1996).

Examining the tables from this dissertation (Gove, 1983) revealed that the challenge lay in predictions concerning the avoidant pattern. Not only were 70% of those predicted to have had the secure pattern in fact secure, but there also was close to 70% accuracy across methods for the resistant pattern. However, those who had been avoidant were just as likely to fit the proposed resistant pattern at age 2. We believe that these findings are a reflection of the challenges of this period, especially perhaps for children of poverty. Negativity, noncompliance, and frustration are strongly pulled forth. Thus, maladaptation commonly takes the "resistant form" at this age. We return to this issue of continuity of patterns in Chapter 7 on adaptation in the preschool, where we see that there is predictability of organization of behavior both for those with avoidant histories and for those with resistant histories.

Predicting Toddler Adaptation from Measures of Maltreatment and Temperament

Parental maltreatment of the infant was clearly related to toddler outcome. Mothers in our maltreatment groups (see Chapter 5) had a great deal of difficulty during the toddler period (Erickson & Egeland, 1987). Interview data revealed that they had a lack of understanding of the toddler's negativism and age-typical ambivalent feelings, often taking such characteristics personally. Not surprisingly, this often led to entrenched conflict. There was a moderate correlation between Physical Neglect and the Experience Scale, and modest but significant correlations for both Psychological Availability and Verbal Abuse. Maltreatment was also significantly related to a variety of specific toddler scales; maltreated toddlers showed lower levels of persistence and enthusiasm, and higher levels of inattention and negative affect (Egeland, Sroufe, & Erickson, 1983). All maltreated groups were more angry, frustrated, and noncompliant than those receiving adequate care. Combining any or all of these early care measures with the attachment security variable incremented the prediction of toddler experience to some extent. Thus, the *cumulative history of care is a more powerful predictor of outcome than quality of attachment alone.* Such a finding was to be repeated over and over in our study.

Maltreatment in the early years was related to other aspects of toddler functioning as well. One striking finding concerned performance on the Bayley Scales of Infant Development. We had, in general, noted some decline in performance between 9 and 24 months. But this decline was most dramatic for those in the Psychologically Unavailable group. These children, on average, showed a decline of 40 points in developmental quotient, reflecting the ongoing influence of such unsupportive care.

The picture derived from our array of early temperament variables was decidedly mixed. The Carey Infant Temperament Questionnaire (ITQ) at 6 months, for example, was unrelated to either the toddler Experience in the Session Scale or the overall Child Rating Scale; it did, however, show some relations to ratings of caregivers. We interpret this to mean that temperament scales like these may be as much measures of caregivers as measures of infants (see also Vaughn & Bost, 1999). One of five factors from the Brazelton Neonatal Behavior Assessment Scales (NBAS) was related to toddler Experience. While Orientation, Irritability, Motor Maturity, and Consolability were not related to toddler Experience, Physical Ability showed a very modest correlation, and it was also related to the Child Rating Scale.

At age 3 months, a composite measure of irritability was derived from our feeding observation, the Carey ITQ, and the newborn rating by nurses. This composite was correlated modestly with toddler Experience. It was not, however, significantly correlated with the Child Rating Scale score, which is focused on child behavior alone. Thus, there may be some role for early temperament differences in toddler adaptation, perhaps through their impact on the relationship with the caregiver.

Most important, when we statistically examined whether temperament accounted for the link between attachment security and toddler adaptation, we found that it did not. The simplest demonstration of this involves the use of partial correlation or statistical regression techniques. We first entered a variable, such as the 3-month irritability variable from the feeding observation, which was known to account for some variation in toddler outcome. Nonetheless, when we subsequently entered attachment security into the regression equation, it accounted for substantially and significantly more variance. Thus, the link between attachment and toddler Experience is not explained by temperament alone.

CONTINUITY OF CARE

Just as toddler adaptation is a lawful outcome of the adaptations that preceded it, so too are variations in parenting at age 2 related to earlier quality of care. It is noteworthy that security of infant attachment forecasts quality of parenting during the toddler period. If our view of attachment assessments as capturing the quality of *relationships* is correct, then this must be so. Attachment variations should predict parental as well as child behavior. For the stable attachment group, the correlation with the overall Parent Rating (across all procedures of the 2-year assessment) was strong (.41), and with the quality of parental responsiveness on the tool tasks alone, it was .37. In addition, 12-month attachment security, 18-month security, and 12- and 18-month security combined all were significantly related to these variables, as was the rating of disorganization in attachment. Such links confirm that variation in attachment is not simply tapping a trait of the infant.

Direct measures of quality of care during infancy also were consistently related to quality of care observed with toddlers. A key finding was a highly significant, moderate correlation between nurses ratings of mother's interest in the baby *in the newborn nursery* and overall quality of mothering at age 2 years. Likewise, ratings of Cooperation–Interference and Sensitivity based on our two observations at 6 months yielded impressive correlations (.28 and .34) with overall Parenting Quality, and both correlated moderately with our measure of emotional support (Supportive Presence) in the tool problems (see Chapter 4). Sensitive and cooperative care at 6 months also predicted the degree of guided self-regulation achieved by the toddler, a finding replicated in the large study being conducted by the National Institute of Child Health and Development (2004).

Observed quality of care at 3 months, as well as being placed in any of the four maltreatment groups, also was modestly related to 2-year quality of care. When these measures were combined using multiple regression, the multiple correlation was .37. Thus, there is some noteworthy continuity of parental care. This is one reason why early care would be related to toddler adaptation. Still, when earlier and later care were controlled, attachment security still predicted toddler adaptation; that is, *the quality of toddler adaptation may in part arise from contemporary care, but it also in part reflects earlier care and the attachment it produced, which the infant carries forward.* Regression analyses showed that even after first entering a composite measure of care during the first 2 years, attachment security continued to predict additional variance in toddler outcome.

Generational Boundaries and the Emergence of Seductive and Derisive Care

Demonstrating continuity in the quality of care does not imply that parenting is static. Quality of individual parenting changes (for better or worse), as we discuss in a later section. In addition, at each age, new parenting issues emerge. For example, it had been suggested to us by June Sroufe, based upon clinical work with families in which there was sexual abuse, that certain patterns of sexualized care would become obvious at this time and would be based in the parents' own histories. Such "seductive care" was an issue that we had only glimpsed in infancy, but it did emerge with frequency in the toddler period. Even though it left no physical marks and was not defined by lack of involvement, we came to view this as another pattern of maltreatment.

In viewing our 2-year videotapes, especially during the toy cleanup session, we noted a variety of tactics that seemed to fit a seductive pattern. We observed mothers passionately kiss toddlers; rub their buttocks, genitals, or stomachs in a sensual way; plaintively ask for kisses; bribe with kisses; and whisper or call to them in ways that were obviously sensual (Sroufe & Ward, 1980).

Three things struck us immediately about the organization of this maternal behavior, an organization parallel to that found in cases of physical abuse. First, the behaviors typically occurred when the child was not complying and the parent had been unsuccessful in getting him to comply. Second, the behavior "emerged" in a sequence beginning with subtle, low-level manifestations and proceeding to frank manifestations. Parallel to the sequence of gritted teeth, followed by increasingly angry tones, and then hitting of the child, with seductive behavior there may be a change in voice tone, then more sensual statements and gestures, and finally sexualized touching. Finally, these behaviors had the appearance of a tactic and often occurred in the context of a fluctuating host of tactics (sweet talk, physical threat, bribe, abandonment threat, pleading, plaintive tone, harsh tone, etc.).

Initially, we reported these observations, as well as the reliability of coders in scoring seductive behavior, and the fact that this behavior was directed almost exclusively to boys. We also reported that seductive behavior was related to low scores on setting and maintaining limits, and that it was strongly related to a history of the mother having been treated sexually by an adult male in childhood. The latter finding was based on interviews made completely independent from this study (Morris, 1980). Reviewers of the initial paper complained that we were unfairly judging mothers for simply being warm and affectionate with their children. But we subsequently demonstrated with independent ratings made in other settings that, in fact, mothers using these tactics showed *lower* warmth and higher hostility (and even actual and threatened physical punishment) than other mothers (Sroufe & Ward, 1980). Maternal affection has consistently been a positive predictor in our work. Seductive caregiving behavior really is not affectionate.

The context of occurrence is always critical to our interpretation of behavior. Saying "good job" and putting an arm around the child when he or she has solved a problem is simply sharing the joy of solution and being appropriately encouraging and rewarding. Hugging a child who seeks you out when frustrated is simply being supportive. But interrupting a child who is working on a problem in an effort to get him to be affectionate with you, or promising him a kiss if he will do what you want, or even grabbing him by the genitals, is seductive, not warm. It does not appear warm to observers who witness it. These behaviors are seductive "because, in addition to being insensitive and unresponsive to the needs of the child, they draw the child into patterns of interaction that are overly stimulating and role-inappropriate" (Sroufe & Ward, 1980, p. 1223). The child is placed in the role of meeting parental needs, rather than the parent responding to the child's needs.

We do not view this behavior in narrow trait terms (i.e., that some women just generally behave in sexualized ways) or as the simple imitation of behaviors observed in one's own parents. Rather, we view seductive behavior as a manifestation of a broader relational construct of intergenerational boundary issues that may occur in this particular way with only one child. Mothers behaving this way may have been emotionally or sexually exploited by male parent figures in a variety of ways. But whatever the specific form, it was a pattern based on the proposition that adults can meet needs with a child in a gender-based way. Moreover, the relational learning involves incorporating an entire family system— how the child was treated by a father figure and by the mother, and how the adults treated each other. They have not simply learned a set of behaviors, but a pattern of relating. The women we observed did not do the identical things that were done to them, but rather engaged in culturally dictated female counterparts.

We proposed a hypothesis that followed directly from family systems theorizing but was explicitly counter to explanations based on traits or simple imitation. Again supported by clinical work, we predicted that mothers who behaved seductively toward sons would not necessarily behave seductively toward another son, and would explicitly *not* behave seductively toward daughters; rather, they would behave in a hostile, derogating, or derisive way. The argument was that since families are coherent, whole systems (Sroufe & Fleeson, 1986), when daughters have been sexually or emotionally exploited by father figures, this has implications for other family relationships. In particular, it is likely that father and mother were not meeting each other's needs (Sroufe & Fleeson, 1988), and that mother was distant and/or hostile with daughter (otherwise, the exploitation would not have been accepted or permitted). In the next generation, then, the daughter will not know how to meet needs with an adult partner, may well be seductive with her son, and will be hostile toward her own daughter. "In depreciating their daughters they are depreciating themselves, and they are reconstructing a relationship pattern that they know" (Sroufe, Jacobvitz, Mangelsdorf, DeAngelo, & Ward, 1985, p. 319).

Our research enabled us to test these propositions empirically. Since we included in our study the first 75 siblings born in our families, we were able to have independent coders rate the mother's behavior with another child, when she had been seductive with a sibling, along with a comparison group of siblings. When this second child was a boy, target mothers were no more likely to behave seductively than were comparison mothers (i.e., this is not a trait, and this relational niche was occupied). This was not likely due to sloppy coding, because the overall correlations across the siblings for general parenting qualities (such as Supportive Presence) were in the .50s. Finally, when the sibling was a daughter, these mothers were indeed significantly more likely to be derisive. While the numbers were small, there was almost no overlap in the distribution of scores between these cases and comparison cases on our derision scale (Sroufe et al., 1985).

In subsequent work, we broadened our assessments of boundary dissolution to include peer-like behavior and role reversal, as well as competitiveness, derision, and seductive behavior. This is because parent–child boundary dissolution, more broadly defined, occurs frequently with both girls and boys, whereas maternal seductive behavior is directed primarily to boys and is therefore germane only to predicting their problems. Behaviors such as giggling with a child who needs to be settled, pleading with children as though they are in charge, and letting children be in charge when they need direction are readily distinguished from periods of play and appropriately following the child's lead. In each case, the parent is abdicating the parental role and the child is being treated as a partner, agemate, or caregiver. We developed two scales to capture these behaviors, one labeled Nonresponsive Physical Intimacy and the other, broader scale labeled Generational Boundary Dissolution. We scored them at both 24 and 42 months. The broader scale proved to be most pertinent at 42 months. The underlying construct showed high stability across this age period (Hiester, 1993). The construct also was significantly related to Cooperation–Interference (intrusiveness) at 6 months. As we report later, these early boundary measures also predict parent–child boundary issues at age 13, as well as important aspects of child functioning through childhood and adolescence.

We emphasize this construct here because such parenting issues seem especially important for toddlers. Toddlers, perhaps more so than any other age group, need a calm, steady, reassuring parental presence. Especially when their arousal threatens to exceed tolerable limits and they approach losing control, toddlers need parents to provide a clear, firm boundary and to help them reduce stimulation. When parents be- have in the ways we are capturing with these scales, they are doing pre- cisely what the child does *not* need. Moreover, since such unduly stimu- lating behaviors occur most often at times when the child already is overtaxed, they promote loss of control and lack of confidence in retain- ing or recapturing control. Among other things, this appeared to us to be an initiating experience for arousal modulation problems, such as are re- flected in what is called attention-deficit/hyperactivity disorder. We pres- ent confirming findings regarding this proposition in Chapter 12.

The Context of Care

Having just described patterns of parenting that are linked to later child- hood problems, we again want to be clear that there should be no ten- dency to cast blame on parents. Parenting occurs in context. In fact, one of our first findings was that when parents behaved seductively, they more likely had a history of sexual abuse or other forms of sexual ex- ploitation by parents or relatives than did other parents in our sample. This history is part of the context for parenting. And, as we reported in Chapter 5, when the cycle of mistreatment is broken, this, too, is related to context, either adult support in childhood or current support. The mothers we studied who behaved seductively with their children were in every case without a current viable means for meeting their own emo- tional needs.

We conducted an extensive study of a subsample of our participants ($n = 36$) to explore the historical context of parenting in detail (Morris, 1980). Each of these women completed an extensive life history inter- view, lasting several hours. In terms of content, this interview could be thought of as a forerunner of the Adult Attachment Interview (George et al., 1985), covering much of the same early family relationship material, although it was not coded for narrative characteristics. Rather, this inter- view was aimed at obtaining a great deal of information about the facts of daily life (eating dinner together, responsibility for household chores, discipline practices), the parents' marriage quality, sexual development, and many other features of life growing up, as well as early parent–child relationship quality. From the voluminous interviews, three major scales were created and coded based on a list of specific descriptors: (1) Spousification (e.g., "daddy's girl" when young; perceives self as being like father, poor marital harmony); (2) Chaos (e.g., poor household or- ganization; harsh punishment; more than five siblings; mother or father alcohol problems or mental illness); and (3) Positive Identification with a Competent Mother (e.g., high maternal emotional presence; wants to be more like mother; positive feeling tone toward one's mother). Judges' ratings on each of these constructs significantly predicted outcomes in the next generation at age 24 months, based on the Experience in the Session Scale. Thus, quality of the primary caregiver–child relationship and degree of chaos in one's childhood, as well as emotional exploitation by father figures, was a foundation for parenting problems in our mothers.

We also routinely examine aspects of the current context of parenting at each age, especially the life stress and social support being experienced by parents. In Chapter 5, we reported that changes in life stress partially accounted for changes in attachment security between 12 and 18 months. We did not have a life stress variable at 24 months, but we did measure social support, including supportive adult relationships. Both the quality of emotional support available to the caregiver at 12 months and the cumulative support available across the second year were significantly related to ratings of the mother's Supportive Presence, Quality of Assistance, and overall quality of parenting in the 2-year tool problems assessment. Moreover, when we entered the cumulative support variable into a regression analysis following entry of infant security of attachment, support accounted for additional variance. This implies that support in part accounted for change in quality of parenting and the caregiver–infant relationship across this interval. As support for the parent becomes more available, quality of parenting improves. In our study, we found repeatedly that changes in stresses and supports predicted changes in parent–child relationships and child functioning.

CONCLUSION

As some children move forward from the toddler period, they do so with a deepened sense of confidence in the availability of support and a beginning sense of confidence in themselves. Having been entrained in flexible control and emotional modulation during this period of "guided self-regulation," they will be well served as they move out into the broader world of peers and the preschool, and as they are given increasing responsibility for self-management in a variety of contexts. Research suggests that this process of entraining operates on every level, from regulation of overt behavior, to regulation of emotions, and to balancing of excitatory and inhibitory systems in the central nervous system (NICHD, 2004; Schore, 1994; Siegel, 1999; Sroufe, 1996). All of these are critical for the developmental tasks ahead.

Other children, often those who already lack confidence regarding care, leave this developmental period even more challenged than when it began. In the face of harsh, inconsistent, or inept support and discipline practices, they may either be easily overaroused and frustrated, unable to contain impulses and doubting in their ability to do so, or they may have adopted rigid strategies for coping with feelings and desires that will handicap them in the rapidly fluctuating circumstances of the pre-school social world. None of these children will have the foundations for genuine empathic engagement and reciprocity that are essential for competent peer relationships. Some of them are filled with malevolence, which often leads to rejection by peers. Finally, they will all face difficulties in self-management and flexibly coping with problems.

Such trajectories are by no means fixed. Strengthened support in the next period, perhaps especially in combination with islands of earlier support, can help children overcome early difficulties. There certainly are many opportunities for change in the preschool period. Still, by age 2, there are discernible developmental trajectories. They represent a force in subsequent development.

CHAPTER 7

Adaptation in the Preschool Period
The Emergence of the Coherent Personality

> In becoming internalized, adopted strategies which first
> characterized regulatory relationships with the interpersonal
> surround will now function as features of self-regulation and
> eventually characterize personality idiosyncrasy.
> —SANDER (1975)

The preschool years are a momentous period of development. It is no exaggeration to say that the person emerges at this time. Not all of a sudden, and not out of nowhere, but nonetheless a new level of organization in the child apart from caregivers is apparent. Such a statement is justified both by the greater coherence in the organization of various characteristics of the individual and by the greater stability and stronger predictive power of individual variations from this time forward. While there is little that we can measure *in the child* prior to this period that powerfully predicts later outcomes, variations in preschool behavior and adaptation often do. A person has emerged from out of the relationship matrix.

To capture the organization of development in the preschool period, several themes seem critical. Important among these are the rise of

121

self-direction, agency, self-management, and self-regulation. Erikson (1950/1963) aptly named the issue at this age "initiative versus guilt," to capture some of these themes, as well as the notion of internalized standards of behavior. Clearly, one sees a more self-reliant, purposeful, and self-guided child at this time. But it is also a time of expanding social competence and, typically, a time of broadening social relationships. Important roots of successful peer relationships are established (e.g., Vaughn, Colvin, Azria, Caya, & Krzysik, 2001). All of these are themes in this chapter. We also discuss how various characteristics fit together in different children, and how coherent, organized patterns of behavior derive from developmental history and current circumstances.

Another critical topic during the preschool years is the internalization of the relationship history; that is, how relationships in the early years are incorporated by the child and carried forward as prototypes for subsequent relationships with others, becoming the roots of alienation or empathy (Zahn-Waxler, Radke-Yarrow, Wagner, & Chapman, 1992). For the first time, we examine relationships with peers, and with adults outside of the family, examining links with earlier parent–child relationships, as well as data our study provides concerning the processes by which such connections occur. One reason behavior is more coherent at this time is that the child has more cognitively elaborated representations of self and others for guidance. We explicitly assessed such representations through play and narratives.

At age 3½, we observed the child with the primary caregiver (using an age-appropriate series of teaching tasks), and also, *for the first time*, we observed the child when the caregiver was not present. In this Barrier Box Situation, the child was pressed to get a set of attractive toys out of a box that was virtually impossible to open, thus maximally challenging the child's regulatory capacities (see Chapter 4). Observations of children away from parents provide critical tests of the proposition that relationship experiences are carried forward and provide the foundation for personality organization. It could well be argued that the continuity of adaptation we demonstrated at prior ages (Chapters 5 and 6) fails to provide evidence for this notion, because the same caregiver is present across all assessments. Thus, perhaps the caregiver is a "discriminative stimulus" for certain child emotions and behaviors or, alternatively, perhaps it is the caregiver's consistently expert or inept handling of each situation that accounts for the apparent continuity of child behavior. Indeed, we ourselves argue that in the earlier assessments, we are really measuring the relationship and not the child. But by age 3½, we made the judgment that it was time to assess the child independently, or at least without the caregiver in the room.

Even though the mother or other primary caregiver was not present in the Barrier Box Situation, this assessment still was not completely free from current caregiver influence. Since the Barrier Box Situation assessment always directly followed the teaching tasks, it is possible that difficulties there (or notable experiences of support) would carry over into the second assessment. Such a possibility was ruled out in the assessments we made at ages 4½ and 5 years. In a laboratory assessment, all children were observed with only an experimenter present at age 4½, and 96 of the children in our sample were also studied in preschool settings. For 40 of these 96 children, we ran the nursery school, and our staff provided transportation to and from the school. After the very first week of the program, parents very rarely attended, so these children were observed for 3 months outside of the direct, immediate influence of parents.

We begin by presenting results on continuity of adaptation to the various assessments in the preschool period. The plan is to present first predictions from attachment history, followed by data based on other aspects of early care and adaptation, toddler adaptation, and then data on contemporary predictors. This ordering is not because we view infant attachment as more important than support provided during the toddler period, but because theoretical predictions are most clear for attachment history.

ASSESSMENTS AT AGE 3½: THE PERSON EMERGES

Assessments with the Caregiver Present

As was the case at age 2 years, assessments in the teaching tasks (tower building, naming things with wheels, form board, and maze tracing) were focused on parental behavior, child behavior, and the relationship (see Chapter 4). We used combinations of child and parent scales achieved through factor and cluster analyses (Egeland & Kreutzer, 1991; Rahe, 1984). For the child, scales such as enthusiasm, persistence, compliance, affection for mother, and reliance on mother were combined into factors tapping cooperation and enthusiasm. The most robust description of child functioning made use of cluster analysis. This technique forms groups of children using information from all of the child scales. As often happens, in this case, four groups emerged: one very competent cluster of 70 children (high on enthusiasm, persistence, compliance, and affection for mother), a very incompetent cluster of 25 children (high on negativism, low on compliance and affection), and two clusters that fell in between.

Attachment history (both stable attachment cases and 18-month attachment considered separately) significantly predicted child functioning in the teaching tasks (Rahe, 1984). Significant differences were obtained on the enthusiasm factor score and on the persistence, enthusiasm, and compliance scales separately. Those with *anxious–resistant* (C) histories were rated significantly lower than the other two attachment groups in each case. At the same time, the anxious–resistant group was rated significantly higher on dependency on their mothers. Likewise, those with anxious–resistant histories more often fell in the least competent cluster group and less often fell in the most competent cluster group. In fact, only 13% of the anxious–resistant group were in the most competent cluster, compared to 45% of those with secure or avoidant histories. Clearly, in this situation, it was a history of anxious–resistant attachment that put children at a disadvantage. Those with avoidant histories were only rated lower than those with secure histories on affection toward mother and on enthusiasm, and these trends fell short of significance.

Other aspects of early care also were related to adaptation in the teaching tasks at 42 months. For example, the summary score for Ainsworth's (1970) Cooperation–Interference Scale at 6 months correlated moderately with a scale of global Experience in the Teaching Tasks and modestly with child compliance with mother. A history of maltreatment in the early years was also predictive of the child's behavior in the teaching tasks. Both those in the "physical abuse" group and the "psychologically unavailable caregiver" group (see Chapter 5) showed a significantly higher level of negativism and noncompliance than did comparison children (Egeland et al., 1983). The psychologically unavailable group was distinguished by avoidance of, and anger toward, their mothers. Those in the physical "neglect" group (see Chapter 5) were primarily lacking in persistence and enthusiasm.

The quality of the caregiver–child relationship, child behavior, and caregiver support in the tool problems at age 2 years all were related to Teaching Task outcomes a year and a half later (see Table 7.1). The child's Experience in the Session at age 2 correlated moderately with Ex-

TABLE 7.1. Correlations between Toddler Experience (24 Months) and Child Behavior with the Caregiver in Early Childhood (42 Months, N = 171)

	Early childhood (42 months)	
Toddler period (24 months)	Experience in session	Compliance
Child experience in session	.32***	.32***
Overall parenting quality	.34***	.24*
Overall child rating	.22*	.24*

$* p < .05; ** p < .01; *** p < .001.$

perience in the Session in the teaching tasks, as did the overall parent rating at age 2 and, to a lesser degree, the overall child rating. These three variables also predicted the child's degree of compliance in the teaching tasks, and they also distinguished the teaching task cluster groups. Measures of the child's persistence, frustration, and anger at age 2 were especially good at discriminating between most competent and least competent groups (Rahe, 1984). Similarly, both the caregiver's supportive presence and quality of assistance at age 2 discriminated among these 3½-year cluster groups. Finally, based on Caldwell HOME Inventory scale observations at age 30 months, mothers of children in the most competent cluster were rated as most responsive and involved.

Each of the measures of care added significantly to attachment history in predicting teaching task outcomes. For example, Experience in the Session at age 2, the most integrative measure of the toddler–parent relationship, more than doubled the variance accounted for in the teaching tasks. *Thus, here, and in general, cumulative history of adaptation is the best predictor of outcome.*

Developed assets of the child also predicted competent functioning in the teaching tasks, especially achievements in the cognitive arena. Those who had been developmentally more advanced in the toddler period (on the Bayley Scales of Infant Development), who had more advanced language skills at age 3½, and those whose tested IQ at age 4 was higher on the Wechsler Preschool and Primary Scale of Intelligence (WIPPSI) performed significantly better in the teaching tasks.

In summary, continuity of functioning from both the infancy and toddler periods was apparent in the teaching tasks at age 3, and at the levels of the relationship, the child, and the caregiver. Personal assets of the child also contributed to performance on these tasks, in contrast with results in the Barrier Box Situation (Arend, 1984; see below). Consequently, we interpret this to be due to the specific demands of the teaching tasks. We describe in Chapter 8 how well the teaching task variables predict to functioning in elementary school.

Assessment without the Caregiver Present: The Barrier Box

The Barrier Box Situation was quite challenging for the children (see Chapter 4). They could see the attractive toys in the box, but it was almost impossible to open. Only after 10 minutes did the experimenter open it for them. Still, many children coped well with this situation. They tried hard to open the box (Agency), took a variety of approaches to the problem (Flexibility), stayed focused (low Distractibility), did not give up (Withdrawal, Persistence), managed their affect (Positive, Negative Affect); and, in general, were involved, purposeful, and confident, as reflected on our Projected Self-Esteem scale. Other children had a more difficult time, one way or another (Arend, 1984). As predicted, the stably secure attachment group was significantly higher on the integrative Projected Self-Esteem scale than those with histories of anxious attachment. This difference was also significant for the comparison between those who were secure and anxious at 18 months.

We also formed cluster groups based on Barrier Box Situation performance (Arend, 1984). Those who had been secure at 18 months and those who had been stably secure were more frequently in the most competent cluster group (high self-esteem, positive affect, flexibility, and agency; low on negative affect). In fact, for those with stable attachment histories, 40% of children in the secure group were in this cluster, compared to *none* of those with avoidant or resistant histories.

A history of maltreatment, a more extreme measure of early, poor quality caregiving, was consistently related to poor functioning in the Barrier Box Situation, which varied with type of maltreatment (Egeland et al., 1983). Children in all maltreatment groups were rated significantly lower on self-esteem and agency than comparison children. Those in the physical abuse group also were rated significantly higher on distractibility and negative affect, while those in the neglect group were most uniquely distinguished by very high passivity (e.g., high withdrawal from the task).

The Barrier Box Situation outcomes also were predicted by child adaptation at age 24 months. Many of the individual ratings (noncompliance, anger, frustration, coping) at age 2 distinguished the competent clusters in the Barrier Box, all in the expectable direction and at high levels of significance. Moreover, when composite positive functioning at 24 months (the Gove profiles; see Chapter 6) was combined with 18-month secure attachment, this stably competent group accounted for 70% of the competent cluster in the Barrier Box assessment, although they comprised only 42% of the children ($p < .01$). In contrast, those with poor adaptation at both 18 and 24 months accounted for 75% of the two incompetent clusters, though only 18% of the children had shown this history of consistently poor early adaptation. It is indeed possible to predict child functioning by age 3½ from prior relationship history and prior adaptation, *even when the caregiver is not present.*

ASSESSMENTS AT AGES 4½–5 YEARS: THE COHERENT PERSON

In the laboratory and preschool assessments at ages 4½–5 years, we were able to assess the full range of pertinent constructs, generally using multiple venues, multiple methods, multiple sources of data, and multiple observers. We assessed curiosity, personal agency, and self-confidence; self-management and behavior problems; self-reliance and self-esteem; and interpersonal empathy, social skill, and popularity. During this age period, we found that these characteristics were highly intercorrelated, even though they were assessed using completely independent observers and methods. This suggests great coherence in the functioning of individuals at this time. Thus, children with high self-esteem also tended to be highly curious, self-reliant rather than emotionally dependent, flexible in coping with challenges, positive in initiating contacts and in responding to others, empathic, and socially skilled (Erez, 1987; Sroufe, 1983). We return to this issue of coherence later in the chapter, but first we overview our findings on the developmental origins of these various characteristics.

Curiosity

A major assessment of curiosity was carried out in the laboratory. The child was presented with a complicated contraption having numerous things to pull on, open, manipulate, and explore (the Curiosity Box; Banta, 1970). It was unusual looking and, certainly in the late 1970s, outside of the experience of our child participants. They were told they could play with it as they wished. Various observations and ratings were made of the child's delay to start, number of manipulations, level of involvement, quality of play, positive and negative affect, agency, and self-esteem. As was done at 42 months, four cluster groups were formed to reduce and summarize all of these data (Nezworski, 1983). Those in the most competent group were characterized by high scores on rated self-esteem, agency, level of involvement, and positive affect, and by low scores on frustration/anger. The least competent group was distinguished by low scores on self-reliance and self-esteem, and a low quantitative score on time playing with the box.

The stable attachment score, the security score across the 12- to 18-month interval, and the 18-month attachment assessment alone all distinguished the competent from incompetent cluster groups (Nezworski, 1983). Based on the 18-month assessments, for example, 84% of the most competent group at age 4½ had been securely attached. Once again, as had been the case in the Teaching Tasks at 42 months, those with histories of *anxious–resistant* attachment fared worst in this situation. Not only were they overrepresented in the least incompetent cluster, but they were also rated significantly lower than those with secure and avoidant histories on scales reflecting positive emotionality.

Barrier Box Situation cluster groupings at 42 months strongly predicted cluster groupings based on the Curiosity Box at age 4½, while child scores from 24 months were less predictive. This is in accord with the proposition that, across this period, the stability and coherence of child functioning is increasing. When early caregiving quality (6 months), attachment history, and 24-and 42-month variables were combined in a discriminant function analysis, prediction was improved over caregiving history or attachment alone. The child's cumulative history again was the best predictor.

Flexible Self-Management, Self-Control, and Behavior Problems

The child's capacities regarding regulation were assessed both in the laboratory and in the preschool. We assessed the constructs of ego control and ego resiliency of Block and Block (1980) using a battery of laboratory procedures described in Chapter 4. Ego control refers to the degree of restraint or expressiveness (undercontrol) of impulses, while ego resiliency refers to flexibility in modifying self-restraint as the setting requires or permits. Thus, ego resiliency is a premier measure of the capacity for self-regulation.

Composite variables for ego control and ego resiliency were made by combining measures. An undercontrol composite was created from initiation time in the Curiosity Box assessment, the delay score in a delay of gratification task (restraining oneself from opening a brightly wrapped gift until after a series of tasks), a structure rating from designs created from the Lowenfeld Mosaics Test, and the number of forceful solutions on the Preschool Interpersonal Problem-Solving Test (PIPS). Ego resiliency or flexibility was based on a composite of scores for the total number of solutions on the PIPS, the imaginativeness rating from the Mosaics, the exploration score from the Curiosity Box, and the number of correct responses on a task of competing sets and a dual-focus task, each of which required divided attention (see Chapter 4).

For the 96 children from our sample who were in any preschool, ego-control and ego-resiliency scores also were derived from composited teacher Q-sorts (based on correlating the Q-sorts of a particular child with ideal Q-sorts of the two constructs made by experts). While there was moderate accord between laboratory and preschool measures for ego resiliency ($r = .34$, $p < .001$), agreement was positive but nonsignificant for ego control (Troy, 1988).

As we found in a previous study (Arend et al., 1979), history of secure attachment was most clearly related to ego resiliency. For example, those with secure histories at 12 months scored higher on resiliency than those with resistant or avoidant attachment histories, and this held for both the laboratory composite and the preschool Q-sort data. For the

18-month attachment variable, only the preschool data yielded a significant prediction, with the secure group again showing significantly greater flexibility than those with either avoidant or resistant histories.

The predictive power of attachment history was even more impressive when we examined the 40 children participating in the University preschool (Sroufe, 1983). These teachers were highly experienced (though completely blind to child history and to hypotheses), and we were able to combine the Q-sorts of three teachers for each child. Thus, the outcome data here are quite reliable. We found that those who had secure histories were described by the teachers via these Q-sorts as dramatically more resilient than those with histories of either resistant or avoidant attachment. The average correspondence (based on correlations) of the children with secure histories with the ego-resiliency criterion was +.50, and the correlation was positive for all 18 children. The average correlation for those with resistant histories was +.07. For the avoidant group, the average was −.13, and 9 of the 11 children had a negative correlation. Thus, there was virtually no overlap in the outcomes of the avoidant and secure groups, with those in the avoidant group showing a rather uniform lack of flexibility in adjusting their behavior and expressiveness to fit circumstances.

These strong findings were supported by observational measures of coping made in the preschool classroom (Erez, 1987). Using ethological methods (Charlesworth, 1979), 901 examples of "social problems" (in which a child's goal was blocked by another child) were culled from 108 classroom and outdoor videotapes. The child's reactions and effectiveness of actions were coded. A key variable was flexibility; that is, the degree to which the child altered strategy when a first effort was not successful. This variable correlated .37 with Q-sort ego resiliency and .52 with our sociometric measure of peer popularity, attesting to its validity. In addition, even though those with histories of secure attachment encountered fewer social problems, they were rated significantly higher on this measure of self-management than those with anxious attachment histories. Taken with the findings on attachment and ego resiliency, this is striking confirmation of the thesis that *dyadic regulation during the infancy period is an important foundation for later self-regulation.*

As is routinely the case with our data, not only attachment but also other aspects of early care and adaptation predicted these outcomes. Cooperation–Interference and Sensitivity ratings of parents at 6 months were modestly but significantly related to both laboratory and Q-sort composites of ego-control and ego-resiliency. Caregiving that was intrusive and insensitive was related to greater undercontrol and less flexibility at age 4½ (see also NICHD, 2004).

Quality of caregiver support in the tool problems at 24 months also related to ego control and ego resiliency (correlations ranging from modest for the laboratory measures of ego control to moderate for the Q-sort ego-resiliency measures), as did quality of caregiver responsiveness on the Caldwell HOME Inventory at age 30 months (r's mostly in the .30s). Measures of caregiving quality at 42 months were even more consistently related to the 4½-year-old self-management measures, with correlations sometimes now strong (in the .40s). For example, the Experience in the Session score at 42 months (the molar scale designed to capture the overall quality of the parent–child relationship) and Q-sort ego resiliency was .42. In addition to these findings, an early history of physical abuse was strongly related to undercontrol (both laboratory and preschool Q-sort measures), and psychological unavailability predicted low resiliency. In summary, quality of care at each previous age was linked to self-management, with measures assessed closer to the outcome showing stronger relations.

Prior measures of child competence likewise were predictive of self-management capacity at age 4½, with relations becoming stronger as the child got older. There was very little prediction of ego control from age 24 months, and correlations with later ego resiliency were generally in the .20s. By 42 months, child behavior predicted self-management at age 4½ quite strongly. For example, every child scale from the teaching tasks was significantly related to the Q-sort ego-resiliency index, with several in the .40s, and they also were consistently related to the laboratory ego-control battery. Moreover, those children with avoidant attachment histories and poor teaching task performance scored dramatically lower on ego resiliency than other children (Rahe, 1984). Again, we take these findings as support for the growing stability in organization of child behavior.

Our early temperament variables were not often related to these self-management measures, and when they were, correlations were quite low. For example, none of the five Brazelton factors from the newborn period was significantly related to any measure of ego control. Regarding ego resiliency, 2 of 10 correlations were significant but very modest. Likewise, none of the 9 dimensions from the Carey Infant Temperament Questionnaire (ITQ; Carey, 1970) at 6 months was related to ego control, while 4 of 18 correlations were very modestly predictive of ego resiliency. (None was significant utilizing 3-month Carey ITQ measures.) The one strong finding was a link between the 6-month Carey ITQ "adaptability" and resiliency ($r = .31$). While isolated, this is a sensible connection. The four dimensions of the Emotionality, Activity, Sociability, and Impulsivity (EASI) Temperament Survey (Buss & Plomin, 1975) at age 30 months produced two significant but very modest associations with ego control and one modest correlation with resiliency (.28). Most important, none of the findings regarding the predictive power of quality of care was altered when accounting for temperament variation (Troy, 1988); that is, the influence of care was not confounded by (or accounted for by) variations in child temperament.

One reason for the weakness of our temperament results may be that the measures themselves were not strong, though they were "state of the art" in the 1970s. Certainly, there are better-designed questionnaires and numerous behavioral and physiological measures available today. We do not conclude that temperament is unimportant. However, we have conducted the kind of research that would be required to truly reveal the importance of temperament. To show that temperament is a driving force in development or a powerful determinant of parenting, observational studies of similar comprehensiveness to ours are needed. When further studies are done, they may find, as have we, that the primary importance of temperament lies in its interaction with other factors (see Chapter 12; see also Bates, 1989; Kochanska, 1997; NICHD, 2001).

Performance on the four subscales of the Wechsler Preschool and Primary Scale of Intelligence (WIPPSI) given at age 4 did correlate consistently with the laboratory battery measures of ego control (correlations in the .20s), and the laboratory and preschool measures of ego resiliency (correlations ranging from .26 to .46). The strongest correlations were with the laboratory measures, some of which may well have an IQ component. A standard interpretation of this finding, that child capacities are important in these tasks, seems reasonable. We would also point out that IQ at these ages is in part based on social and emotional factors, including capacity to engage the experimenter. We found, for example, that those with histories of anxious–resistant attachment had the lowest IQs. This, too, seems reasonable given their general difficulties engaging novelty and challenges. In Chapter 8, we present further findings on the role of social factors in IQ and IQ change.

Nonetheless, because of the IQ findings, we examined our caregiving variables with child IQ controlled (Troy, 1988). This had little impact on the relationships between caregiving and the self-management scores. For example, with the 42-month quality-of-care variables, it did make the correlations with ego resiliency lower, but they remained significant. It actually made the correlations with ego control *higher*. For the ego-control Q-sort variable, every 42-month maternal scale was now significantly related, with correlations reaching the .30s. So while child IQ appeared to be important in these assessments, it was not so at the expense of caregiving history; rather, it is an independent predictor.

Before leaving the topic of self-management, we want to briefly present some findings on behavior problems in the preschool period.

There is a more complete discussion of the origins of disturbance in later chapters. Deportment and behavior problems, either withdrawal or acting out, are closely related to self-management capacity. For example, the Q-sort composites of ego undercontrol and ego resiliency correlated −.58 and .53, respectively, with teacher ratings of compliance, and .43 and −.64, respectively, with total number of behavior problems on the Preschool Behavior Questionnaire (Behar & Stringfield, 1974). These are so high, in part, because the same teachers made all ratings. However, preschool ego-control and ego-resiliency ratings also were significantly related to behavior problem scores provided by kindergarten teachers the next year (r's from .22 to .40).

Attachment history proved again to be an important antecedent, with the avoidant group showing the most behavior problems at preschool (Erickson et al., 1985). Those with avoidant histories were less compliant, scored higher on hostility and isolation, and had a greater number of total problems. Based on factor analyses of two behavior problem questionnaires, an effective group of children, with very minimal problems, and three problem groups (acting out, withdrawn, and inattentive) were formed. For children who had been anxiously attached at both 12 and 18 months, only 12.5% were in the effective group at preschool, compared to 68% of those who had been secure at both ages. Of those with mixed histories (once secure), 40% were in the effective group. These dramatic findings were highly significant. Both 12-month and 18-month security considered separately also were significantly related to behavior problem group status.

Likewise, early measures of maltreatment were strongly related to behavior problems (Egeland et al., 1983; Erickson & Egeland, 1987; Erickson, Egeland, & Pianta, 1989). Each maltreatment group showed significantly more problems than comparison children. Children in both the physical abuse and psychological unavailability groups were rated higher on negative affect and were undercontrolled and noncompliant. Those in the neglect group were rated high on these problems as well, but they were also very dependent, anxious, inattentive, and lacking in initiative and good work habits. Retention or special education services were recommended for 65% of these children. Such problems forecasted and laid the foundation for academic problems throughout the school years that we describe in later chapters.

Our caregiving measures in the 24-month tool problems, at 30 months (the Caldwell HOME scales), and in the 42-month teaching tasks also predicted behavior problems. Each of these accounted for additional variance beyond attachment. One way we have illustrated this is by examining those children who had been securely attached but later had problems, and those who had been anxiously attached but later did not have problems (Erickson et al., 1985). Secure infants with later problems had caregivers who provided less support at 24 months, were less involved at home at 30 months, and less consistent, firm, and confident in the teaching tasks than caregivers of secure children who continued to thrive. Likewise, those with anxious histories who were doing better than expected at age 4½, compared to those who, as expected, had problems, had caregivers who were rated as significantly more involved at home at 30 months and significantly higher on *every* scale at age 42 months. *Thus, while quality of attachment represents an important starting place with regard to later problem behavior, change remains possible, and caregiving is important in each period.* We have much more to say about change throughout the remainder of the book.

Self-Reliance, Self-Esteem, and Self-Confidence

Our most extensive data on self-reliance, or independence, came from the University preschool study of 40 children in two classrooms, drawn from our larger sample (see Chapter 4 for selection criteria). For these children, we had extensive, independent observational data on contact between children and teachers, as well as ratings, rankings, and Q-sorts on a variety of dependency indices composited across three teachers. Self-reliance received such attention from us because of the specific and crucial predictions made regarding this characteristic from attachment theory. Those with histories of anxious attachment are expected to be very dependent later. This includes those with histories of avoidant attachment, even though they failed to go to caregivers when stressed by the brief separations in the infant assessments. Having early needs met in a consistent fashion, not "precocious independence," is the foundation for later self-reliance.

General findings regarding attachment history and dependency were quite clear (Sroufe, 1983; Sroufe, Fox, & Pancake, 1983). On teacher overall rankings, only 12% of children with secure histories (Group B) were ranked in the top half of their class on dependency, compared to 90% of those with an anxious attachment history (Groups A and C). The exact ranks, from highest to lowest dependency, were as follows for the larger class: C,C,A,A,C,A,C,A,A,B,C,A,C,B,B,C,B,B,A,A,C,B,B. On numerous ratings of dependency, including frequency of seeking help in self-management or social management, seeking help in negative ways, overall dependency on three different scales, and a compilation of dependency items from the Q-sort, those with secure histories were always strongly and significantly less dependent than those with histories of either resistant *or* avoidant attachment. Four- and 5-year-olds, even those with secure histories, are of course still dependent on adults for many things. But for children who are developing well, there is a shift toward "instrumental dependence." One goes to adults when one's own resources are exhausted, or when a problem is obviously too difficult. One does not rely on adults for continual guidance, direction, and emotional support.

The teacher ratings were corroborated by observations made during "circle times" (for stories or songs) and during general classroom observation. Those with secure histories sat next to teachers less and leaned against or sat on the teacher's lap dramatically less often than those with histories of resistant or avoidant attachment. An overall proportion of contact index strongly and significantly distinguished those with secure histories from the two groups with anxious histories (.24 versus .71 and .86, respectively). The correlation between this measure and the teacher dependency ranking was .62. Likewise, observations of total contact with teachers and amount of contact initiated by teachers distinguished secure from anxious groups. Teachers initiated much more contact with those with anxious histories, for discipline or for care. Thus, as hypothesized by Bowlby (1973), *the foundation for self-reliance is a history of responsive care and the secure attachment to which it leads.*

Completely parallel to these data were rankings and ratings of self-esteem and agency, or self-confidence (Sroufe, 1983). The highest ranked children on self-esteem (see Appendix E) were virtually all those with histories of secure attachment, while those ranked near the bottom were nearly all those with anxious attachment, with very little overlap. Likewise, children with secure histories were rated significantly higher on self-confidence.

Social Competence, Interpersonal Emotion, and Empathy

Preschool teacher rankings of social competence and ratings of social skills showed that children with histories of secure attachment were more socially effective than those with resistant and avoidant histories. This was true for both the larger group of all of our participants who attended preschools (Erickson et al., 1985) and for the 40 children in our two University preschool classes (Sroufe, 1983). For the latter group, we also had available teacher rankings on number of friends and child sociometric ranks on popularity (see Chapter 4). In both cases, those with secure histories were found to be most competent. Additional validation of these findings comes from the correlation between the teacher competence ranking and the completely independent child sociometric popularity scores (average correlation across the two classes = .71), as well as the child's observed receipt of attention from others in the classroom (LaFreniere & Sroufe, 1985).

Teacher ratings and detailed behavioral data regarding emotional expression and empathy allowed us to better understand the dynamics of social behavior that promoted popularity with peers and teacher judgments of competence. In general, children with secure histories showed more positive affect and less negative affect than those with anxious histories, as rated by teachers (Sroufe, 1983). Moreover, detailed observational data indicated that those who had been securely attached more often initiated contacts with other children with accompanying positive affect, and they more often responded to the initiations of others with positive affect as well (Sroufe et al., 1984). The composite of the frequency of all affectively positive interactions was highly significant. Moreover, members of the secure group less often were aggressive, less often fussed or whined, and in general showed less negative affect across all settings observed. Having experienced a relationship with an emotionally responsive adult in the early years, securely attached children bring forward positive expectations regarding encounters with others; they exhibit fewer negative behaviors in these interactions, and they bring an enjoyment and an enthusiasm to the exchanges. All of these characteristics make them attractive play partners.

Empathy and prosocial behavior also likely promote a child's popularity with other children and positive regard by teachers. We created a "mega-item" or scale for empathy using pertinent items from the Q-sort (e.g., "tends to give, lend, and share"; "considerate of other children"; "empathic"; see Sroufe, 1983). The average placement of these items in categories 1–9 from most characteristic to least characteristic of the child became the empathy score. Results were dramatic and significant for attachment group. In fact, the average item placement suggested that empathy was "very characteristic" for those with secure histories and "uncharacteristic" for those with avoidant histories, with the resistant group falling in between (Sroufe, 1983). We discuss these differences further and provide some actual examples of behavior in the section on internalizing relationships later in this chapter.

Summary

At age 4–5 years, as before, positive adaptation builds upon the history of care and prior adaptation. When outcome measures are highly reliable and based clearly in theory (e.g., self-reliance, self-regulation, and competence with peers in the nursery school), empirical support for continuity in functioning is quite strong. This is especially true when attachment history is combined with other predictors. We now turn to the question of organization and patterning in individual adaptation.

PATTERNS OF ADAPTATION

In our study of personal development, we were interested not only in predicting levels of competence but also in tracing the emergence of patterns of adaptation or personality, which we believe arise in the organization of early caregiving relationships; that is, we wanted to understand the particular patterns of problems or strengths that different children have, not just whether they are doing well or not. The differences in nursery school behavior that we have just described—on empathy, popularity, dependency, ego resiliency, and so forth—have simply established that those with positive histories in general fare better than those with less supportive histories. Note that no differences in level were revealed on these measures between those with avoidant and resistant histories, nor should they actually have been expected. Neither of the anxiously attached groups have histories that would support flexibility, self-reliance, empathic capacity, or social skill. Rather, differences should be in how, when, and the way in which such problems are expressed; that is the organization of this problem behavior.

There are, for example, lots of ways to become unpopular or to show dependency. Our theory implies more than the fact that some children will have problems with peers and others will do well, and that some will be highly dependent, while others are more self-reliant. It also implies that different children will manifest their peer problems or dependency problems in particular ways and in particular circumstances, and that their sets of difficulties will be organized or patterned in different ways.

Demonstrating such patterns is extremely difficult. First of all, development and change, and the twists and turns of each life, make each individual unique. To discern patterns and to verify them quantitatively, it must be possible to group individuals, that is, to see commonality in organization despite variability. The developmental principle of differentiation increases the complexity of this task. With development, there likely is branching of patterns. For example, no one should expect all children with avoidant histories to reveal the *same* pattern of adaptation at age 4–5, even given continuity. At best, there should be a family of patterns that derives in a coherent way from the original pattern. These patterns retain some common core aspect but are not identical.

The seven boys in our University nursery school who had histories of seductive care (see Chapter 6) illustrate these problems. Based on our observation, this history was revealed in each child's behavior but in a variety of ways: Three boys were impulsive and anxious; two boys were characterized by "tension bursts" (e.g., sudden, rapid hand jiggling), extensive masturbation, and infantile behavior; and two boys were the outstanding favorites of female teachers, spending more time with these teachers than with children. Almost none of the 21 boys in our preschool without histories of seductive care showed any of these three kinds of problems. After the fact, each of these patterns seems to be a reasonable outcome from a history of overstimulation and sensualized care. But we did not specify them in advance, and we expect that other patterns exist. Such observations prompted us to explore whether we could demonstrate quantitatively distinctive families of patterns of adaptation for those with avoidant and resistant attachment histories.

Situational Variations

There were solid reasons for believing that the avoidant (A) and resistant (C) groups evolve different patterns of adaptation. For one thing, we found repeatedly that certain situations do not pose particular problems for one group or the other, and even reveal positive aspects of adaptation. One may observe, for example, a child with an avoidant history playing contentedly with Legos for a sustained period, or a child with a resistant history sitting quietly on a teacher's lap and looking at a book. Different situations likewise reveal the difficulties of each group, and such situational variations are part of what is meant by the organization of behavior. Situations of novelty, high stimulation, object mastery, and cognitive challenge are especially difficult for those with resistant histories. Thus, for example, only the C's looked incompetent dealing with the Curiosity Box, which was not at all challenging or stressful for the A's, and only the C's were heavily challenged by the teaching tasks. Only the C's had low performance on the WIPPSI. Furthermore, when we observed the children as toddlers one time in a playroom with an unfamiliar partner (Pastor, 1981), only the C's were incompetent in this novel situation.

On the other hand, for those with avoidant histories, it is intimate social encounters that most readily reveal problems. In initial social encounters, such as the first day of nursery school, the A's are quite socially active and forward (even more so than those with secure histories, who watch and explore). Later, as *relationships* started to form, they had difficulty and removed themselves from social commerce, becoming increasingly isolated (Sroufe, 1983). In our nursery school, each child was assigned a play partner, and these pairs had 14–20 sessions together in a playroom. From videotapes, coders with no knowledge of the children's histories made ratings of "depth of relationship" (degree of reciprocity and shared emotion) and hostility (Pancake, 1988). In this context, the difficulty of children with histories of avoidant attachment stood out; pairs containing even one member with such a child were significantly more distant, with little overlap with the ratings of the other pairs, and they were characterized by significantly more hostility. One anecdote from the classroom, among countless such examples, illustrates the issue of isolation for some of these children. ET one day noticed a "space capsule" the teachers had set up (a large, foil-covered cardboard barrel with a cutout for entry). With interest, he made his way across the room and started to approach it, but as he drew near, he saw that two boys were already playing inside. He turned and walked away. This type of close encounter with others was not attractive.

The Organization of Dependency, Coping, and Peer Behavior

We can further illustrate differences in the organization of behavior of children with different attachment histories with observations of dependency and problems with peers. For example, children with histories of avoidance were not as direct in expressing their dependency needs as those with resistant histories. Thus, while members of neither of these groups were self-reliant, they showed their dependency in different ways. Whenever children in the resistant group were upset, disappointed, or anxious, all of which happened easily and often, they went right to a teacher. They "wore their hearts on their sleeves." Those with avoidant histories tended to seek contact obliquely, as did ET upon entry into the classroom. He walked in a series of angles, like a sailboat tacking into the wind. By approximations, he eventually wound up near the teacher; then, turning his back toward her, he would wait for her to contact him. In keeping with their history of rebuff when needy, these children generally would explicitly *not* go to the teachers when they were injured or acutely upset. For example, one day, when ET bumped and obviously hurt his head, he went off into a corner by himself. Another child sat by himself on the last day of class, until a teacher came, put her arm around him, and suggested that he was feeling bad; then he burst into tears.

Children with histories of avoidant and resistant attachment also showed distinctive patterns of coping with social problems in the classroom (Erez, 1987). In the face of problems, the members of the resistant group were less persistent and more often used the coping strategy of leaving the situation than did members of the A or B groups. It is interesting to note that these children were injured with significantly greater frequency than those in the other groups. All of this is in accord with the tendencies toward immaturity and passivity previously noted. The avoidant group was distinguished, in contrast, by being less flexible than the other two groups.

Likewise, the two groups with histories of anxious attachment showed very different kinds of problems with peers. The C's did not isolate themselves as did the A's. They were oriented toward peers, often hovering near a group of children or attempting, but failing, to maintain one-on-one interactions (Sroufe, 1983). They had difficulty controlling frustration or modulating arousal during sustained interactions. If the C's were aggressive, it was when they flailed out in reaction to some provocation or perceived slight, but they did not engage in systematic, unprovoked aggression or bullying, as did the A's. Thus, the A's were seen as more aggressive than the other attachment groups (see Erickson et al., 1985). In terms of formal sociometric analyses, children with resistant histories more often fit the "neglected" pattern; that is, they were not named as being liked, but neither were they named as being disliked (Rubin, Bukowski, & Parker, 1998). The A's were more frequently named as being disliked, and common reasons given by the children were "She's mean" or "He hits" (Sroufe, 1983).

Profile Analysis

We used several methods to group children in terms of profiles of behavior, which allowed quantitative statistical tests of distinctions between those with A and C histories. We first created hypothetical profiles of expected preschool outcomes, three for A's (avoidant) and two for C's (resistant). The patterns for Group A were centered on isolation, emotional disengagement, and malevolence, while those for Group C were centered on lack of control, immaturity, and passivity (see Table 7.2). These were done a priori. There was no prior research on what these patterns should be. We knew our profiles could only be approximations and that there likely would be more than five patterns, yet at that time, these were our best guesses regarding patterns that might evolve.

The first test of the pattern hypothesis involved having three teach-

TABLE 7.2. Hypothetical Profiles Derived from Insecure Attachment History

Avoidant groups

A_a Hostile/mean, aggressive, antisocial (lying, stealing, devious).

A_b Emotionally insulated, asocial, isolated.

A_c Disconnected, spaced out, psychotic-like. May be oblivious or bizarre, or just not know what is going on.

Resistant groups

C_a Overstimulated (hyper), easily frustrated, tense, or anxious.

C_b Dependent, passive, weak, helpless, teacher-oriented.

Note. From Sroufe (1983). Copyright 1983 by Erlbaum. Reprinted by permission.

TABLE 7.3. Teacher One-Phrase Descriptions of Individual Children

Group A (Avoidant)

1. Mean to other children, kept things that didn't belong to her. The most dishonest preschooler I have ever met. Mean lying—everything is hers.
2. Very mad, "I hate myself!" An unhappy and angry kid. Terrible self-concept. Angry, unhappy.
3. So mean—lack of respect for humans. Angry, mean, playing with cars. Out of control, trying to do better.
4. Sad, depressed, and withdrawn child. By himself. Coy, looks like a baby.
5. "She's not my friend," spaced. Affable but mentally slow. Inappropriately, highly impulsive and vulnerably good-natured.
6. An angry, withdrawn, rigid person. Attached to Kate (teacher). "I love you, Kate." So frail but gutsy.
7. Dominant, self-reliant. Sweet/funny and responsible, yet not always fair or kind.
8. A very nice kid—level-headed, capable of taking care of himself. Warm, responsive. Loving, calling for Sarah (child), Jane (teacher).

Group B

1. Ideal kid, good looking, OK. Well-coordinated, agile, competent. Very solid kid. Vulnerable to life changes, positive and negative.
2. Happy, rising star in the group—looked better all of the time. Agile, coordinated, jumping around room. Shy, but gutsy, with care group.
3. Spunky sleeper—more powerful than meets the eye. Competent, quiet. So funny, cute, elf-like.
4. Very nice kid—sensitive and somewhat moody. Quiet, drifted at times, kept to herself. Depressed, withdrawn, easily hurt.
5. Queen bee, to Lonnie (child), "I'm not done yet!" Sparkplug. Competent, yet overstimulated other kids at times. Dominant, had trouble waiting her turn. Excited other kids.
6. Very competent, yet unsure of self—oversocialized female. Feminine. Dressed up, sucking finger, coy.
7. A mystery—looks OK, but never in places where it was "scary." "I don't feel good. I'm sick."
8. Always up high—attached to Kate (teacher). Up high—look at me. Very confusing to me. A spacy, undersocialized kid.
9. Don't know him. Seemed OK, yet rigid and somewhat tight. Evasive. "Boys can't wear those shirts."

Group C

1. Play with yellow truck. Trouble dealing with stress. Confusing—OK outwardly, yet sad and prone to self-recrimination/guilt. Falling down in dramatic scene—an actor.
2. Bright but impulsive and tense. Frustrated easily in play situations, inconsiderate of children. Holding "gun," saying it is his.
3. "High"—difficult to settle and difficult to concentrate. High (hyper). An operator—popular and fast (very elusive).
4. Running around being Batman. "Bullshit," angry, Batman, didn't like self. A confused and angry kid doing the best he can.

(continued on next page)

5. Immature and unwilling to take a risk/loves Jean (student). Lacks initiative, looking for Jean, controlled. A baby, can't tolerate kids.
6. "Kate (teacher), push me," "Where's Karyn (teacher)?" Dependent, liking Lorenzo (student). Happy–sad—is competent but does not handle disapproval or stress well.
7. Always going part way up and then down the loft ladder. Weird mouth, sunken eyes, tiny. A sleeper, knows more than her withered appearance lets on.

Note. From Sroufe (1983). Copyright 1983 by Erlbaum. Reprinted by permission.

ers independently contribute descriptive phrases that they thought captured the essence of each child. Our coders, blind to history, were given these descriptions, with cases in a random order vis-à-vis attachment. The coders dramatically more often placed children with avoidant histories in one of the three "A" profiles, and children with resistant histories in the "C" profiles ($p < .006$). The reader may wish to try this. The actual descriptions for the second class are in Table 7.3, grouped by attachment history for convenience.

In the second method, we asked coders to examine the 10 Q-sort items that the teachers had placed in the "most characteristic" and "least characteristic" piles for each child. Based on these items, coders again were significantly more likely to place those with A histories in one of the "A" profiles and those with C histories in one of the "C" profiles, again with no prior knowledge of the identity of the child.

Finally, we had judges select items from the Preschool Behavior Questionnaire that would seem to be characteristic of each of our five profiles (see Table 7.4). Children receiving highest scores on one of the three "A" sets of items more often in fact had avoidant histories, while those whose highest scores were on one of the "C" sets of items more often had been resistant (Sroufe, 1983). In Chapter 12, we again discuss how specific attachment histories forecast different kinds of problems, in particular, different psychiatric diagnoses.

INTERNALIZING THE CAREGIVING RELATIONSHIP

We believe that an organized personality emerges in the preschool years, and that this process reflects the internalization and carrying forward of the organization in primary caregiving relationships. The links between attachment history and the profiles of behavior just discussed support this thinking. There were two other ways we sought to examine these propositions: first, by examining the patterning in the preschool child's relationships with peers and teachers; and second, by looking at the way the social world was represented in the child's mind.

TABLE 7.4. Hypothetical Preschool Profiles and Associated Items from the
Preschool Behavior Questionnaire (Behar & Stringfield, 1974)

Pattern A_a: Hostile, mean, aggressive, antisocial (lying, stealing, devious)
  Tells lies
  Bullies other children
  Blames others
  Inconsiderate of others

Pattern A_b: Emotionally insulated, asocial, isolated
  Tends to do things on own; rather solitary
  Stares into space
  Fails to play with most other children
  Is shy, bashful
  Has flat affect—rarely expresses positive or negative feelings directly

Pattern A_c: Disconnected, spaced out, psychotic-like
  Has twitches, mannerisms, or tics of the face and body
  Stares into space
  Demonstrates little interest in things and activities in environment
  Daydreams frequently
  Rocks, sways, whirls, or does other repetitive whole body movements

Pattern C_a: Overstimulated (hyper), easily frustrated, tense or anxious, impulsive,
    flailing out, rather than hostile
  Restless; runs about or jumps up and down; doesn't keep still
  Squirmy, fidgety child
  Has poor concentration or short attention span
  Is impulsive, acts without thinking
  Is easily upset by failure
  Is tense or jittery in everyday situations or activities

Pattern C_b: Dependent, passive, weak, helpless, teacher-oriented
  Tends to be fearful or afraid of new things or new situations
  Gives up easily
  Is hypersensitive, easily hurt
  Stays close or clings to mother or adult
  Acts overly fearful and cautious
  Lacks initiative, is passive and easily led

Note. From Sroufe (1983). Copyright by Erlbaum. Reprinted by permission.

The Quality of Relationships with Peers

We found extensive evidence for attachment history–based differences in
the quality of peer relationships both in the play pairs and in the classroom of our University nursery school. In the play pairs (see page 137),
coders described a pattern of behavior called "victimization" (Troy &
Sroufe, 1987). The presence of a noninteractive experimenter thwarted
most physical aggression, so in most cases this involved sarcasm, deri-

sion, rejection of overtures, or other verbal hostility or hostile gestures (e.g., sticking out the tongue), but in each case it was systematic. Such a pattern was observed in 5 of 19 pairs, with 100% agreement between independent coders. In each case, the victimizing child always had a history of avoidant (A) attachment, and the victim always was another child with an anxious history (either C or A). The convergence of two anxious histories was required. When a secure child was paired with an A, either the two of them would engage in counterassertiveness or a mutual distance was maintained. Those with secure histories tended to form nurturing relationships with C children; they in no case victimized them. When two C's were paired, the play may have been very low level, but there was not victimization. When the partners were both A's, the weaker child was exploited. In keeping with our position that the whole relationship is internalized (Sroufe & Fleeson, 1986), it made sense that A's could be both victims and victimizers, given the history of rejection in relationships that they had known.

Our empathy data also revealed qualitative differences for the attachment groups in relating to peers (Kestenbaum, Farber, & Sroufe, 1989). From voluminous video recordings, we culled every occasion in which a child was injured or upset. Independent coders recorded the behavior of each child present during these video segments, and these were placed into three categories. Sometimes children were concerned and helpful (e.g., going to get a teacher); that is, they were genuinely empathic and prosocial. This was the most common reaction of those with secure histories. Some children seemed to lose the distinction between themselves and the distressed child. They would become very upset themselves, perhaps going to a teacher for comforting. This reaction is common in younger children (Zahn-Waxler, Radke-Yarrow, Wagner, & Chapman, 1992), and it was most common among the C's in this assessment at age 4½. Finally, some engaged in "antiempathy," a category of behavior forced upon us by the observations: They would explicitly do something to make the child feel worse (e.g., teasing a crying child; poking a child in the stomach who said he or she had a stomachache). Those with avoidant histories were distinctive from both other groups in engaging in this behavior. Having experienced rejection and hostility, the child was now rejecting when another was in need.

The Predictability of Teacher–Child Relationships

We also used classroom videos to investigate relationships between the two principal teachers and children with varying attachment histories (Motti, 1986; Sroufe & Fleeson, 1988). We catalogued the contents of each tape and made use of a grid consisting of the teachers and every child. We were able to create summary tapes of at least 50 episodes in which one of the teachers was present and the child in question was also on camera. Coders, blind to all other information, reviewed these tapes numerous times, then made ratings of the teacher's behavior regarding the child on scales created for this study. These scales included Engagement, Affection, Control, Anger, Nurturance/Support, Tolerance, and Expectations for Compliance. The last three scales require some explanation. Nurturance is distinguished from affection, in that it involves caregiving behavior, comforting and taking care of the child's physical and emotional needs. Typical 4- to 5-year-olds would not tend to elicit frequent behavior of this type. Tolerance refers to the degree to which the teacher makes allowances for the child, that is, tolerates or permits immature behavior or rule infractions. We assume that teachers do this because they do not see the child as capable. Finally, Expectations for Compliance are inferred from the way the teacher gives directives, and the timing and extent of follow-up. When the teacher asks a child to do something, then immediately turns to other business, it can be assumed that he or she believes the child will comply. In contrast, if a directive is immediately followed by a repetition or other supporting action (perhaps even before the child could have responded to the initial directive), this conveys doubts about the likelihood that the child will comply (see Sroufe & Fleeson, 1988, for more detail on these scales).

Although rating such scales seems complex, coders were able to rate these relationship qualities quite reliably (Motti, 1986). In a special test of reliability, we even gave coders independent sets of 50 teacher–child episodes, and they still agreed well. This conveys not only reliability of the coders but also reliability of the particular relationship.

Results of this procedure were dramatic and similar for ratings based on each of the two teachers (Sroufe & Fleeson, 1988). With children with secure histories, teachers were engaged and affectionate (as they were with the other two groups as well), but they also treated them in a respectful, age-appropriate, matter-of-fact way. They were rated high on Expectations for Compliance but low on Control, Anger, Nurturance/Caregiving, and Tolerance (i.e., they held out high standards for these children). Such a relationship would support and expand the child's emerging competence. With children with resistant histories, the teachers were rated low on Expectations for Compliance, but high on Nurturance, Tolerance, and Control; that is, they treated the children as one might treat younger children, no doubt in response to the neediness they perceived. In a separate analysis, teachers were observed to initiate significantly more contacts with those with resistant histories than they did with the other two groups (Sroufe et al., 1983). Such a relationship might consolidate their immaturity. With the A's, the teachers were also high on Control and low on Expectations for Compliance, but they were low on Tolerance and low on Nurturance/Caregiving. Moreover, children in this group were the only ones observed to elicit anger. When one saw a teacher so upset with a child that she wanted to remove him from the classroom, the child was an A (who, without exception, had done something very hurtful to another child). The history of rejection experienced by these children was to a degree recapitulated by our teachers, even though they were incredibly compassionate individuals.

Since the procedure involved the same two teachers, they were a constant. The variation in a teacher's behavior with particular children is characteristic of the relationship with that child, not a trait of the teacher. Relationship histories are carried forward and are powerful influences on subsequent relationships. This is one reason for continuity in individual adaptation.

Measures of Representation in the Preschool Years

We assessed representation in two ways during the preschool years. The first was the PIPS (Shure & Spivak, 1970), a measure of representation, as well as a procedure that provides indices of ego control and ego resiliency. When children are asked questions about interpersonal conflict and the ways that it might be addressed, they reveal their expectations and beliefs about relationships, that is, the contents of their minds. We rated positive expectations regarding the caregiver, flexibility of problem solving, and positive expectations regarding peers. Children with secure histories across the 12- to 18-month period were rated higher on all three scales ($r = .40$, $.42$, and $.33$, respectively; Carlson et al., 2004). Early caregiving sensitivity and cooperation also correlated modestly with all three scales.

Our second approach to representation involved looking at the content of the play of children in the playroom. In addition to the quality and elaborateness of the play, we looked at two specific aspects of content: (1) the presence of people in the fantasy play; and (2) when there were themes of conflict in the play (which was common in all groups of children), were the conflicts generally brought to a successful resolution (Rosenberg, 1984)? We found that not only was the level of play more elaborate for children with histories of secure attachment, but also they significantly more often showed successful conflict resolution than those with avoidant or resistant histories. An example of this might be, "Uh oh, he got his leg broke by a truck. . . . Here come the ambilens. They take him to the hospital. . . . They fixed it!" Both the secure and the resistant groups showed richly peopled play, with interpersonal situations abounding. Consistent with their observed isolation, the fantasy play of those with avoidant histories was almost entirely devoid of people, a significant difference from those with other histories.

These were only the beginnings of our attempts to probe the inner world of the child. In later chapters, we describe our work with representational measures based on drawings, projective techniques, and narratives.

CONTEXT AND CHANGING ADAPTATION

As was the case during the toddler period (Chapter 6), the surrounding context continued to be important for the caregiver–child relationship and for the child's adaptation. Two supports that have appeared to us to be most consistently important are the involvement and support of the maternal grandmother and a stable, supporting adult partnership for the primary caregiver. For example, a woman's dissatisfaction with her partner relationship predicted higher boundary dissolution scores between herself and her son at age 42 months. Other family members and friends have also been important, and measures of overall social support often were the strongest correlates of positive outcomes. Such surrounding support generally was related to child adaptation at each age, and also often accounted for changing adaptation from the infancy or toddler periods. Two examples follow.

The competent and incompetent cluster groups based on the Curiosity Box ratings were consistently discriminated by level of overall support from family and friends, on every assessment between infancy and preschool (18, 24, 30, 42, and 48 months), with results being statistically significant at three of these time periods, even considered separately. Moreover, when the combined support measure was entered into a discriminant function analysis with attachment and other early predictors of competence, predictability was improved (Nezworski, 1983). As Bowlby (1973) has argued, adaptation is always a product of cumulative history and current circumstances.

Behavior problems in the preschool also proved to be best predicted by a combination of prior history and support in the intervening years (Erickson et al., 1985). Many children who had been anxiously attached showed behavior problems in the preschool, but there was a group of children that we referred to as "exceptions." Parents in the group of children whose behavior had improved were rated as having significantly more support from family and friends, and significantly less stress at 42 and 48 months. Level of family stress is in general an excellent predictor of child behavior problems in the preschool period (Egeland & Kreutzer, 1991). Moreover, mothers of the formerly anxiously attached children, now with a low level of behavior problems, had significantly more often formed a stable, intact relationship with an adult partner during the intervening years. In turn, during the teaching tasks, these mothers, compared to mothers of children whose problems persisted, were judged to be more respectful of the child's autonomy and desire for exploration, while still providing structure. Without intruding on the child, they nonetheless provided clear, consistent limits. They were more warm and supportive. The converse was true for those children who moved from secure attachment toward a pattern of behavior problems in preschool. Such findings testify both to the possibility of change and to the lawfulness of change. As parental circumstances improve, so do parenting and child adaptation during this period.

CONCLUSION

As suggested by other theorists, children in our study had formed coherent personalities by 5 years of age. Characteristic ways of regulating and managing themselves and of dealing with the object and social world had emerged. Such coherence was demonstrated in the way various behaviors clustered together in individual children, and in the way their behavior varied from situation to situation in the face of different challenges and opportunities. Not simple frequencies of behaviors but the organization of behavior within and across situations best characterized individual children.

Our data strongly suggest that such organized patterns of behavior are the offspring of variations in care and patterns of parent–child relationship organization that preceded them. From this point on, the central questions for our study became more elaborate. Added to our interest in early origins of behavior were questions concerning the predictive power of these preschool patterns of adaptation and processes that govern continuity and change in adaptation across the years.

CHAPTER 8

Adaptation in Middle Childhood
The Era of Competence

> INTERVIEWER: Well, what if you had an argument or a fight with your friend? Could that make your friendship end?
> SERENA (*age 11, after thinking for a moment*): No, really you would probably be better friends afterwards, because you would understand each other better.

The expansion of the child's world continues at a rapid rate during middle childhood, roughly ages 6–11 years. To be sure, during the preschool years, the child's social world expanded, as did the settings in which the child developed. But during middle childhood, increasing hours are spent away from home, and in interaction with peers rather than family members. It is also the age when most children participate in organized groups and activities that do not involve parents. Most notably, this is the era in which full-time formal schooling begins, and when the child is given more responsibilities.

The importance of middle childhood has been recognized by many scholars. This includes contemporary researchers (Collins & van Dulmen, in press) and scholars such as Erikson (1950/1963) and Sullivan (1953) in the middle of the previous century. Erikson described the period in terms of "industry versus inferiority," because he believed it was so important to establish oneself as a responsible, agentic, hardworking, serious minded person at this time. One must become competent, not in the fantasy play world of the preschooler, but in the real world of tasks and accomplishments. In our culture, children must do well in school, must handle responsibility for self-guidance and proper deportment, and must develop skills and talents about which they feel positive. As emphasized by Sullivan (1953), they also must make major advances in relationships with peers, including developing close, loyal friendships. To Sullivan, such special friendships were the hallmark of this period. Also of great importance is the capacity to function in the more organized peer groups of middle childhood, and to coordinate friendships with group functioning (see Chapter 4). Many changes are happening in the inner world as well, as children evolve a more coherent, integrated view of themselves (Harter, 1998).

Thus, competence in middle childhood is a multifaceted phenomenon, involving both personal and social components, and developments within the self and in the social world. Nonetheless, our thesis remains that however complicated capturing the quality of adaptation now becomes, it is based upon, and grows out of, what has gone before. The confidence that the child can now show in the self derives from the confidence in responsive care present from the child's earliest months. The capacity for proper deportment and self-regulation is built step-by-step upon the foundation of caregiver, dyadic, and guided self-regulation that came before. And the competence with peers derives from both the attitudes and support of parents, and the experiences and training in regulation that occurred in the world of preschool companions. The hours of working on sustained interactions allow the construction and maintenance of loyal friendships now, and the hours spent learning how to play with others allow successful functioning in formal groups. Competent, positive adaptation is a developmental construction, calling upon all of one's past experience.

This view of adaptation as a developmental construction leads us to a change of emphasis in this chapter. In predicting toddler and preschool outcomes, we emphasized variations in infant attachment security. This made sense in light of the short time span, the theoretical specificity, and the need to validate toddler and preschool measures against the well-established attachment measures. And attachment continues to be part of the predictive picture. Especially for certain outcomes, where theoretical ties remain uniquely strong (e.g., dependency and certain qualities of peer relationships), we even continue to evaluate attachment separately. This is the case when we return to the problem of profiles of adaptation, because, theoretically, attachment variations are not only variations in degree of competence but also prototypes for qualitatively different patterns of personality organization. However, for many analyses to be presented, our predictors are the history of care across the early years, as well as prior child adaptation at each age, and ongoing measures of developmental context. In keeping with the developmental construction viewpoint, the broader history of care and support, and cumulative measures of adaptation, are consistently stronger predictors of later adaptation than is attachment or any other single index of care or child functioning.

Of course, it is the case that aspects of parenting outside of the attachment system and after the infant period also are important in the child's development (Sroufe, Egeland, Carlson, & Collins, 2005). In addition to providing a secure base, parents provide stimulation for the child that may or may not be appropriately modulated. They provide guidance, limits, and interactive support for problem solving. Moreover, they support the child's competence in the broader world, for example, by making possible and supporting social contacts outside the home. Many relationships with those other than parents (siblings, peers, and teachers) are important as well.

Thus, we use our data on adaptation in middle childhood to illustrate four critical themes in our work. First, in general, it is not experience at any one age that provides an understanding of developmental outcomes, but the totality of the person's history. As powerful as attachment variations are in predicting certain outcomes, there is much more to development than attachment, or even all aspects of care in the first year or two of life. Second, the whole array of important relationship experiences must be considered, not just experiences with parents. Certainly, this includes relationships with siblings, peers, teachers, and other supervisory adults, as well as adults who may move in and out of the home. We assessed each of these. Third, it is not only the history of care and support that is the foundation for current functioning, but also the history of child adaptation itself. While controversy swirls around how much of individual functioning is endogenous, there is general agreement that children become increasingly active forces in their own development with age. They seek out, engage, interpret, and react to opportunities and challenges in different ways, based upon previous integrations of experience. Finally, as always, adaptation is a product of cumulative history *and* current circumstances. Current challenges and supports impact functioning and may even transform established patterns of adaptation. At the same time, the impact of new experience is modulated by expectations and capacities based on history. Fundamental change is possible in new contexts, even though history is not erased.

PLAN FOR THE CHAPTER

During the elementary years, we had broad measures of adaptation on all 180 participants, based on teacher evaluations in the school setting and formal testing of academic achievement. In addition, a subsample of 47 children participated in a series of 4-week summer camps at age 9 or 10 years. This included 39 of the children who participated in our preschool (see Chapter 4 for descriptions). The summer camps provided the highest quality, most reliable data for several reasons. First, ratings were made by highly trained counselors, with ample opportunity to observe the children in a variety of settings. Moreover, they could compare the children with each other, since all campers were project participants. (In contrast, elementary teachers generally had only one participant in their class and perhaps only one at their school.) Finally, we were able to support the counselor data with copious amounts of behavioral observation and extensive videotape recordings. Many questions could only be answered with camp data, such as what were the histories of those who became friends and how do children coordinate their friendships with the demands of group functioning? Thus, the camp data were the strength of our middle childhood social competence data. Still, classroom teachers provided data on all of our participants in the critical school setting and allowed us to corroborate many of our camp findings with the broader sample. In addition, they provided valuable data on behavior problems.

We first overview the findings from our summer camp study, with an emphasis on competence with peers. Then, we present our data for all participants on four indices of adaptation at school: (1) Emotional Health/Self-Esteem, (2) Competence with Peers, (3) Deportment, and (4) Achievement. A great deal of information was obtained during these years. Our goal is to overview this information sufficiently to convey the coherence of adaptation from early life to middle childhood, and to illustrate the developmental processes that underlie such continuity. In many cases, accessible publications can provide further detail for the interested reader. These are cited where appropriate.

THE SUMMER CAMP STUDY: CONSTRUCTING SOCIAL COMPETENCE

The middle childhood summer camp component of our project well illustrates several of the critical developmental themes outlined earlier. By filming and using multiple teams of observers every day for 4 weeks, and by using four highly trained counselors as participant observers and raters, we were able to obtain convergent validity for key constructs and highly reliable composites of outcomes. It was also possible to uncover many details regarding the social world of peers for these 47 ten-year-olds.

One of the main points illustrated by the obtained data was the importance of the cumulative history of experience and adaptation. As we describe, it was indeed the case that attachment history (and the sensitive and cooperative care that preceded it in the first year) was significantly related to major outcomes 8–10 years later (e.g., Elicker et al., 1992). Still, in most cases, both the more extensive measures of history of care across the first 3½ years (attachment history plus parenting measures between 24 and 42 months) and the history of competence across this same period (attachment plus child ratings) predicted camp outcomes notably more strongly. Usually, the latter composites accounted for twice the variance of attachment alone. Likewise, prior functioning in the preschool peer group accounted for variance over and above attachment or early care in predicting social competence. Some examples follow.

In accord with numerous later studies (Schneider, Atkinson, & Tardif, 2001), we found that attachment security was significantly related to the broadest measures of competence at camp, such as the counselor ratings and rankings of social competence, self-confidence, and emotional health/self-esteem (see Chapter 4). As an illustration of the size of these relations, the average social skills rating was 4.5 (on a 7-point scale) for those with secure histories and 3.4 for those with anxious histories, a one standard deviation difference (Sroufe, Egeland, & Carlson, 1999). The average social competence rank of those with secure histories was 6 (out of 16 children in each camp), whereas the average rank of those with anxious histories was 10, a notable difference. Specific behavioral observation measures confirmed these findings. Those with secure histories were significantly more frequently in the company of peers, and less frequently isolated or in the company of adults alone. These independent measures correlated with the counselor ratings of child social skills in the .60s. Finally, there was great convergence among multiple measures with regard to the formation of close friendships, the "hallmark" of middle childhood (Sullivan, 1953). Reciprocal nominations of "best friends" by children, counselor judgments of who were close friends, and observed association "friendship" scores all were in high agreement. The "friendship" score followed from the notion that individuals who were close friends would often be in each other's company (Ladd, 1983). Thus, one's highest proportion of time with another becomes a score. This score averaged 39% for those with secure histories, and 25% for those with anxious histories.

As impressive as these findings were, they generally pale in comparison to those based upon a broader history. For example, in correlation terms, the association between attachment and global social competence was .18 (3% of the variance). For the 12- to 42-month care composite, the comparable correlation was .39 (14% of the variance). Attachment history was more strongly related to the friendship score, as might be expected, due to the emotional closeness component. Here, number of times secure in the 12- to 18-month assessments was positively correlated with friendship ($r = .30$; 9% of the variance), an impressive finding 9 years later. However, the correlation with an early care composite was .55 (30% of the variance; Sroufe, Egeland, et al., 1999).

Similarly, when adaptation in the preschool peer group was considered along with early care, even stronger predictions resulted. Using preschool teacher ratings of social skills, the resulting multiple correlation was .62, accounting for fully 40% of the variance. In general, individual measures of preschool adaptation predicted well to later summer camp functioning. For example, ego resiliency in preschool correlated moderately (.35) with ego resiliency at summer camp (Urban, Carlson, Egeland, & Sroufe, 1991). In almost every case, preschool measures added to early care in predicting middle childhood outcomes. Thus, not only is social competence constructed on the foundation of attachment and other aspects of the history of care, but it is also based in prior experiences in the peer group. We elaborate this theme further in Chapter 9.

There was one camp variable for which the relation to attachment history was dominant. Maintaining boundaries between genders is a normative occurrence in middle childhood. Only 6% of observed interactions were with children solely of the opposite gender in our camps (Sroufe, Bennett, Englund, Urban, & Shulman, 1993). In some cultures, adults enforce separation between genders in preadolescence, perhaps by removing the boys to a separate place. But in Western, industrialized countries, children must maintain these boundaries themselves. When children interacted with members of the other gender in our study, they did so with the "protection" of same-gender partners or had some other form of "cover" (a counselor made them do it, it was inadvertent, etc.), or they disavowed the contact through name-calling or some other form of "borderwork" (Thorne, 1986). Moreover, boundary violations were followed by sanctions (teasing, ridicule, and innuendo) by members of the child's own gender (Sroufe et al., 1993). From videotape records, we were able to reliably score both boundary violations (unprotected contact) and boundary maintenance efforts. The composite of these two variables correlated strongly with other measures of social competence (r's between .37 and .53, all highly significant). Moreover, as we present in Chapter 9, they predicted both competence in the mixed-gender peer group during adolescence and certain kinds of adolescent problems

(Collins et al., 1997; Hennighausen, 1996). Such a prediction followed from our view that gender boundary maintenance is normative and functional (allowing the practice of intimacy in a safe social context) in middle childhood.

The boundary maintenance composite was strongly related to secure attachment (correlation = .48), one of the highest associations we obtained across this time span. Moreover, the correlation was not improved upon by adding cumulative care or preschool competence. We speculated that there is something special about attachment experiences with regard to establishing personal boundaries, perhaps because of the importance of physical proximity and close bodily contact in attachment formation. One other early childhood measure also predicted failure to maintain gender boundaries at camp, namely, parent–child boundary violation at 42 months. Thus, there may be a connection between having self-boundaries violated and later issues with maintaining boundaries with others, including gender boundaries. Anecdotally, children who "crowded" others (e.g., standing or walking too close, touching too often or too much) often had anxious attachment histories, including disorganized attachment, as well as parents who violated parent–child boundaries. Recall also that those preschoolers who became distressed when others were distressed had been anxiously (resistant) attached (see Chapter 7). We will return to this matter of particular areas of importance for attachment history and parent-child boundary violations in later chapters.

Finally, we found evidence for the coherence of social behavior in middle childhood in the interrelations among the various competence indices from the summer camp (Sroufe, Egeland, et al., 1999). For example, measures of self-confidence, agency and ego resiliency were correlated negatively with dependency measures and positively with measures of competence with peers (most often in the .40s). This held even when the measures were totally independent (e.g., counselor ratings on the one hand, and behavior observations on the other). Moreover, there was convergent and discriminate validity in the correlations; that is, variables were most correlated when the independent measures were of the same construct. For example, the counselor ratings of dependency correlated .69 with observed amount of counselor–child contact, and ratings of social skills correlated in the .60s with observational measures of peer effectiveness. High self-esteem, adequate emotional regulation, self-reliance, and effectiveness in the peer group all go together.

The Dynamics of Peer Competence

On the one hand, the camp data, based on a relatively small number of participants, cannot answer certain questions about the interplay of large numbers of variables. On the other hand, the richness and comprehensiveness of the observational and other data allow us to make certain suggestions regarding the dynamics of peer relationships. We were especially interested in variations in how children balanced the complexity of interacting with same- and other-gender children, functioning in groups, and maintaining close friendships. Potentially, a friendship could be a boost to group acceptance and participation, and being in groups could advance functioning in friendships through providing new venues and formats for sharing. Being able to coordinate these tasks smoothly would be an important foundation for the later, more complex networks of relationships in adolescence. We observed a large number of children who achieved balance in these tasks (Shulman, Elicker, & Sroufe, 1994). As just one example, if two friends were chosen to be on different teams in a group game, they nonetheless maintained contact through frequent interaction, compliments on each other's play, and so forth. Observation of such children inspired a new code in our scheme, "pair in group." These same children made sure they were accompanied by their friend or another companion when they interacted with members of the opposite gender. In that way, they maintained boundaries. Almost always, both members of such pairs had secure histories.

For some children, however, the stimulation and challenge of group participation could overwhelm their capacities, making it difficult for them to maintain contact with their friend. It was children with resistant histories who seemed to have such difficulties. In general, their contact with friends seemed more intermittent. We only had one friendship pair consisting of two children with avoidant histories, an interesting finding in its own right. This pair completely avoided group activities when given a choice and played, physically separated from other campers. They were each jealous of overtures by others toward their friend (see A. Freud & Dann, 1951), and on days when the friend was not in attendance, appeared "lost" and isolated (Shulman et al., 1994).

Patterns of Adaptation

Children with histories of supportive care confidently engage the social world of middle childhood, function effectively in the peer group, follow its rules, and maintain close relationships with friends. In addition, they show a sense of agency and confidence by setting goals high and tackling tasks that were challenging. From countless possible examples, we provide a sampling to illustrate these characteristics (Sroufe, Egeland, et al., 1999). For example, a group of secure boys designed a split-level clubhouse structure and actually built it, to the amazement of adult supervisors. (It remained in use by the University nursery school for more than a year.) A group of girls decided that they should set up a store to sell their macramé creations, working hard both at home and at camp to generate adequate inventory. This real-world competence is the stuff of middle childhood, and those with secure histories were remarkable. As another example, we set up a series of challenging tasks (e.g., getting over hurdles) and filmed groups of children who had different histories (not known to those filming or coding) engaging in them. Those with secure histories organized themselves in more effective ways, cooperated well, avoided scapegoating, and performed dramatically better. Finally, in circle meetings, children with histories of secure attachment most often sat next to friends. Those with anxious histories sat next to counselors, members of the opposite gender, random children, and friends in approximately equal proportion, and those with avoidant histories most frequently sat by themselves, apart from the group (Elicker et al., 1992; Shulman et al., 1994).

These descriptions suggest patterning in the organization of social behavior of children with differing attachment histories. As in the preschool (see Chapter 7), there were highly significant overall differences in dependency between children with secure versus those with anxious attachment histories (Urban et al., 1991). This was true both with regard to counselor ratings of dependency and direct observation of the total amount of adult–child contact. Moreover, on these global measures of dependency, there were no differences between children with avoidant and resistant histories. However, as hypothesized, and in corroboration of the preschool findings, there were differences in how dependency was expressed in these two groups. For example, more of the contact was initiated by the adults for those with avoidant histories compared to those with resistant histories. However, for one specific category of adult contact ("support giving"), the resistant group was significantly higher. Thus, the pattern of the avoidant group being indirect in contact seeking and the resistant group receiving undue nurturance from adults was repeated at this age. As happened in the preschool, adults often treated children in accordance with the histories they brought forward.

We also replicated the preschool findings with regard to descriptions based on "most characteristic" and "least characteristic" Q-sort items (see Chapters 4 and 7). When given these descriptions for each child, judges, blind to history, were able to discriminate significantly between those with avoidant and resistant histories, with 19 of 23 children accurately judged. Given the likelihood of change, this is remarkable concordance. It suggests that there is often at least some residual of the earlier prototype organization. When we intercorrelated the entire Q-sort of each child with every other child, we also found that for the secure and resistant groups, the strongest correlations were most likely to be with another child of the same history. This was not significant for the avoidant group.

Thus, we continued to find some evidence for patterning in individual adaptation in middle childhood, and we found substantial evidence for the predictability of social competence from early in life. We turn now to the data on our total sample in the elementary school setting, both to corroborate the findings we have discussed and to illustrate certain themes that require the larger sample. In particular, we use these data to illustrate the role of contextual factors as contributors to development, beyond the role of early parenting.

COMPETENCE IN THE ELEMENTARY SCHOOL SETTING

Broadband Competence Measures

The most integrative measures of adaptation available for the whole sample were the two rankings made by teachers (see Chapter 4 and Appendix E). The first, Emotional Health/Self-Esteem, referred the teacher to the degree to which the child was confident, curious, self-assured, engaging, and eager for new experiences and challenges. This measure tapped the child's overall quality of adaptation in the school setting. The second, Competence with Peers, captured the popularity, social skills, sociability, and leadership qualities of the child. Thus, this ranking captured in a broad way the child's competence with peers, a critical issue at this time. Moreover, Competence with Peers is an integrative construct, calling upon the child's cognitive abilities, social capacities, and regulatory skills. It also draws upon the child's entire developmental history. By collapsing across grades, these two scale scores provided a summary of the child's competence as evaluated by teachers in the school arena.

All major measures of early care—cooperation and sensitivity at 6 months, attachment security at 12–18 months, Experience in the Session at 24 and 42 months, early physical abuse, and the Caldwell HOME scale of environmental stimulation and responsiveness at 30 months— were related positively to these two global measures of competence grade-by-grade in elementary school (e.g., Elicker et al., 1992; Urban et al., 1991). Although modest in size, 75% of the correlations were significant. Moreover, these relations likely are underestimates of true values because they are not corrected for attenuation (unreliability).

Not surprisingly, and in accord with our developmental construction view, much more impressive correlations were obtained when we combined the early care measures and when we collapsed measures across grades. These analyses were done for this book and have not been published previously. For example, when we combined the 6-month sensitivity and cooperation ratings, or when we combined the 24- to 42-

month measures of care and related these composites to the composited grades 1–3 emotional health and peer competence rankings, the correlations became moderate (around .30). A single composite of all early care measures in the first 42 months yielded correlations of .44 and .41, respectively, with our two outcomes. Such singular correlations do not need to be corrected for chance and reflect a degree of continuity from early care to the school years.

These two global competence outcomes may also be used to illustrate the theme of development as the product of history *and* ongoing support and context. We did this by carrying out regression analyses in predicting grades 1–3 outcomes. In the first analysis, we entered a composite measure of 6-month cooperation/sensitivity and attachment security in the first step. This would be a very early care composite. We next entered the grade 1 HOME Scale as a measure of contemporary care. Finally, we entered caregiver life stress and support for the caregiver during the early school years. Table 8.1 shows the results. Early care pre-

TABLE 8.1. Summary of Hierarchical Regression Analysis Predicting Emotional Health and Peer Competence from Infant Experience, Home Organization, and Maternal Life Stress and Support (Grades 1–3, N = 171)

Variable	Model 1			Model 2			Model 3		
	B	SE	β	B	SE	β	B	SE	β
Emotional health									
Infant experience	7.87	2.16	.27***	5.70	2.30	.19*	5.76	2.25	.20*
HOME score				.40	.15	.21	.27	.17	.14
Life stress							−5.10	2.39	−.17*
Maternal support							1.54	2.02	.07
R^2 change	.07			.04			.04		
F for change in R^2	12.90***			7.09			3.73**		
R	.27***			.33***			.38***		
Peer competence									
Infant experience	7.92	2.16	.27***	6.42	2.30	.22**	5.76	2.25	.20*
HOME score				.28	.15	.14	.14	.17	.07
Life stress							−6.38	2.37	−.22**
Maternal support							1.16	2.00	.05
R^2 change	.07			.02			.05		
F for change in R^2	13.44***			3.40			5.18**		
R	.27***			.30***			.38***		

Note. Infant experience (6–18 months); HOME store (grade 1); life stress (grades 1–3); maternal emotional support (grades 1–3).
*$p < .05$; **$p < .01$; ***$p < .001$.

TABLE 8.2. Summary of Hierarchical Regression Analysis Predicting Emotional Health and Peer Competence from Early Experience, 42-Month Relationship Experience, Home Organization, and Maternal Life Stress and Support (Grades 1–3, N = 163)

	Model 1			Model 2			Model 3		
Variable	B	SE	β	B	SE	β	B	SE	β
Emotional health									
Early experience	11.05	2.58	.33***	8.37	2.84	.25**	7.35	2.83	.22*
Relationship experience	1.53	.60	.20*	1.37	.60	.18*	1.38	.59	.18*
HOME score				.36	.17	.18*	.25	.18	.13
Life stress							−4.41	2.34	−.15
Maternal support							1.62	1.99	.07
R^2 change	.19			.02			.03		
F for change in R^2	18.95***			4.67*			3.11*		
R	.44***			.47***			.50***		
Peer competence									
Early experience	10.04	2.55	.33***	8.89	2.81	.27**	7.62	2.78	.23**
Relationship experience	1.15	.59	.15*	1.02	.59	.13	1.07	.58	.14
HOME score				.28	.16	.14	.18	.17	.09
Life stress							−6.16	2.26	−.21**
Maternal support							.80	1.95	.04
R^2 change	.17			.01			.05		
F for change in R^2	16.34***			2.81			4.96**		
R	.41***			.43***			.48***		

Note. Early experience composite (6–30 months); relationship experience (42 months); HOME store (grade 1); life stress (grades 1–3); maternal emotional support (grades 1–3).
*p < .05; **p < .01; ***p < .001.

dicted both emotional health and peer competence, but even with early care taken into account, the Grade 1 HOME scores and the caregiver stress–support variable accounted for additional significant variance. In another analysis (Table 8.2), we used a broader early care index and got similar results and an even more powerful overall prediction (R = .50). Competence in elementary school is a product of early care, later care, *and* the current family supports and challenges.

Researchers always wonder whether results such as those above are due simply to variations in IQ. We conducted a series of regressions to control for differences in early intellectual development using WIPPSI scores. This is a harsh test because early care predicts IQ, which is thus not independent of care. Nonetheless, after controlling for IQ, history of care and caregiver stress and support still significantly contributed in predicting emotional health and peer competence (Table 8.3). This also was true when mother's IQ was controlled. Thus, our psychosocial measures do not predict adjustment at school simply because they are correlated with IQ.

Early childhood competence, which we argue can be properly assessed by age 42 months, produced an array of results quite parallel to those for early history of care. This was especially true for ratings of the child with the mother present in the teaching tasks. Each of the child ratings in the 42-month teaching tasks correlated significantly with grade school emotional health and peer competence, in each case .23 or more. Child compliance and child persistence (two variables with high relevance for school) yielded stronger correlations (from .30 to .38).

Deportment at School

Later, we devote an entire chapter to the origins and course of various forms of psychopathology. However, since certain kinds of behavior problems and deportment issues are so critical for school functioning and are a key manifestation of competence during the school years, we overview some general findings here. The presentation is parallel to that for emotional health and peer competence just discussed.

The primary measure of deportment problems we used was the Child Behavior Checklist—Teacher Report Form (CBCL-TRF) of Achenbach and Edelbrock (1986). The CBCL yields a number of scales, as well as summaries of externalizing, internalizing, and total behavior problems. To reduce the number of analyses, we will focus on the total score here, and we again collapse measures across grades. We did not include parental reports of problem behavior in these analyses, since parents were the source of our life stress and social support data. In the analyses below, the observation-based measures of care, the child tests, the interview-based stress and support data, and the teacher reports are all independent.

As was true for the emotional health and peer competence outcomes, the more history of care we cumulated, the stronger the prediction became (see Table 8.4). Measures of care in infancy, and during the toddler and preschool years, were significantly related to behavior problems in grades 1–3, especially when combined. Early care significantly predicted behavior problems, even after controlling for child IQ on the WIPPSI.

Major contextual variables also were significantly related to total behavior problems in elementary school (e.g., Jimerson, Egeland, & Teo, 1999; Renken, Egeland, Marvinney, Sroufe, & Mangelsdorf, 1989).

TABLE 8.3. Summary of Hierarchical Regression Analysis Predicting Emotional Health and Peer Competence from WIPPSI, Early Experience, 42-Month Relationship Experience, Home Organization, and Maternal Life Stress and Support (Grades 1–3, $N = 163$)

Variable	Model 1			Model 2			Model 3			Model 4		
	B	SE	β	B	SE	β	B	SE	β	B	SE	β
Emotional health												
WIPPSI	1.20	.20	.42***	.77	.23	.27***	.75	.23	.26***	.79	.23	.28***
Relationship composite				10.16	2.97	.28***	7.11	3.22	.20*	5.57	3.20	.15
HOME score							.37	.16	.18*	.27	.17	.13
Life stress										−5.16	2.22	−.18*
Maternal support										1.49	1.89	.07
R^2 change	.18			.06			.03			.04		
F for change in R^2	34.64***			11.71***			5.25*			4.33*		
R	.42***			.49***			.51***			.55***		
Peer competence												
WIPPSI	.97	.20	.35**	.05	.23	.19*	.51	.23	.19*	.56	.22	.20*
Relationship composite				10.61	2.96	.30***	8.24	3.23	.24*	6.42	3.17	.18*
HOME score							.29	.16	.15	.17	.17	.09
Life stress										−6.64	2.20	−.23**
Maternal support										1.13	1.88	.05
R^2 change	.13			.07			.02			.06		
F for change in R^2	22.81***			12.85***			3.15			6.33**		
R	.35***			.44***			.46***			.52***		

Note. WIPPSI; Relationship experience composite (6–42 months); HOME store (grade 1); life stress (grades 1–3); maternal emotional support (grades 1–3).
*$p < .05$; **$p < .01$; ***$p < .001$.

These included the grade 1 HOME score, total life stress, relationship support for the mother, parental involvement at school ($r = -.40$), and SES, all assessed in grades 1–3. It should be pointed out that since all of our participants were living in poverty at the time of the child's birth, the SES range is constricted. In general, SES is known to be a powerful predictor of behavior problems and school performance. As always, when contemporary measures of care and the surrounding context were combined with history of care, predictions of behavior problems were increased (see Table 8.4).

Child maltreatment and witnessing parental violence also have proven to be important in our work for predicting externalizing problems for boys in the elementary years (e.g., Erickson et al., 1989; Yates, Dodds, Sroufe, & Egeland, 2003). In recent analyses, neither IQ nor SES was predictive, but child physical abuse accounted for 14% of the variance ($r = .38$). Even with physical abuse controlled, witnessing violence in the home at this time accounted for an additional 6%, another highly significant finding. The impact of witnessing violence is discussed further in Chapter 9.

In one of our early reports, we focused in particular on aggression in grades 1–3 (Renken et al., 1989). In this analysis, history of care included physical abuse and maternal hostility at 42 months, because of strong links in the literature between such variables and aggression. The hostility–abuse composite was significantly related to aggression for boys ($r = .44$). Even so, the prediction was improved when we included measures of life stress, support for the parent, and increases in economic

TABLE 8.4. Summary of Hierarchical Regression Analysis for Variables Predicting Behavior Problems (Grades 1–3, $N = 161$)

Variable	Model 1			Model 2			Model 3		
	B	SE	β	B	SE	β	B	SE	β
Early experience	−2.37	1.04	−.19[*]	−1.36	1.14	−.11	−.96	1.14	−.08
Relationship experience	−.62	.24	−.21[*]	−.56	.24	−.19[*]	−.57	.24	−.19[*]
HOME score				−.14	.07	−.18[*]	−.11	.07	.14
Life stress							2.01	.94	.18[*]
Maternal support							−.29	.80	−.36
R^2 change	.11			.02			.03		
F for change in R^2	9.32[***]			4.19[*]			3.06[*]		
R	.33[***]			.36[***]			.40[***]		

Note. Early experience composite (6–30 months); relationship experience (42 months); HOME store (grade 1); life stress (grades 1–3); maternal emotional support (grades 1–3).
[*]$p < .05$; [**]$p < .01$; [***]$p < .001$.

hardship (r = .58, a highly significant increase in variance explained). In all, it is clear that contextual factors, as well as history of maltreatment and unsupportive care, are of great importance.

Finally, earlier low child competence, especially at 42 months, also predicted behavior problem measures in elementary school (Egeland, Kalkoske, Gottesman, & Erickson, 1990). An integrative early child incompetence measure correlated moderately with grade 1–3 total problems. It also correlated significantly with both externalizing and internalizing scores. However, none of these correlations remained significant after controlling for WIPPSI IQ. Thus, during the preschool period, IQ and child competence may well be part of the same construct.

Of course, one of the strongest predictors of behavior problems in elementary school was a history of behavior problems in the preschool years. There was notable stability across this time period (r's in the .40s). Those with clear, early behavior problems were more than twice as likely to be troubled in elementary school and less than half as likely to be competent as those without a history of problems (Egeland et al., 1990). Problem behavior in preschool also predicted problems with peers and 10-point lower average achievement scores on the Peabody Individual Achievement Test (PIAT).

Continuity and Discontinuity in Behavioral Problems

Data on change (increases and decreases) in behavior problems from preschool to elementary school were very useful for illustrating the ongoing role for context. Some children showed dramatically fewer problems at the later age. This "exceptions" group was marked by a more supportive environment for the child at school entry (the HOME scales), lower parental life stress during the elementary years, and lower maternal depression in first and second grades (Egeland et al., 1990). In a similar way, those whose problems increased between preschool and elementary school had lower HOME support scores, higher life stress, and high and increasing maternal depression. Level of maternal depression seemed to affect directly the quality of care the mother provided and to affect indirectly the quality and organization of the home environment. Both of these then were related to child functioning. Such relations suggest the importance of intervention to improve family circumstances and parental well-being (see Chapter 13).

School Performance

The risk status of our sample was clearly confirmed by our school performance data (Egeland & Abery, 1991). In each of the first three

grades, approximately half of the students were referred for special educational services or continued services from the preceding year. By third
grade, 20% had failed to pass a grade. At the same time, we documented
a substantial range of school performance.

Performing well in school is a complicated business. It involves
more than native intelligence. Our work has underscored the importance
of psychosocial factors, including peer relationships and early and ongoing support from parents. The data we have obtained on achievement
clearly illustrate the theme of cumulative history and the interplay between parental care and child competence over time (Englund, Luckner,
Whaley, & Egeland, in press; Teo, Carlson, Mathieu, Egeland, & Sroufe,
1996).

Both caregiver sensitivity and cooperation at 6 months and infant
attachment security were related to math and reading performance
across the school years (e.g., Egeland, Pianta, & O'Brien, 1993; Mathieu,
1990). For example, the correlation of the early caregiver sensitivity
composite with combined grade 1–6 achievement was .41. A cumulative
early history variable yielded correlations in the .40s, grade by grade,
and family life stress during the school years added to these predictions
(e.g., Egeland & Sroufe, 1986). These findings remained significant after
taking IQ into account.

IQ measured in preschool correlated in the .40s with elementary
school tests of achievement, while IQ assessed in grade 3 yielded correlations in the .60s; yet attachment and other early care measures do not
predict achievement because of a relation with IQ. In fact, attachment
security is not significantly related to WISC IQ in third grade. So why
are secure attachment and other measures of early care related to reading and math ability in school? We argue that these links are indirect,
through their impact on attitudes and motivation concerning school and
the capacity for positive social relationships. The central outcomes of attachment security and early supportive care are a basic sense of social
connection, positive expectations concerning self and others, and the capacity for self-regulation, but these can have wide-ranging implications
for functioning.

In any case, school achievement was forecast long before school entry, and we report this to be the case for later school outcomes as well
(Chapters 9 and 10). Furthermore, quality of the home environment at
school entry (total HOME score at age 6) consistently predicted achievement scores, as did measures of peer competence and adjustment in the
school setting itself (Teo et al., 1996).

In another analysis, we focused on parental expectations for achievement assessed during the school years and parental involvement at
school, as rated by teachers, as well as the quality of parental instruction

in the teaching tasks at 42 months (Englund et al., in press). We used teacher ratings of actual classroom performance as the outcome.

We found that all three parental variables were consistently related to classroom performance. Positive parental expectations regarding achievement and parent involvement with school were moderately related to each other. When these two measures were combined and averaged across the school years, they yielded a strong correlation with classroom performance. Moreover, this composite measure predicted achievement in the third grade after controlling for earlier achievement. Thus, ongoing parenting and the context of care, not just early care, are relevant to competence in the school setting.

Quality of parental instruction in the 42-month teaching tasks remained significant even after controlling for IQ. Moreover, it predicted IQ (WIPPSI) itself ($r = .46$), and path analysis revealed that it had an indirect effect on school performance through IQ. This suggests both that achievement is based on more than IQ, and that IQ is not simply an endogenous variable. In other analyses, we showed that early family stress predicted IQ, with boys with high-stress mothers being three-fourths of a standard deviation lower than boys whose mothers experienced low stress (Egeland & Sroufe, 1986). We also predicted change in IQ from preschool to elementary school as a result of both quality of care during the preschool years and social support available to the mother across these years (Pianta & Egeland, 1994).

In our study, we also systematically examined predictors of change in achievement test performance over time (Jimerson et al., 1999). Some students, for example, were achieving at a higher level in sixth grade than would have been predicted based on their trajectory in grades 1–3. Three factors were clearly related to such changes: (1) the quality of the HOME at school entry, (2) parental involvement at school, and (3) SES. SES accounted for 5% of the variance after every other variable, including earlier achievement, had been entered into the equation. It is a very powerful contextual factor (see also Sameroff, 2000).

Finally, we have found that psychosocial variables are important for placement in special education. The 42-month teaching variables, both ratings of maternal behavior and child functioning, were especially strong, rivaling and adding to IQ and achievement test scores as predictors of special services (see, e.g., Pianta, Erickson, Wagner, Kreutzer, & Egeland, 1990, for more detail).

The Transition to School

We have emphasized developmental transitions in our theorizing and in our assessments on this project. Transitions often tax the organizational capacities of the child and, in doing so, maximize individual variation and predictive relationships over time (Waters & Sroufe, 1983). The transition to the formal school setting is a major challenge for children in Western culture, and it certainly proved to be so for the children in our study.

First grade is generally the onset of full-time schooling and the beginning of more formal academic demands. Not surprisingly, it was a difficult year for many of our participants. It was interesting to note that measures of early care and prior child adaptation often predicted more strongly to grade 1 than to grades 1–3 or 1–6 combined, despite the fact that the latter, based on psychometric principles, should be more reliable. Although the differences in the correlations generally were not significant, almost every major measure of early care, and every combination of measures, predicted grade 1 more strongly. For example, caregiver intrusiveness at 6 months predicted a one standard deviation difference in achievement for boys in grade 1 (Egeland et al., 1993).

Child ratings at each age predicted first-grade achievement strongly as well, with child behavior in the 42-month teaching tasks being the strongest (see Table 8.5). Both caregiver life stress and relationship support in the early years also predicted well to grade 1 emotional health and peer competence, and when these were combined with the early care or early competence measures, we obtained correlations in the .50s. We interpret this set of findings as indicating that this transition to school amplified the patterning in individual child adaptation.

Kindergarten, of course, also is a transition by some criteria, although in these days of widespread day care and preschool, it may not

TABLE 8.5. Correlations between Early Adaptation Variables, Context, and Socioemotional Functioning in Middle Childhood (N = 170–191)

Variable	Social competence		Emotional health		Behavior problems	
	Grade 1	Grades 1–3	Grade 1	Grades 1–3	Grade 1	Grades 1–3
Teach Task (42 months)						
Compliance	.38***	.29***	.40***	.33***	−.40***	−.36***
Persistence	.36***	.30***	.46***	.38***	−.37***	−.33***
Enthusiasm	.30***	.24***	.36***	.29***	−.30***	−.23**
Experience in the Session	.25***	.22**	.31***	.26***	−.36***	−.27***
Maternal life stress (12–54 months)	−.24***	−.23**	−.26***	−.24***	.17*	.18*
Maternal support (12–54 months)	.27***	.25***	.25***	.23**	−.27***	−.27***

$^*p < .05$; $^{**}p < .01$; $^{***}p < .001$.

be as dramatic a transition as that represented by first grade. Nonetheless, we again found strong predictability to kindergarten outcomes, especially from 42-month child behavior. Individual behavior in the Barrier Box situation, which often did not significantly predict outcomes for grades 1–3, was consistently related to kindergarten outcomes (Ashley, 1987). Moreover, child functioning with the parent in the teaching tasks strongly discriminated among children with and without difficulties in kindergarten, based on emotional health, peer competence, and total behavior problems indices.

In general, we found that children with a history of maltreatment began school already at a disadvantage. This was especially the case for our neglect group (see Chapters 4 and 5). These children entered school with poor language skills and a lack of school-relevant competencies, such as the ability to follow directions, to work independently, and to be persistent (Egeland, 1988; Erickson, Egeland, et al., 1989; see Chapter 7). Early neglect predicted achievement problems throughout the school years, even controlling for the consequences of SES.

Finally, caregiver intrusiveness, *measured at 6 months of age*, was strongly related to inattentiveness and hyperactivity at school entry (Egeland, Pianta, & O'Brien, 1993). As we discuss further in Chapters 9, 10, and 12, this set of problems was related not only to later clinical problems but also to academic success.

THE DEVELOPMENTAL PROCESS

Later, we devote an entire chapter to issues of developmental process, that is, we discuss the dynamic way in which myriad influences, historical and contemporary, work together to shape individual adaptation over time. Here, we introduce three topics that we pursue in depth later. They are well illustrated by findings from middle childhood.

The Ongoing Interplay of Multiple Influences: Historical and Contemporary Factors, Risk and Protection, Assets and Liabilities

We have been emphasizing that history alone does not determine later functioning; rather, later experience and later context also contribute to development. At times, such later influences even seem to alter a previously established course, as in the data just presented on behavior problems and achievement. Life stress, for example, has clear relevance for these outcomes and routinely adds to predictions made from history alone.

However, these later influences do not occur in a vacuum. The impact of later adversity in part depends on prior history. In a number of analyses, we have explored factors that protect individuals from the consequences of stress; that is, some individuals in the face of high stress do not show low achievement or an elevation in behavior problems, and such discordances are predictable. As it turns out, chief among the array of protective factors is a history of supportive care and of early competence (see Nachmias, Gunnar, Mangelsdorf, Parritz, & Buss, 1996).

In one study, we found that children experiencing high stress during the early elementary school years, but who nonetheless were functioning well at that time, were distinguished by a combination of secure attachment at 12–18 months, plus adequate functioning in the 24-month tool problems situation and the Barrier Box situation at 42 months (Egeland & Kreutzer, 1991). Both boys and girls with such positive histories demonstrated greater competence with peers in elementary school than did children in high-stress families who did not have positive histories. In addition, boys protected by a positive history were dramatically less likely to show externalizing problems in the face of high stress. Likewise, in another analysis, responsive care at age 6 (HOME scores) was a protective factor vis-à-vis stress, as was caregiver relationship stability (Pianta, Egeland, et al., 1990). In other words, high stress experienced by a family did not necessarily increase child behavior problems, if the parent had adequate support and was able to provide stable support for the child.

Established child competence itself also served as protection from the influences of high stress (Pianta, Egeland, et al., 1990). Boys who functioned in a competent manner in the 42-month mother–child teaching tasks (i.e., were compliant, persistent, and positive) and showed more advanced language ability at that time were less impacted by later stress. IQ per se was not protective for boys, but it, as well as language ability, was protective for girls.

For girls, maternal characteristics, such as education level, IQ, and personality characteristics, also were important. Having a mother who portrayed competence and confidence has repeatedly proven to be an important feature in the development of *girls* in our study (Sroufe & Egeland, 1991). Apparently, having a mother who is a positive reference point is critical. (We discuss the impact of men and fathers on boys, in particular, in Chapter 9.)

Indirect Effects: Attachment, Peers, and Siblings

Another feature of the developmental process is the dynamic way in which competence is constructed. At times, certain aspects of care or competence lead to a process or way of functioning that itself has implications for further development. These are often referred to as *indirect effects*; that is, the initial feature had its impact on a later outcome by creating favorable intermediate conditions.

Such an effect already has been implied in our previous discussion of attachment and preschool peer experiences. Competence with peers in preschool was a reliable predictor of summer camp social competence outcomes. Had our study begun in preschool, one might have come to see such experiences as causal in a simple way. However, preschool competence itself was predicted by infant attachment security and other aspects of earlier care, which, in turn, were predicted by even earlier caregiver sensitivity. A more appropriate view of the construction of social competence begins in infancy. Certain attitudes, expectations, and regulatory capacities are acquired in the first years. These are foundations for early peer encounters, which then provide additional foundation for competence with peers in middle childhood. It is complicated, because for some aspects of peer competence in elementary school (e.g., "friendship," gender boundary maintenance), attachment continues to predict, after preschool experience is taken into account, or predicts outcomes even more powerfully than preschool measures. Sometimes, attachment history is no longer a significant predictor; that is, all of its predictive power is indirect through its impact on preschool functioning. We discuss such complexities further in Chapters 9 and 10 (see also Sroufe et al., 2005).

Our data on sibling relationships provide another example. Secure early relationships with parents are important for the development of healthy sibling relationships; yet relationships with siblings are important in their own right. Our theoretical perspective begins with the notion that there are unique developmental functions for relationships with siblings (Sroufe et al., 1992). Sibling relationships are among the most enduring relationships. At the same time, these relationships can be thought of as hybrids, like and yet unlike both parent–child and peer relationships. There are often strong emotional features, as with relationships with parents, yet in most cases, the age gap more closely approximates that with peers. Still, except for twins, there is an age difference. Sibling relationships are a perfect format for learning to stay involved in the face of emotional conflict (one cannot just get a new sibling or discard an old one) and to practice leadership and following.

Available resources enabled us to study the first 75 sibling relationships that were formed by our participants. In an initial study, we found that in 53% of the cases, the second sibling had the same attachment classification with the caregiver as had the first (Ward, Vaughn, & Robb, 1988). With the three-category Ainsworth system, this is a significant finding, but, as can be seen, there also was substantial discordance. We next set out to examine the sibling relationships themselves.

Previous studies often simply drew variables from peer studies (e.g., positive and negative affect) to investigate siblings. Given our functional developmental view, we emphasized more dynamic constructs that were largely unique to this relationship (Marvinney, 1988). We expected a mix of feelings in a well-functioning sibling relationship. We expected bickering, with the older child trying to boss the younger, and the younger child complaining. In brief, we assessed the degree to which the relationship exhibited appropriate *asymmetry*, with the older child clearly in the leadership role, but without being exploitative. Based in our relational view (Sroufe & Fleeson, 1986), we would argue that both members of the pair learn a great deal about both roles from such a relationship.

We videotaped 30 of the sibling pairs in a laboratory setting when the older child was 7 or 8 years old and the younger sibling was at least 5. We used a set of cooperation and competition tasks designed by Millard Madsen (1971). For example, in one task, siblings had to control a stylus by separate strings that they each controlled. They could only be maximally successful by cooperating, thereby getting to each person's goal. Since we were scoring very difficult constructs (asymmetry, role violations), we used pairs of coders who conferenced their ratings. Reliability was established by using an independent pair of coders for a subset of the cases.

We found that the "appropriately asymmetrical" sibling pairs were indeed predicted by histories of secure attachment (Marvinney, 1988). Moreover, for first-borns, the asymmetry score predicted subsequent teacher rankings of peer competence at school ($r = .46$, $p < .05$). We think this finding is especially important, because it suggests that relationships with siblings, as well as those with parents, contribute to the development of peer competence. The sample size was not large enough to test formally the pathway from attachment through siblings to peers, but this would be an important task for future research. We expect that siblings made unique contributions (see also DeHart, 1999; Dunn & Kendrick, 1982).

A developmental scientist would not ask the question (cf. Harris, 1998), "Are parents or peers or siblings more important for the child's development?" In light of the findings discussed earlier, it is obvious that all three sets of relationships are important. Moreover, the contribution of peers and siblings to social competence in no way trivializes the importance of parents; rather, it highlights their role in a complex developmental process (Sroufe et al., 2005).

Internalizing and Carrying Forward Experience

Vygotsky (1978) argued that cognitive developmental capacities may first be seen in relationships before becoming capacities of children. We believe that this also applies to personality organization (e.g., Sander, 1975; see also Chapter 2, this volume). Primary relationship patterns (rooted in parental experience and personality) are prototypes for emerging self-organization. This has been the thrust of our argument in seeking meaningful patterns of adaptation as outcomes of infant attachment relationship groups. But there are other examples as well.

One interesting example for us was the unfolding of the impact of a chaotic relationship history that some of our mothers had with the men in their lives (Pianta, Hyatt, & Egeland, 1986). This proved to be a powerful variable, but its influence was not immediately obvious. In our 24-month tool problems assessment, this variable was related to the mothers' behavior (lower emotional support and poorer quality of assistance), but it did *not* predict child behavior. By age 42 months, child behavior (as well as maternal behavior) was predicted, but only in the dyadic teaching tasks situation. Even at this age, when the child worked on the Barrier Box, without the mother present, there was no demonstrable impact of maternal chaotic relationships on the child. However, by grade 1, children from families with a history of such instability were rated by teachers as having dramatically more social, emotional, and behavioral problems than children whose mothers had stable relationships.

Similarly, we would argue that the data on the link between secure attachment and self-esteem, self-confidence, and agency in our preschool (see Chapter 7) and in our summer camps in middle childhood are in accord with the internalization proposition. That attachment relationship history is internalized is also suggested by our data on the total sample using the Harter Perceived Competence and Acceptance Scale (Harter, 1979), completed by the elementary school teachers. These measures of self-development showed a dramatic difference between children with avoidant attachment histories and the other attachment groups (Loewen, 2004). The chronic emotional unavailability and rejection that underlies the formation of avoidant attachment does not provide a solid foundation for forming strong self-attitudes (see Kim & Cicchetti, 2004).

Finally, we specifically attempted to assess internalization of experience through measures of representation, such as family drawings, projective tests, stories, and other narratives. For example, when asked to draw family pictures, third-grade children who had histories of secure attachment more often drew figures that were well grounded and centered on the page (Fury et al., 1997). Their pictures showed connection among family members, positive affect, and appropriate placement and spacing of figures. The self was well proportioned, complete, individuated, and in connection with others. Those with avoidant histories tended to draw people with stiff, rigid postures, missing parts, lack of individuation, and distance between them. The drawings of those with resistant histories reflected vulnerability (e.g., excessively small self). Raters, blind to history, significantly discriminated among drawings by all four attachment groups (including disorganized), using either global judgments or more formal scoring of groups of indicators, based on a system first developed by Kaplan and Main (1986; Main et al., 1985). Such distinctions were not accounted for by differences in IQ.

Furthermore, in sentence completions, stories, and other narratives, children with secure histories more often portrayed a sense of confidence about the availability and responsiveness of parents and peers, and about their own self-worth and social competence (Carlson et al., 2004). For example, those with avoidant histories often told stories in response to Thematic Apperception Test (TAT) pictures that reflected less positive engagement and more negative expectations, including anger, between characters (McCrone, Egeland, Kalkoske, & Carlson, 1994). Likewise, sentence completions conveyed differences in expectations based on attachment history (Ramirez, Carlson, Gest, & Egeland, 1991). Completing the sentence stem, "My mother always . . ." with "yells at me" conveys a very different set of expectations than "likes to do things with me." Likewise, completing "Other kids . . ." with "are fun to be with," conveys a very different viewpoint concerning self and other than does "always pick on me." When summary scales from both procedures were combined, they correlated moderately with a summary attachment history variable. Moreover, each was related to contemporary measures of peer competence. When combined, the correlation with social competence at summer camp was very strong (.66).

We have much more to say about the internalization of experience and representation in Chapter 11 on the process of development. Following Bowlby, it has been our hypothesis throughout this project that representation is the carrier of experience, but at the same time, later experience can alter representations. Thus, there is an ongoing interplay between functioning in the world (and the potential for new experiences this engenders) and representations based on past experience.

CONCLUSION

Ten-year-old children have been preparing their entire lives for the competence they show now. Their reasoning skills are supported by years of wrestling with cognitive problems in their real and fantasy worlds. Their impressive agency is underpinned by secure-base exploration in infancy and emotionally supported and guided curiosity in the preschool years, and by recognition and lauding of their accomplishments by significant others at every point. Finally, effectiveness in the organized peer group and the capacity for loyal friendships build upon foundations of struggle and accomplishment in preschool peer interactions, and upon the parental support for interpersonal connection and emotional regulation in the early years. Development is a logical, coherent process.

The coherence of development is amply demonstrated in our middle childhood data. Within the age period, the characteristics of individuals are arrayed in meaningful ways. This was illustrated in our section on the dynamics of peer competence and is manifested in the high intercorrelations among variables at the summer camp. Children who were rated high on agency and ego resiliency, for example, more often sustain close friendships, more often function effectively in the group, and less often are isolated.

Development also is coherent over time. When measures are carefully assembled and highly reliable (as in our camp data), when measures are combined, when both relationships with parents and others are considered, and when both history and current context are taken into account, prediction of individual variation can be substantial (with multiple R reaching .60 and beyond). Individual adaptation is constructed in the context of care, which itself takes place in a broader context of supports and challenges. Even when individual measures of early care are used and correlations are small, we argue that they are nonetheless theoretically meaningful; that is, they follow from the perspective that the organization of individual behavior is based upon the relationship organization that preceded it.

We have been impressed over the years with the consistency of our findings. Correlations often may be small, and sometimes they are not significant. However, they are virtually never in the "wrong direction." History of physical abuse, at the group level, is never related to positive outcomes. A history of secure attachment is virtually never related to lower competence in our data. This is not to say that no individuals with negative histories later thrive, or that children with early secure attachments never have problems later. Of course they do. Our point is, however, that such change too is lawful. Reasons for such changes, again at the group level, can be found in other early supports, later support, and/or changes in the challenges being faced. This is what we mean by the coherence of development.

CHAPTER 9

Adaptation in Adolescence
Autonomy with Connectedness

INTERVIEWER: What did you think about Thomas?

SERENA (*age 15*): Well, he was kind of obnoxious and always doing rude things . . . but he's one of us, so we accepted him.

INTERVIEWER: And Veronica?

SERENA: You see she was kind of upset a lot. See, she liked Henry and he kinda liked her. But he *has* a girlfriend and. . . . Well, you know Lena? She's his girlfriend's cousin and she would tell if he did anything, so he's not gonna, so that's why Veronica was mad.

These vignettes reveal some of the emerging complexity of thought and personhood of adolescence, as well as the capacity for more complex relationships within a peer network. As sophisticated as Serena was at age 11 (see the opening vignette for Chapter 8), she has a much more elaborated understanding of social relationships at 15. During adolescence, young people become able to see inconsistencies in themselves and others, can reflect on multiple possibilities (including how things *could be*, in addition to how they are), and can think about the future in sophisticated ways. There are new ways of thinking, a new impetus toward autonomy, and notable physical changes at this time.

These dramatic changes bring with them important opportunities for psychological growth, but they also can bring about both crises within the young person and conflicts with parents and others. The changes of adolescence can lead to important advances in relationships and to a new level of self-integration later in the period (Anderson, 1999). For many young people, this is a period of personal consolidation and social expansion. It can be a period of discovery, commitment to social ideals, and intimacy in relationships. Likewise, for some young people, conflicts with parents are short-lived and are followed by a new alignment. Struggles with inconsistencies in the self give way to a more complex integration and a pulling together of past and present, in anticipation of the future (Erikson's [1950/1963] sense of identity). For others, on the other hand, it is a period of significant troubles. It is the case that more children have problems, and more serious problems, during adolescence than during middle childhood. Such difficulties are most common early in adolescence (see Collins & Steinberg, in press, for a review).

In our view, the explanation for why some young people thrive and others seriously falter during this challenging period lies substantially in developmental history, a history that now covers more than a decade, as we review our data. A basic sense of inner worth, of connection with others, and of others as available and supportive remains critical. So too do the capacities for flexible emotional regulation, agency, persistence, restraint, and ego resiliency, and the confidence these capacities engender. All of these are the legacies of the earliest years of life. The fruits of exploratory and problem-solving successes in the preschool period, as well as positive encounters with peers, all serve the young person well now. Finally, the sense of competence, mastery of peer group challenges, and experience in close friendships during middle childhood provide a foundation for negotiating the challenges of adolescence.

As in earlier periods, positive adaptation in adolescence is best viewed as a developmental achievement. Consider, for example, the capacity to be involved in intimate relationships, with their high demand for emotional sharing and self-disclosure, and attendant feelings of vulnerability. Intimacy, which characterizes adolescent friendships much more so than friendships at earlier ages, is a classic developmental phenomenon. "Intimacy has 'emergent properties' that are not fully specified by earlier capacities, but that evolve from those precursors through a series of transformations, each of which builds on the previous ones" (Collins & Sroufe, 1999, p. 127). Such a complex capacity does not simply emerge de novo in adolescence, though it does represent a profound accomplishment. Rather, such a capacity is rooted in the history of early care, ongoing support from parents, and the entire cumulative history of experiences with peers. Intimate relationships clearly have trust components and emotional regulation components that are nurtured in the family from the earliest years forward. In addition, they require capacities for mutual give and take, negotiation, and staying together through conflict. While family experiences are important here as well, there is a clear role for experiences with peers. As we laid out in Table 4.2, there is a progression of challenges and accomplishments in the world of peers. For example, from sustaining interactive bouts and maintaining organization in the face of arousal in the preschool years, to sustaining friendships and tolerating a wide range of emotional experiences in middle childhood, the young person is prepared for commitment in relationships and the emotional vulnerability that comes with intimacy. Thus, some of the required capacities may arise in the family, and these support later social relationships, but they are linked together and practiced in the world of peers, with each phase supporting the next.

The same themes we saw in middle childhood development surface again in adolescence. For example, as in earlier periods, adolescent outcomes are better predicted by the cumulated history of care or the history of competence than by measures from any single time period. Adolescent social sophistication and preparation for adulthood build upon the agency, close friendships, and peer group functioning of middle childhood, just as middle childhood competence built upon peer group engagement and movement toward self-management in the preschool period. Moreover, we can predict more reliably adolescent outcomes when relationships with peers, as well as caregivers, and men as well as mothers, are considered. Indeed, the role of men in the lives of our (primarily) mother-reared children is more clearly evident in adolescence than in earlier periods. When care, and the context of care, current circumstances, and history are considered together, the coherence and predictability of adaptation are more apparent. Several interesting examples are presented in which contextual variables in early childhood (e.g., witnessing violence between adult caregivers) have more predictive power for adolescence than for middle childhood. We take this as both confirming the enduring importance of early experience and as perhaps pointing to special vulnerabilities during the adolescent period.

PLAN FOR THE FOLLOWING CHAPTERS

A number of important developmental tasks face adolescents. Our assessments, as always, derived from a consideration of these tasks. We examined how our teen participants negotiated the complexities of an expanded, mixed-gender peer network, evolved further the capacity for intimacy, and realigned relationships with parents. We also assessed their educational achievements and whether they had formulated a plan for advanced education or work. More generally, we wanted to know how well they had integrated past development and were projecting themselves into the future. Finally, were they avoiding the many potential snares of adolescence, such as drug or alcohol abuse, or early pregnancy?

Three assessments, taking place between early and middle adolescence, are discussed in this chapter. When children were age 13, we carried out a laboratory observation of parents and teens. This included 175 mothers and 44 men, who were fathers of the teenager or partners of their mothers. It was important to assess quality of parenting at this time for two reasons. First, this is a critical time for parents and children, and the quality of available support likely impacts the course of adolescence (Collins, 1995; Collins & Laursen, 2004; Collins & Steinberg, in press). Second, given our theoretical interest in early care, it was important also to have later measures of care, to see not only whether they supplanted early care but also how they supplemented early support, and to examine how the various measures worked together to forecast later development. We had no doubt that both early care and care at this age were important, but no one had previously studied how they work together.

Our second assessment, with children age 15, entailed a series of weekend reunions with 41 of the young people who had attended our summer camps in middle childhood. As was true for the earlier camp study, the reunions allowed us to see our participants in interaction with each other; moreover, they allowed us to composite the ratings of multiple counselors and to coordinate multiple sources of information: ratings, behavioral observations, and interviews with the teens. An additional benefit was the opportunity to film the teens in both informal and formal group settings, participating in activities and tasks we designed.

A third major assessment was carried out on all of the participants at age 16. This assessment was comprehensive and included lengthy interviews with the teen, covering family relationships, friendships, dating, work and school, activities, and other aspects of personal development. The young person also completed a life stress interview, a wide-ranging Adolescent Health Survey (which included, among other things, questions about drug and alcohol use, and suicidal ideation), and a self-report behavior problem checklist. Mothers were interviewed regarding stress, social support, and their ongoing lives, and they also completed the checklist of child behavior problems. Teachers provided this information as well. School records data also were obtained this year and every year until graduation or age 19, whichever came first.

In examining the camp reunion and high school data, the presentation strategy again derives from our "developmental construction" viewpoint. With particular outcomes, where theoretical ties are compelling, we look at the legacy of attachment history, but our major focus is on cumulative history. As we did in Chapter 8, in our formal analyses we first report how early measures and later measures independently predicted these adolescent outcomes. Then, using statistical regression techniques, we successively examine later measures in chronological order, describing how adaptation is created, age by age. Regression used in this way allows one to ask whether later measures add to the prediction of earlier measures. We again show that cumulative history is most powerful, and that contemporary circumstances, as well as history, are important considerations for understanding the young person's functioning. Later, in Chapter 11, we present some analyses in reverse chronological order. This allows us to demonstrate that early experience remains important, even after taking into account more contemporary influences.

Information that we obtained at age 17½ from an extensive clinical interview is presented in a separate chapter (12) on psychopathology. Comprehensive assessments between ages 19 and 21 are presented in Chapter 10 on the transition to adulthood.

QUALITY OF CARE IN EARLY ADOLESCENCE

Our assessments of parents and 13-year-olds were keyed to the realignment struggles that may arise at this time (see Chapter 4). Thus, having parent and teen plan an antismoking campaign tapped the partners' capacity for a new level of collaboration, wherein the child had some special expertise. Having the child direct the blindfolded parent in the construction of an object pulled forth the issue of transfer of control. Other tasks (discussions, a Q-sort) provided a good look at their openness and confidence concerning each other, and their ability to resolve conflicts. In all, we were able to code scales capturing (1) spontaneity–security, (2) support and scaffolding, and (3) ease and efficiency of working together, as well as emotional tone, conflict resolution, and parent–child boundary problems. We viewed these as relationship scales, and only later did we make individual ratings of the child (which are discussed in later chapters). As described in Chapter 4, the first three scales, referred to as "balance scales," may be thought of as measures of the overall quality of the relationship, whereas the summary scale of boundary violation was viewed as possibly pathogenic; that is, as reflecting serious distortions in family structure that might be associated with later behavior problems.

Our initial task was to validate these scales with our participants. The scales were first correlated with sixth-grade outcomes. These school measures preceded the 13-year assessments; however, they were close enough in time to be a meaningful test of concurrent validity. The balance scales were moderately but significantly correlated with all of the major outcomes for sixth grade. In addition, they were validated against summer camp data from age 10–11. Balance I, the 13-year variable having to do with security and spontaneity in the relationship, showed especially strong relations with summer camp measures. The correlations with emotional health and peer competence ranks in the camps were .45 and .47, respectively. Finally, the balance scales also were related to the composite early care variable ($r = .26$) and to quality of home support and stimulation at age 6 (.33).

As predicted, parent–child boundary problems at age 13 were significantly related to behavior problems in sixth grade, especially to problems such as inattentiveness (Hiester, 1993). Moreover, such boundary problems were significantly related to a history of sexual exploitation of the mother when she was a child, to dissatisfaction with her current adult relationship, to alcohol or drug abuse by her partner, and to general quality of support from partners. These findings were especially strong for mothers of boys. Thus, as was the case in early childhood, contextual factors were implicated in the maintenance or breakdown of boundaries between parent and child.

Finally, there was substantial continuity between measures of parent–child boundary violation across time, with correlations of .34 and .45 between boundary dissolution at 42 months and boundary dissolution and seductiveness, respectively, at age 13 years (Hiester, 1993). We noted anecdotally, and later confirmed, that an interesting transformation occurred in boundary violation across this period (Shaffer & Sroufe, in press). Whereas, earlier, this variable was keyed to parental behavior, by age 13, boundary problems were notable in the child's behavior as well. The child may have, for example, been unduly attentive and solicitous toward the parent, as in the case of a child noticing the slightest hint that his mother was cold (as she hunched her shoulders a bit). "Are you cold?" he asked. "Oh, just a bit," she said. "Should I go (back out to the car) and get your coat?" This was only one of many examples in their interactions that contained many other spouse-like behaviors. Further validation of the 13-year-old care measures is presented below and in subsequent chapters. These measures predicted important outcomes later in adolescence and in early adulthood.

THE CAMP REUNION STUDY

As described in Chapter 4, the weekend camp reunions were intense social experiences, including outward bound–type activities, meals together, a party planned by the young people, an overnight stay in cabins, and recreational activities the following day. As usual, there were multiple counselors, and a fleet of observers was present at all times. Almost everything was filmed with four cameras, and much reliable information was obtained in this short period. All counselors and observers were blind to child developmental history.

As predicted, social competence in the camp reunion reflected the platform of competence established earlier. Both the friendship score and the general social competence index from the summer camp at age 10 correlated strongly with teen social competence (.40 and .57, respectively). Likewise, the preschool social competence rating correlated .47 with social competence and .57 with the capacity for vulnerability scale at age 15. These are remarkable correlations over the age spans in question.

The strength of the ties between teen functioning at these camp reunions and measures of early care were equally remarkable (Sroufe, Egeland, et al., 1999). Each measure of care between 6 and 42 months was related to the adolescent outcomes. For attachment history, relations were as strong or stronger than they had been for the preschool and middle childhood outcomes. For example, the correlation between number of times secure and the molar measure of social competence, composited across four counselors, was .46. Moreover, attachment history was significantly related to all ratings and behavioral measures of competence for these 15-year-olds. A variable of special interest, based on our theoretical considerations (Chapter 4), was the rating of capacity for vulnerability. This variable captured the teens' willingness to be emotionally vulnerable and thereby participate in the full range of potentially growth-enhancing experiences at the weekend retreat. It correlated with attachment history (.41).

Teens with secure attachment histories showed a greater capacity for negotiating the complexities of the adolescent peer group than did those with anxious histories. Mutually consistent sociograms constructed by the counselors revealed the presence of an organized "crowd" (Dunphy, 1963) at each of the three retreats. This was a discernible group of mixed-gender youth who consistently interacted together. The crowds were constituted by securely attached teens far beyond chance. Moreover, all eight campers involved in couples (as agreed upon by youth sociometrics and counselor judgments) had histories of secure attachment and were prominent in the mixed-gender crowd at their camp. Such findings underscore the consistent link between early attachment security and later close relationships that appears in our work.

We also conducted a formal assessment of leadership and effectiveness in the group (Englund, Levy, Hyson, & Sroufe, 2000). Small groups, and then larger groups, of teens were given the problem of utilizing an additional $150 for the party or for recreational activities the next day. But they had to come to an agreed-upon solution, and they could not simply divide the money. Following their decision, they elected a spokesperson for the discussions with the next larger group (all the boys or all the girls, then all boys and girls). We rated leadership, involvement, self-confidence, and overall social competence, all with high reliability. These ratings correlated remarkably well with independent counselor ratings; for example, the counselor rating of social competence correlated .70 with the observed competence rating, and the two self-confidence ratings correlated .74.

Children with secure attachment histories were distinguished from those with anxious histories on each of the ratings, with more than one standard deviation difference on the overall competence rating. Thus, those with secure histories tended to be involved in the discussions, were skillful in interactions, drew the attention of others in positive ways, were effective in both negotiating and persuading, and, in general, guided and facilitated the process. They were significantly more likely to be elected spokesperson at some level of the process; 13 of the spokespersons had been secure (out of 24), whereas only 3 (of 16) had anxious attachment histories, a statistically significant result. Even when not chosen to be spokesperson, they often were influential in electing the spokesperson. This was a subcomponent of the leadership scale.

Remarkable as these findings were, it is not just attachment or early care that is the foundation for adolescent competence. It is the cumulative history of care and adaptation, and much of the strength of attachment comes through its links with peer competence at prior ages. For example, 13-year-old parent–child relationship variables not only were related to social competence in adolescence (r's mostly in the .30s), they sometimes added significantly to early care measures.

Likewise, preschool peer experiences and middle childhood peer functioning added to attachment history in predicting adolescent competence, with multiple correlations (R) often in the .50s and .60s. With attachment and preschool data entered, middle childhood camp data did not add to the results. This attests to how much basis for social competence had been established by the end of the preschool period. Partly, it also reflects overlap in the situational demands of our preschool and camp. When we used teacher ratings from elementary school for our middle childhood measure, it did add to early history and nursery school adaptation, and the multiple R increased to .69 (see Table 9.1 and Sroufe, Egeland, et al., 1999, for details).

The 13-year-old family measures generally did not add to predictions of adolescent social competence with the middle childhood camp

TABLE 9.1. Summary of Hierarchical Regression Analysis Predicting Adolescent Social Competence from Early Childhood Experience, Preschool Experience, and Middle Childhood Social Competence ($n = 35$)

Variable	Model 1			Model 2			Model 3		
	B	SE	β	B	SE	β	B	SE	β
Infant attachment	7.14	2.57	.44**	6.04	2.37	.37*	5.94	2.17	.36*
Social competence (preschool)				4.27	1.53	.41**	1.60	1.72	.15
Social competence (middle childhood)							.27	.10	.43*
R^2 change	.19			.16			.12		
F for change in R^2	7.72**			7.83**			7.08*		
Multiple R	.44**			.59***			.69***		

Note. Infant attachment security (12–18 months), preschool social competence teacher ratings (4.5 years), middle childhood social competence teacher ratings (grades 3 and 6), and adolescent social competence (15 years).
*$p < .05$; **$p < .01$; ***$p < .001$.

measures controlled. There was one interesting exception. When the outcome was "Capacity for Vulnerability," Family Balance I (the spontaneity–security scale) accounted for an additional 8% of the variance. Thus, secure relations with parents continued to influence aspects of peer relationships centered on freedom to experience emotion and emotional closeness (Sroufe, Egeland, et al., 1999).

There was one final facet to our camp reunion study. We found that generally those with secure attachment histories were the most socially competent and were interested in, and knowledgeable about, the peer social network. Thus, variations in such social perception were not very great or very informative for those with secure histories. However, it proved to be quite important for those with anxious attachment histories. Those with anxious histories who were nonetheless socially perceptive, based on our extensive exit interview, were much more likely to be socially competent than their less socially aware and less socially interested counterparts (Weinfeld, Ogawa, & Sroufe, 1997).

AGE 16 ASSESSMENTS

At age 16, data on all participants ($N = 175$) were collected from teachers, parents, and the young people themselves. Measures of social competence and behavior problems were obtained from each of these three sources. Measures of school performance were obtained from teachers, school records, and formal testing. And we gathered data on friendships, dating, and positive and negative aspects of self-development, using extensive interviews with the teens.

Social Competence

We begin our discussion with the broadest measure of social competence at this age, in which we were able to combine three independent measures from separate sources. One was a ranking on competence made by the teacher who knew the child best (often a "homeroom" teacher or English teacher). Another was the Social Problems Scale from the Child Behavior Checklist, completed by the mother. Finally, this same checklist was also completed by the teenager. As was true for the camp reunion data, we found that, using this composite index, social competence at age 16 built upon competence in the preceding periods. The composite competence index was significantly predicted by preschool ratings ($n = 78$), elementary (grades 1–6) teacher competence rankings, social competence ratings from the summer camp at age 10, and ratings from the camp reunion at age 15, with many correlations in the .40s. Moreover, the 6- to 42-month early history of care variable, as well as severity of physical abuse correlated with the social competence at age 16, more than 13 years later (.35 and −.29, respectively).

As was true in middle childhood, the more features of history that were combined, the stronger the predictions. Quality of parental care at school entry added to early care in predicting social competence at age 16, as did stress–support and peer competence in the elementary years. When just early care and elementary school competence were entered into a regression analysis, the multiple correlation was .40. Moreover, path analysis revealed partial mediation. The beta for early care dropped substantially after elementary competence was entered, and this elementary measure was significant above and beyond the earlier measure (Ostoja-Starzewska, 1996). We interpret this to mean that some of the impact of early care on adolescent outcomes derives from the influence of early history on prior peer competence. Table 9.2 shows the strength of prediction from early care, care at school entry, early elementary peer competence, and life stress and relationship support up to the third grade. The multiple correlation was .48, a substantial prediction across an 8-year period.

Friendship

Another important measure of social competence was derived from a friendship interview with the adolescent. Questions centered on the quality of the relationship with a best friend. The primary rating scales

TABLE 9.2. Summary of Hierarchical Regression Analysis Predicting Adolescent Social Competence from Early Childhood Experience and Home Organization, and Middle Childhood Peer Competence, Maternal Life Stress, and Social Support ($N = 160$)

Variable	Model 1			Model 2			Model 3			Model 4		
	B	SE	β	B	SE	β	B	SE	β	B	SE	β
Early experience	2.93	.57	.38***	2.53	.66	.33***	2.02	.67	.26**	1.89	.66	.24**
HOME score				.04	.04	.10	.03	.04	.08	.03	.04	.01
Peer competence							.04	.02	.21**	.04	.02	.20*
Maternal life stress										.61	.51	.10
Maternal support										1.27	.43	.25**
R^2 change	.14			.01			.04			.04		
F for change in R^2	26.67***			1.44			7.08**			4.31**		
Multiple R	.38***			.39***			.43***			.48***		

Note. Early experience composite = maternal sensitivity/cooperation (6 months), attachment security (12–18 months), toddler experience in the session (24 months), early childhood experience (42 months); HOME score (grade 1); peer competence teacher rank (grades 1–3); maternal life stress and emotional support (grades 1–3).
* $p < .05$; ** $p < .01$; *** $p < .001$.

184

tapped disclosure, closeness, and "coherence of transcript," which was inspired by work on the Adult Attachment Interview (e.g., Main & Goldwyn, 1998). The latter two scales were composited to form the major variable, "friendship quality," for analyses at this age. This composite was first validated against contemporary measures. It correlated significantly with the Harter self-report friendship scale, with the mother and teacher competence measures, and with camp reunion competence rank (r's from .27 to .42). Correlations for girls considered alone were consistently higher, ranging from .31 to .56, for these same measures. It was clear to us that the friendship interview was not as useful for our males. Minnesota males, and perhaps even more among our subpopulation of youth, are "men of few words."

When we looked at antecedents of friendship quality in adolescence, we again found that correlations with preschool teacher rankings, elementary school rankings, and summer camp competence rankings all were significant. Remarkably, the "friendship" score from summer camp correlated a robust .55 (.64 for girls). This is powerful confirmation of the validity of the friendship quality measure at age 16, and strong evidence for the stability of competence in this domain. We also found that early history of care was significantly but modestly predictive of teen friendship quality.

Regression analyses again showed that middle childhood elementary school competence added 6% to early childhood care history in the prediction of friendship quality. There was again evidence for partial mediation, with a substantial drop (to nonsignificance) in the power of early childhood competence after elementary school competence was entered.

Dating

Our final analyses of social functioning at age 16 centered on dating relationships, also derived from our extensive interviews of the teens. The platform of earlier peer competence was again in evidence. Measures of earlier peer competence, especially those derived from the summer camps, were consistently related to dating outcomes. For example, the observation-based "friendship" score significantly related to felt security in one's dating relationship (Schmit, 1995).

Several analyses targeted more specific, theoretical questions. A number of important findings centered on gender boundary violation or maintenance while children were at the camps (Collins, Hennighausen, Schmit, & Sroufe, 1997). Recall that from our view of developmental organization and complexity, maintaining clear gender boundaries in middle childhood is a mark of competence, because it denotes adherence to peer group norms. Violating such norms is *not* a sign of precocious social maturity, and boundary violators were predicted (paradoxically, in terms of linear theories) to later be less competent in dealing with mixed-gender relationships. In accord with this, it was boundary maintenance, not violation, that predicted general competence in adolescence, as well as the capacity for vulnerability (r's = .31 and .48, respectively). In general, it was related to more effectiveness in the mixed-gender peer group crowd at the reunions, as well as to a greater capacity for intimacy in friendships at age 16 (Ostoja-Starzewska, 1996).

What were the implications of boundary violations in middle childhood for adolescent dating? Were such young people precocious? In fact, they were not; there was no relationship between this variable and age of onset of dating. Moreover, those who violated gender boundaries in middle childhood, compared to those who maintained them, were *less* secure in their dating relationships (r = .47)

There also is an obvious intimacy component to dating, so we returned again to a focus on attachment history. We found first that both teens with secure attachment histories and those with avoidant attachment histories commonly had dating experience by age 16. Only those with resistant histories lagged behind in this area. This is consistent with prior findings of social immaturity, dating back to the preschool years. Recall, for example, that these children as a group hovered near the preschool teachers and were unduly nurtured and indulged by them. Children with secure and those with avoidant histories were not distinguished by whether or not they dated; rather, they were distinguished by whether their dating relationships had any longevity. The measure we used was a duration of 3 months, and those with secure histories who dated were significantly more likely to have such a relationship than those with avoidant histories who dated. This supported our general hypothesis regarding the challenge of intimacy for those with anxious–avoidant attachment in infancy.

Achievement and Adjustment at School

At age 16, achievement test scores were well predicted by historical and contemporary psychosocial variables and by academic measures (see Teo et al., 1996, for details). The summary early care variable correlated .41 and .42 with math and reading, respectively. Quality of care at school entry (grade 1 HOME) also was significantly correlated with high school achievement, as was a history of child maltreatment. Severity of early neglect, for example, was significantly correlated with both math and reading achievement (Egeland, 1997). Neglect remained a significant predictor even after controlling for SES, a rigorous control, since SES correlates with neglect and predicts reading and math achievement substantially (Egeland, 1997).

Math and reading achievement tests scores at age 16 were predicted strongly by measures of achievement at each earlier grade (all correlations in the .50s and .60s). They also were predicted by IQ. This is not surprising, since such a relationship is built into the design of the tests. However, even with IQ (or earlier achievement) controlled through prior entry in regression analysis, the early care variable accounted for additional significant variance in predicting math and reading achievement. These are rigorous tests and, overall, the power of the early measures of care was impressive.

Obviously, connections between early care and later achievement cannot be direct. Having a secure attachment relationship in infancy does not likely change one's "math brain." Rather, we find links through variables such as more regular school attendance, parent involvement with school and schoolwork, and positive child–teacher relationships (Carlson et al., 1999; Jimerson et al., 1999). Regular attendance and ongoing work is required to keep up with math. Such factors probably explain why the correlation between attachment and math achievement is higher than the correlation between attachment and reading comprehension.

In grade 11, we also assessed a broader measure of school adjustment. Ratings were made of overall school functioning on a 7-point scale, based on records of attendance, grades and credits earned, class standing, history of discipline problems, alternative placements, and history of grade retention (Carlson et al., 1999). At the high end of this scale, the student was making good progress, was at or above grade level for age, had good attendance, and had no record of discipline problems. Given the fact that our participants were in 90 different schools, we viewed such a rating as superior to more discrete, quantitative measures such as days of attendance, grade point average, or achievement test scores, for a variety of reasons. For example, some schools did not keep accurate attendance records, and some students were in settings where attendance was compulsory (e.g., incarceration or residential treatment). Some schools did not assign grades, and grading standards varied widely. Achievement tests are strongly related to IQ, whereas our rating correlated with IQ only .30. Moreover, some aspects of achievement (e.g., reading comprehension) reflect earlier work as much as current work. Finally, we found that our adjustment rating correlated with dropping out of school much more highly (.65) than did IQ or achievement test scores (.30s). Thus, it proved to be an excellent measure of school functioning. (We discuss dropping out in Chapter 10).

The high school adjustment measure was well predicted by antecedent measures, especially those obtained in the early elementary school years (Carlson et al., 1999). All major measures in early elementary school (grades 1–3) yielded highly significant predictions of the high school adjustment outcome. For the emotional health ranking, the peer competence ranking, and the total behavior problem score, all of the correlations were substantial (ranging from .35 to .52). Family life stress in the first three grades also was highly significant. Each of these correlations was higher than the correlation between achievement test performance in early elementary school and grade 11 adjustment (.27). Moreover, even after we controlled for achievement using regression analysis, early elementary school psychosocial functioning added 20% to the variance accounted for in predicting adjustment. Finally, behavior problems in grade 6 strongly predicted grade 11 school adjustment (.52).

High school adjustment was quite well related to our cumulative early history variable (.32). In this case the 24- to 42-month support variables alone showed a similar correlation. The quality of home stimulation and support at school entry (the grade 1 HOME) added to these early measures, and a regression in which they were combined yielded a multiple correlation of .37. Thus, by the time of school entry, 14% of the variance in the high school adjustment outcome could be predicted. When the 13-year family measure concerned with working as a team and marshaling resources to deal with external demands (Balance III) was added to the equation, the multiple R was .39. Finally, early care still predicted high school adjustment after taking into account early achievement or IQ (Carlson et al., 1999).

Behavior Problems in Adolescence

Because of their theoretical and practical significance, we have thoroughly analyzed behavior problems in adolescence (e.g., Egeland, Pianta, & Ogawa, 1996). We have examined an especially broad array of psychosocial risk factors; that is, those conditions, early and contemporaneous, that make behavior problems more likely. Although we will discuss risk, protection, and psychopathology more thoroughly in later chapters, we want to provide an overview of key antecedents of troubled behavior here. Our work on teen behavior problems once again underscores the importance of considering a range of factors. SES, life stress, interparental conflict, and family disruption all have proven to be important, in addition to the quality of care directly experienced by the child.

We begin with the early care summary variable, which was significantly correlated with total behavior problems at age 16, based both on the teacher alone and on the combination of teacher, parent, and adolescent. The measure of care at school entry (grade 1 HOME) yielded a significant but small correlation. Measures of competence in elementary school all yielded stronger correlations (.30s), as did relationship support for the mother at that time. Behavior problem history was, of course, quite predictive; for example, externalizing in grades 1–3 correlated .42 with teacher-rated problems at age 16. We were able to show, however, that experiences within the family still were important, even after taking behavior problems into account; for example, parent–child boundary dissolution at age 13 predicted change in behavior problems between grade 6 and age 16 (Nelson, 1994).

Maltreatment History and Adolescent Behavior Problems

At earlier ages, we found that maltreatment affected core adaptational issues at each age, from attachment in infancy to self-regulation in the toddler period, and to the later movement to self-management (e.g., Erickson et al., 1989; see also Chapters 5–8). Thus, "by the time the young maltreated child reaches adolescence, the major differentiation and integration of the social, emotional, cognitive, and other systems that occur during this period are severely affected" (Egeland, 1997, p. 429).

Our assessments of abuse history in the preschool years were indeed consistently related to adolescent behavior problems (Egeland, 1997). In fact, membership in any of the maltreatment groups—physical abuse, psychological unavailability, neglect, and sexual abuse—was in each case related to significant problems, and in each case predicted the likelihood of some psychiatric treatment. As we discuss further in Chapter 12, fully 90% of these children qualified for at least one psychiatric diagnosis by age 17. Measures of severity of physical abuse and severity of neglect were both significantly related to total behavior problems and to an array of more specific types of problems. Sexual abuse was related to the broadest range of problems, ranging from withdrawal, anxiety, and attention problems to aggression, delinquency, and heavy drug use. Even with SES controlled, various forms of maltreatment history added to the prediction of various kinds of problem behavior.

Every form of maltreatment was related to delinquency, with a history of psychological unavailability being the strongest predictor. We reasoned that this was because of both the legacy of anger, negativity, and defiance in these children, and the lack of monitoring provided by their parents in adolescence. It is likely that, for the latter reason, neglect also predicted delinquency, even though these children tended to not be aggressive or defiant (Egeland, 1997).

As was the case at earlier periods (e.g., Erickson et al., 1989), there was some patterning to these links between maltreatment and behavior problems. Even though most of the groups had a range of problems, in accord with the principle of "multifinality" (Cicchetti, & Rogosch, 1996), patterns of consequences could be seen (Egeland, 1997). Membership in the neglect group was the only predictor of school achievement problems, once SES was controlled, and neglect did not predict aggression, cutting school, or heavy drug use, as did a history of physical abuse. The neglect group did use alcohol more than controls, but they did not get into trouble with it. Physically abused children later were distinguished by heavy drug use and were frequently in trouble, including being defiant, aggressive, and often truant from school. Those in the psychologically unavailable group were distinguished by the pattern of aggression, social problems, and isolation, as manifested in elevated suicide attempts.

While these data indicate substantial continuity from early abuse to adolescent problems, there was evidence for change as well. Some children with histories of maltreatment were doing relatively well. A case analysis revealed that many of the same factors associated with positive change earlier were apparent here as well (Egeland, 1997), including an early history of support and competence, an alternative available caregiver, a good school, and an organized home environment.

Witnessing Violence

Not only direct maltreatment of the child but also *witnessing* violence between parental figures (usually father or boyfriend being violent with the child's mother) was important. We obtained summary measures for this variable from interviews with mothers for both the preschool and middle childhood periods (Yates, Dodds, et al., 2003). Previous studies had reported correlations between witnessing violence and child behavior problems, but not with the array of controls available in our study. Controls are important, since such a correlation may be obtained because children who witness violence also are more likely to be abused directly, experience more stress in general, or live in impoverished conditions. Behavior problems may be the result of these factors and not witnessing violence per se. In fact, these variables were correlated with behavior problems in our study, and with witnessing violence. Life stress correlated strongly with witnessing violence in the preschool years (.48). Nonetheless, we were able to demonstrate a contribution to behavior problems, even with all of these variables and child IQ controlled (Yates, Dodds, et al., 2003).

Our first finding was that witnessing parental violence in the preschool years was significantly but modestly correlated with internalizing and externalizing problems during adolescence. The findings were stronger when both gender and type of problems also were considered. For boys, witnessing violence in the preschool period predicted *externalizing* problems at age 16 (.31); for girls, it predicted *internalizing* problems (.29). These results are consistent with the notion that psychosocial risks may push girls toward internalizing problems and boys toward externalizing problems.

Follow-up regressions confirmed that witnessing violence was at least partially independent of other predictors. With IQ, SES, stress (which itself was highly significant), child abuse, and neglect already controlled, early witnessing of violence was still significant in predicting externalizing problems at age 16 for the total sample and for boys. In these analyses, witnessing violence in middle childhood was not significant, although it was previously related to problems in middle childhood (see Chapter 8). The adolescent data are another bit of evidence concerning the special role of early experience. *Witnessing violence in early childhood leaves a legacy that appears during the adolescent years, especially in boys.*

The Role of Men

Other important contextual factors in predicting adolescent behavior problems centered on the role of men in the lives of our participants. Adult male presence could be considered either as a risk factor (if frequent comings and goings of men were disruptive to family stability) or as a "promotive" factor (Sameroff, 2000), if male presence marked additional support for the child or mother. For example, a key variable in the literature with regard to adolescent behavior problems has been "monitoring," that is, the degree to which parents are aware of, and keep track of, their teen's activities and companions (e.g., Pettit, Bates, Dodge, & Meece, 1999). We did not have enough stable male presence to consider "father" monitoring alone, but we did find that parental monitoring during adolescence was in general higher when there was stable male presence, and that higher monitoring was associated with lower behavior problems for boys (Pierce, 1999; Sroufe & Pierce, 1999).

From systematic review of interviews with mothers on 17 occasions over the years, as well as six teacher interviews and three interviews with our adolescent participants, three key "father" variables were examined: (1) disruptiveness of males in the home; (2) supportiveness of the child by men, and (3) family structure (Pierce, 1999). The first two variables were summary ratings made for early childhood, middle childhood, and adolescence. In families with a high score on disruptiveness, the mother was involved with multiple partners, and there were numerous moves by men into and out of the home. For families with high ratings on support, the man was available, attentive, and involved with the child in an ongoing and supportive way. The third measure was categorical, based on whether the child lived with the mother alone, the mother and the biological father, or the mother and a stepfather from age 3 to first grade.

In keeping with the findings on witnessing violence presented earlier, disruptive male presence predicted adolescent externalizing problems most powerfully from the early childhood period ($r = .31$). Disruptiveness was still predictive based on middle childhood assessments (.21), but was not significant when measured during adolescence. Moreover, early childhood disruptiveness (men coming and going) accounted for additional significant variance in externalizing even after life stress and direct support of the child by the mother were taken into account.

Direct support of the child by available men, assessed in early and middle childhood, and adolescence, all predicted lower externalizing (correlations in the .30s). In regression analyses, support in adolescence proved to be the strongest variable. *The combination of early disruption and low adolescent support was a strong combination, especially for boys.*

With regard to the impact of type of early family organizational structure, there was an interesting significant interaction with gender. For girls, externalizing was highest when they had lived in a stepfamily in the early years. For boys, externalizing was highest when they had lived with their mothers alone, especially when externalizing was measured in middle childhood. In general, stable supportive male adults proved to be a positive influence for our male participants; notably, unstable adult male presence was worse than no man involved at all.

General Social Support and Cumulative Risk

Recently, we extended our view of social support available to the child beyond the father (Appleyard, 2004). These additional supportive persons could be not only other partners of the caregiver but also grandparents, other relatives, or family friends. The quality of this support in early childhood was rated (including the dependability and affective involvement of the person), as were disruptions in social support. These measures predicted peer competence and adjustment at various ages, all the way up to adolescence. For example, quality of support in early childhood predicted both lower internalizing and externalizing behavior problems at age 16, even after controlling for the quality of maternal care. Such findings again testify to the role of context and the impact of cumulative resources for the child.

Finally, we completed an analysis in which we examined five major risk factors concurrently: SES, life stress, child maltreatment, witnessing parental violence, and family disruption (Appleyard, Egeland, van Dulmen, & Sroufe, 2005). The variables were assembled for two developmental periods—early and middle childhood. Because we were interested in cumulative risk, we dichotomized each variable and created a risk index from 0 to 5 at each period. The risk index for each period was entered into a regression analysis to predict internalizing and externalizing problems at age 16. In accord with findings for separate risk factors described previously, early cumulative risk predicted both internalizing and externalizing, and it did so more strongly than did middle childhood risk. Moreover, when middle childhood risk was entered first, early risk continued to predict at a significant level. These latent effects of early risk represent an important developmental phenomenon. We also found a significant linear trend (but not a significant quadratic trend) in a follow-up to an analysis of variance. This means that as each risk is added, there is an increase in the likelihood of behavior problems. This was true for both internalizing and externalizing problems.

ADOLESCENT RISK BEHAVIOR

Terrie Moffitt (1993) has pointed out that, for many teenagers, a period of acting out can be relatively benign. Such problems simply reflect the young persons' striving to find themselves and to define their place in the adolescent peer group. Many leave their problems behind when they move into adulthood. However, even for these youth whose problems have not been chronic, there are potential hazards. Moffitt refers to these as "snares," behaviors that in and of themselves can produce lasting problems. Three of these snares that we discuss here are (1) risky sexual behaviors (e.g., early, unprotected sex), (2) drug or alcohol abuse, and (3) association with deviant peers. Everyone is familiar with the potential social, economic, and health consequences of such behavior patterns. We focus our attention on the antecedents of such risky behavior.

Risky Sexual Behavior

When adolescents engage in frequent sexual activity, especially with multiple partners and without adequate use of contraception, they place themselves at risk for both health and economic problems. Early age of first intercourse is another serious risk factor, in part because it also tends to be associated with these other factors and with early pregnancy. Such sexual practices increase both the likelihood of contracting life-altering and life-threatening diseases, and the risk of pregnancy out of wedlock. In our data, for example, for boys, both age of first intercourse and number of partners predicted getting someone pregnant (Levy, 1998).

Giving birth early and without a stable partner leads to economic hardship and places the newborn child at risk for developmental problems. Our data confirm that single status of the mother at the time of the child's birth is a risk factor for behavior problems (Aguilar et al., 2000; Carlson, Jacobvitz, & Sroufe, 1995). For example, it was the single strongest predictor of attention/hyperactivity problems in elementary school (see Chapter 12). Moreover, single status of the mother at birth predicted drug and alcohol problems and risky sexual activity in the next generation. Thus, risky sexual behavior plays a role in a cycle of disadvantage across generations: from disadvantage to sexual acting out and other problems, to disadvantage again.

Just as was true for competence and earlier behavior problems, risky sexual behavior was predictable from a variety of psychosocial antecedents (Siebenbruner, Zimmer-Gembeck, & Egeland, 2005). These are not problems that simply spring up in adolescence without a history. Lawfulness of emergence was found both when we looked at specific variables, such as age of first intercourse and number of partners, and when we defined groups of high-risk teens, based on combinations of frequent and unprotected sexual activity.

For example, having first intercourse at later ages was significantly predicted by history of early positive care, peer competence, low behavior problems, and low family life stress in elementary school. Number of sexual partners was predicted (in reverse) by most of these same variables and by parent–child boundary distortions at age 13.

Our high sexual risk group was characterized by poor support on the grade 1 HOME, negative emotional climate in the family at age 13, poor parental monitoring during adolescence, and lack of motivation in school beginning as early as first grade (Siebenbruner et al., 2005). Consistent with a large literature (e.g., Jessor, 1984), sexual risk behavior was strongly related to drug and alcohol problems, other behavior problems (past and present), expulsion from school, and conflict with dating partners. When measures up to age 8 were combined, 16% of the variance was explained. The measures of behavior and support up to age 12–13 accounted for 27% of the variance. Finally, when all psychosocial measures used in this study were combined, well more than half of the variance was predictable.

Other findings regarding sexual risk behaviors were more specifically tied to theory. One analysis concerned gender boundary violation in middle childhood. Gender boundary violation was associated with age of becoming sexually active for this whole subsample, and quite dramatically for females (.75), although it should be noted that the sample size here was only 23 girls. For girls, gender boundary violation also was significantly related to a failure to use contraception; the correlation between boundary maintenance and contraceptive use was −.49. For males, boundary violation was significantly related with number of sexual partners. Thus, gender boundary violation in middle childhood does not forecast capacities for greater closeness in relationships or general social competence, as discussed earlier in this chapter. Rather, it predicts early and more frequent unprotected sexual activity for females, and promiscuity for males.

Heavy Use of Alcohol and Other Drugs

As in other samples, heavy use of alcohol and heavy use of other drugs were related in our study, and they have many of the same antecedents. Not surprisingly, given the intertwining of teen problems, these antecedents also greatly overlap with those that predicted sexual risk behavior. For example, lack of motivation in school in grade 1 predicted heavy drug use ($r = .31$), with about the same strength that it predicted risky sexual behavior.

In the case of drug and alcohol use, even more so than with sexual behavior, it is important to distinguish between heavy participation and experimentation. Teens experiment with "adult" behaviors, and such experimentation may well be an important part of self-discovery. At the least, research suggests that those who experiment with drugs or alcohol have more positive backgrounds and are generally more competent and psychologically healthy as teens and later, than those who are either heavy users *or* abstain totally from substance use (Shelder & Block, 1990). Therefore, in our primary analyses of drug or alcohol use, we distinguished between heavy and moderate drinkers. As we reported earlier (p. 189), a history of either sexual or physical abuse was associated with heavy use of drugs (Egeland, 1997).

The major variables we examined as antecedents of alcohol use were parental support and hostility measures from the preschool period and at age 13 (Englund, Hudson, & Egeland, 2003). Both parental hostility in the preschool period and hostility at age 13 discriminated heavy drinkers. These measures also correlated with how often the teens became drunk or high on drugs, as did attachment security and behavior problems in elementary school.

Associating with Deviant Youth

Associating with troubled youth, or "hanging out with the wrong crowd," is often given credit for all the problems of young people, especially in popular writing (e.g., Harris, 1998). In some ways, this is completely understandable. Associating with deviant peers is related to serious problem behaviors, such as drug and alcohol abuse, risky sexual behavior, and early pregnancy. These relationships were very strong in our own data, with correlations ranging from .28 to .52. Indeed, having friends that are troubled was far and away the strongest predictor of criminality in late adolescence (O'Brien, Huston, Egeland, & Duggal, 1998). At the same time, blaming all of the problems of youth on deviant friends is too simplistic. First of all, it would be just as valid to say that a strong network of *positive friends* is a protective factor for teens. Even more important, it misses the point that having such associates is itself a developmental outcome, however important it is for subsequent behavior. A comparison may be made to anxious attachment. We hope we have indicated clearly that we do not view such variations as *causing* later problems; rather, their importance is their part in a total developmental picture created over time, based on a complex array of factors. We believe that associating with deviant peers should be looked at in the same way.

Indeed, associating with deviant peers, as measured by a combination of teacher, mother, and child reports, was significantly predicted by our summary early care variable, as well as by parental support at grade 1 and parent–child boundary dissolution at age 13. However, these correlations were very small. Measures of earlier competence with peers told us more. Of note, being victimized by peers at summer camp correlated at .39; those who later associate with "troublemakers" have a history of low competence with peers. Recall that in middle childhood, those who were confident in themselves tended to form friendships with other confident and competent children. That meant that others were either left to associate with less competent children or were isolated. Either would make it more difficult to acquire the skills for later social functioning.

Similarly, those who are failing in school, or are expelled or drop out, have mostly others in like circumstances as candidates for association. We found very strong correlations with some of these measures. Most notably, the correlation between the 11th-grade school failure index discussed earlier and association with deviant peers was .55. Which is the chicken and which is the egg here is, of course, difficult to decide. By no means have we fully explained development of the tendency to congregate with deviant peers, but our findings point to an important direction for future work.

In general, our predictions of these adolescent risk behaviors were less strong than our predictions of competence at the same age. This is consistent with the notion that, for some teens, problems are newly emergent, while for others they are long-standing. We more closely examine this idea of two groups of troubled teens in Chapter 12, when we discuss our findings on the origins and course of psychopathology.

CONCLUSION

One of the emergent themes in our work is that the predictive power of variables depends on the particular outcome in question. Put another way, different developmental pictures emerge for distinctive outcomes that are always coherent but with varied patterning of predictors. Thus, for example, we predicted high school failure most strongly from measures of psychosocial adjustment in elementary school. Moreover, the most prominent of the relevant parenting variables were those from the parent–child teaching tasks at age 42 months. This is consistent with our discussion of earlier school outcomes in previous chapters. In predicting behavior problems, in contrast, we found that the strongest predictor was a climate of violence, chaos, and disruption in the home, perhaps especially in the early years. In contrast, supportive adult male presence appeared to be more important in the teen years than in the earlier years. Risky sexual behavior among girls (early and unprotected sex) was by far most strongly predicted by a middle childhood peer measure, namely, gender boundary violation (Collins, Hennighausen, Schmit, & Sroufe, 1997). Attachment history itself, while related to a range of teenage outcomes, was most clearly and strongly related to outcomes tapping intimacy and trust issues. Thus, attachment has its place in understanding adaptive and maladaptive functioning across time, but it is best placed within a broader array of antecedent conditions (Sroufe et al., 2005).

CHAPTER 10

The Transition to Adulthood

In recent months, Elton, age 20, had gotten very involved in soccer. The implications of this were bothering Yasmine. The following exchange took place during our problem-solving interview:

HE: I guess I haven't seen that big of a change, so I didn't think it was that big of a deal, but you feel it has been a big change on your part?

SHE: Yes, I do.

HE: In what way?

SHE: You don't call me as often. I don't see you as often.

HE: Do you think that has hurt our relationship?

SHE: Um . . . no, I don't think it has hurt it right now, but I think if it continues, it could, like I mean next year. 'Cause I feel like we just lose track of what each other feels. I know I love you and you do, that you love me. I just feel that by not spending any time with me, you make me feel like you don't care.

The partners sit facing each other, maintaining eye contact even when the discussion begins to make each of them more vulnerable. They give each other time to speak and respond to what they hear. Neither turns away from the other or becomes defensive at any point.

In Western culture, the end of the second decade of life and the beginning of the third is a time for pulling together past achievements, forging a plan for the future, and assuming more self-direction in one's life. It is also a time to evolve further one's capacity to be involved in intimate partnerships. Such tasks may require the next decade and beyond, but the capacities for intimacy and for integration should be apparent in both the behavior and the representations of the well-functioning person, even at this relatively early age. For many young people, the developmental history contains a solid foundation of emotional support, opportunities for engaging in successful peer relationships in each developmental period, adequate academic preparation, and ample experiences in successful problem solving. They have acquired a sense of themselves as both capable and valued. What remains is to draw upon these experiences in a coordinated way to create a meaningful adult life. For those whose history has been in some way compromised, the task of integration is more challenging, but the cognitive capacities available by the end of adolescence allow a reconsideration of the past and the possibility of setting a new direction. One can see, for example, that negative treatment by parents was not deserved, that people vary in their capacity for caring, and that certain patterns of behavior may punish others but also harm the self.

In more specific terms, one must move toward the possibility of self-responsibility and of life outside of the family of origin. Self-responsibility need not mean financial self-sufficiency, but it should entail some kind of active involvement in preparing for self-sufficiency. Either the individual must be making meaningful forays into the area of work or must be actively pursuing educational or training opportunities that will support work or career. At the same time, developing adult relationships and social support networks, if not emerging, at least should be glimpsed on the horizon, even while individuals continue to draw support from family. Finally, young people must evolve a sense of personal responsibility. This entails knowledge that they are indeed the ones in charge of directing their own lives, as well as the capacity to establish reasonable goals and the ability to appraise their progress toward these goals.

We assessed our participants' negotiation of these transition-to-adulthood tasks, both globally and more specifically. We conducted extensive interviews that covered living arrangements, work, training/education, and relationships with families and friends, among other things (see Chapter 4). We got not only the facts about the young people's circumstances but also information regarding goals and aspirations, the setbacks they had experienced, and what actions they were taking in the face of those setbacks. From interviews at age 19, we were able to make global ratings of the young person's adjustment and quality of the established social support network. We also assessed amount of life stress, physical and emotional health issues, and representation of childhood attachments (the Adult Attachment Interview). Beginning at age 20, for all those involved in romantic relationships, we conducted an observational assessment of the couple and administered an extensive battery of instruments to each member of the couple. Another extensive interview, conducted at age 23, also is used in this chapter as a basis for discussing work ethic and other aspects of work competence.

The differentiation of antecedent–outcome linkages that was apparent earlier is more pronounced in early adulthood. Some outcomes in adult functioning are best predicted by experiences with peers. Some, especially those tapping into capacities for emotional closeness in relationships, are most strongly tied to the history of care and, in particular, to attachment experiences. Others are best predicted by experiences in school. Moreover, the nature of the ties between experience of care and particular outcomes also varies, with effects sometimes being direct, sometimes indirect, through intermediate outcomes in a different setting, and sometimes both direct and indirect.

GLOBAL ADJUSTMENT IN EARLY ADULTHOOD

We begin with results of a rating of "Global Adjustment" at age 19, based on the totality of information from the extensive interview. In addition to considering in a general way the young person's movement toward autonomy, three major criteria guided the rater: adequate progress in the work/training/school area; meaningful relationships with family, friends, and partners; and a functional level of self-awareness.

The first two criteria are straightforward and rather easily judged on a factual level. Are the individuals engaged in a substantial and continuous way (20 hours a week or more) in some combination of work, training, or school? Do they have a stable group of friends with whom they are involved? Can they draw upon family support? Do they have experience with more intimate relationships in some form? The third criterion is more difficult to define in a few words, but in some ways it is the most important at this age. Young people, of course, experience failures and at times do not have truly good options available to them. Sometimes past problems pose obstacles. They may have been mistaken about what they wanted or might change their minds. One may, for example, be in a job that, as it turns out, he really does not like, and because of this, performance is compromised. But if he has some insight into this, if he has formed and is executing a clear plan to change his situation (e.g., "I'm taking a night class in computers at Metro, and I really like it"), he may well be on track for this age. Therefore, to get the highest rating on our 5-point scale did not require that there be no problems, but the person had to "be aware of obstacles he might have to surmount while pursuing his goals." Likewise, another young person might be working full time in a job she does not like and say she has plans to get her general equivalency diploma (GED), so that she can improve her work situation. If this plan is realistic, and if she has taken concrete steps in this direction, she may (given solid relationships, etc.) also get the highest score. But the presence of only a vague plan, with no evidence of putting it into action, would lower the score. Similarly, relationship problems are common; more important is the kind of insight the person has regarding such problems.

In addition to these verbal descriptions and definitions of scale points, the rater was given sample summaries of actual cases that described the scale points. This is an application of Ainsworth's template-matching approach described in Chapter 3. For example, one of three templates for the middle scale point (3) was as follows:

> Participant has dropped out of high school and is now enrolled in an alternative learning center, which he attends a few times a week. He plans to obtain his high school degree eventually but does not appear to be in any hurry. Participant has a part-time job for 10 hours a week. He has no plan for the future, and this is beginning to trouble him a bit due to his 5-month-old relationship with a college-bound young woman who attends the regular high school. He believes that the band he is in may someday "make it big," although they have not yet played for money. Participant has a slightly tense relationship with his mother due to his avoidance of any interaction with her. He is confused by his own behavior. Participant has never connected with his father and is currently not speaking with him. Participant has been thinking a lot about his relationship with his parents and seems to want to make changes. Participant has several close male friends.

A score lower than 3 would be given if there were an even spottier educational and work situation, or if there were fewer social connections. A higher score would require more current involvement in work and/or training and more insight into his situation. We see this kind of rating as a compromise between unspecified subjective judgments and highly reliable, discrete measures, which are not as meaningful. It is a lot easier to say whether someone is working or not, but this simply may not tell us what we want to know about the person's level of maturity. The validity of any procedure is ultimately decided by its correlates. As described below, this rating had notable validity. We believe that it captured well in general terms how well our participants were doing at age 19.

Indeed, adaptation at each preceding age was associated with the global adjustment measure. Peer competence measures in preschool and at each grade in elementary school, and family stress and support during these years, all were highly significant, with correlations in the .30s.

Compositing just peer competence across the elementary school grades, the correlation was .38. Likewise, measures of early care also predicted global adjustment at age 19. Each component of early care, including attachment security at 12–18 months, was modestly correlated with global adjustment at age 19, and a composite early care variable from ages 6 months to 6 years was correlated at .34 with the measure at age 19. When elementary peer competence was combined with early parental care, the resulting multiple correlation was .45. This is substantial prediction across a decade of further development. When we also added the amount of stress and social support that the young person was experiencing in middle adolescence, the final multiple correlation was .55; all of this without including a history of behavior problems. Clearly, adaptation at the edge of adulthood builds on a cumulative history beginning early in life.

It was also interesting to note that measures of emotional health and behavior problems in elementary school were themselves highly predictive of global adjustment. The Total Problems score on the Teacher Report Form across the elementary school years, without being combined with any other measure, yielded a correlation of −.45. This is striking, because emotional disturbance and pathology were not explicitly part of the global adjustment rating (since they were independently assessed). They would enter in, of course, to whatever extent they compromised functioning in the school, work, and relationship areas. Thus, we take these findings as affirmation of the great importance of behavioral and emotional problems in childhood for later adjustment and of their role in social functioning. These data also are further testimony to the coherence of individual development.

Finally, every measure of relationship representation we obtained from preschool through adolescence (stories, drawings, and narratives) forecasted global adjustment, with correlations ranging from .24 to .40. As we explain in Chapter 11, we found the highest correlations when we had multiple measures available at the given age. The point for now is that internalized relationship experiences, as well as assessments of manifest behavior, allow prediction of late adolescent/early adult outcomes.

SOCIAL RELATIONSHIP OUTCOMES

Social Support Network at Age 19

In addition to analyzing this global outcome data, we also examined components of adaptive social functioning, often with more specific hypotheses in mind. One of these, "Richness of the Social Support Network," is discussed next. It is our general hypothesis that each component of global adjustment also is predictable from history. Having a good support network, which one may consider a current asset, is itself a developmental construction. Since this measure was drawn from the interview at 19 years, it was not surprising that it had virtually all of the same correlates as the global competence measure discussed earlier. Moreover, because it may be thought of as one component of the global competence measure, the magnitude of the correlations was generally smaller for this index than for the global measure. There were, however, a few interesting exceptions. For example, relationship support for the *mother* in middle childhood and quality of a friendship of the teen at age 16 predicted age 19 social support as well as they predicted the broader global adjustment measure. These variables all may be specifically related to an underlying capacity to draw strength from the social world.

Thus, not only is having a good social support system a predictable outcome, but also the total array of findings suggests the discriminant validity of both outcome and predictor measures. As we discuss later, this trend is even clearer with certain other early adult outcomes in the school and work arenas.

Observed Romantic Relationships in Early Adulthood

We made direct behavioral assessments on 74 couples between the ages of 20 and 21 years (and these assessments are ongoing). Scales were parallel to those used in the observational family assessments described in Chapter 9 (relationship balance, affective tone, conflict, and conflict resolution scales). A number of analyses await more of our participants' forming partnerships; still, the early findings provided ample support for the developmental construction position regarding adult competence. Some of the findings are complicated, involving analyses of how certain variables impact the relations between attachment history and relationship outcomes, so we provide an interpretive summary after presenting these results.

First, as strongly predicted by theory, infant attachment history predicted numerous aspects of intimate relationship functioning, including a composite relationship process variable (the "balance scales"; see Chapters 4 and 9). Disorganized attachment (e.g., Main & Solomon, 1990) was an especially good predictor, correlating strongly two decades later with the composite process variable (.35), and with ratings of the couple's hostility in interaction (.42). Insecurity composites from 12 and 18 months tended to yield modest or moderate correlations across the range of romantic relationship variables.

The second point is that elementary peer competence measures (teacher rankings in grades 1–3) and parent–child interaction measures at age 13 also were related to the romantic relationship outcomes, and when either or both were added to the infant attachment measure, prediction was often significantly increased (to the .30s or .40s). For example, when a composite of parent support measures at age 13 (Balance I and II; see Chapters 4 and 9) was added to attachment security in predicting the capacity of the romantic couple to resolve conflict, the correlation rose from .27 to .36, with the change being significant. In this case, there was also evidence for partial mediation. Some of the variance explained by infant attachment was due to the measure at age 13, and when it was included, the link to infant attachment was no longer significant. When conflict resolution between parent and child at age 13 was substituted as a predictor, the result was very similar (with the multiple correlation at .39). When teacher-rated peer competence was included in the regression following attachment, there was again a significant increment in predicting couples' conflict resolution, but no evidence for mediation. Thus, attachment history and peer experiences both contributed to young adults' capacity to resolve conflict, but their contributions were independent. With frequency of conflict, in contrast to capacity for conflict resolution, there was some evidence that attachment influence was mediated by later peer experiences (Sroufe et al., 2005).

When couples' observed hostility was the outcome, both parent–child interaction measures at age 13 and elementary school peer competence accounted for significant additional variance, beyond that accounted for by infant attachment. In the case of the peer variable, the contributions again seemed to be largely independent (even though the attachment and peer variables are related); there was no evidence for mediation. Various measures at 13 years also accounted for variance beyond infant attachment in predicting couples' hostility, and in the case of the composite parent support variable at 13 years, there was again evidence for partial mediation. In this case, however, even with the evidence for an indirect effect for attachment, the direct effect also remained significant. Thus, for this emotional aspect of young adult romantic relationships, early attachment seemed to retain a direct influence, in addition to that of its impact through later parenting.

To summarize, the complex capacities required for well-functioning romantic relationships draw upon the individual's entire history of social experience: early emotional closeness with caregivers, ongoing parental support, and history of competence with peers (see Sroufe et al., 2005, for a more complete discussion). This is true even when the variable in question is loaded with attachment relevance, such as hostility in couples' relationships. Precisely how these different aspects of history work together, however, seems to vary with the particular outcome in question. For some variables, such as amount of conflict, peer experiences seem to be most important, and they mediate the effect of early care; that is, early care appears to have its impact through its role in promoting positive middle childhood peer experiences. Thus, perhaps, a secure attachment history promotes engagement and closeness with peers. Then, in that context, one practices skills in negotiated interaction with an agemate that will later serve to mitigate conflict in romantic relationships. For other variables, early attachment experiences, or attachment and later family experiences together, have more predictive strength. Generally, these are emotional tone and trust aspects of relationships.

Reported Relationship Difficulties and Satisfaction

Other measures of romantic relationship quality were derived from interviews and a self-report battery filled out by the couple, producing results that were consistent with those based on our observations (Collins & van Dulmen, in press-a). For example, infant attachment security significantly predicted responses to Hendrick's (1988) measure of relationship satisfaction at age 21 ($r = .32$), as did peer competence in elementary school (a composite of teacher rankings in grades 1–3). Again, there was evidence for partial mediation, and with peer competence in the regression, the link with attachment no longer was significant. This again supports the notion that, at times, attachment prepares the way for successful relationships with peers, and these latter relationship experiences then provide the platform for satisfying romantic relationships in adulthood.

The middle childhood measures also were strong predictors of reported relationship violence. These data were based on the widely used Conflict Tactics Scales (Strauss, 1979, 1990), specifically, the reported frequency of various acts of aggression (e.g., shouting, pushing, hitting, threatening with weapons). Those with lower peer competence in middle childhood were more likely both to use and to be the victims of such actions.

Relationship Representation: The Adult Attachment Interview and the Current Relationship Interview

We first administered the Berkeley Adult Attachment Interview (AAI; George et al., 1985; Main & Goldwyn, 1998) at age 19. As described in Chapter 4, this interview is aimed at capturing the adult's representation of attachments, based on descriptions of childhood experiences with parents. It in part entails providing adjectives or phrases describing caregiving relationships and examples to document these descriptions. The Current Relationships Interview (CRI; Crowell & Owens, 1996), is parallel to the AAI in format but is centered on a current salient relationship with a partner. We administered this beginning at age 20 to our participants (and their partners) who had formed a romantic relationship. The antecedents and correlates of these two procedures are described in this section, beginning with the AAI.

The AAI aims to capture the young adults' "current state of mind" regarding attachment. Like other measures used in our study, this measure is believed to reflect a developmental construction. Thus, while early childhood history is part of this construction, and is often salient because of the preverbal nature of early experiences, it is the entire history of attachment-relevant experiences that is represented. Even though each history contains a variety of experiences, with perhaps quite different relationships with two parents, for example, nonetheless, a singular state of mind typically results. Depending on the cumulated history, qualitatively different states of mind evolve. Some individuals' states of mind are classified as "autonomous" (parallel to "secure" in infancy). These individuals can think freely, openly, and coherently about their attachment experiences, and they recognize the importance of attachment and value such experiences. Note that this does not imply that all of their experiences have been positive. When experiences have been negative, autonomous individuals view them with some understanding and often forgiveness, and see such experiences as nonetheless important in their development. Other individuals manifest a "preoccupied" state of mind, remaining entangled in past angers and disappointments, while still others are "dismissing," either of their own feelings or attachment issues in general. Both of these are considered nonautonomous or insecure states of mind. Finally, individuals who have experienced serious loss or trauma may be categorized as resolved or unresolved regarding these experiences. This is independent of primary state of mind regarding attachment, but being unresolved is considered insecure. (See Chapter 4 for more complete descriptions of all these categories.)

Our findings on the relationship between AAI status and other measures of representation throughout childhood and adolescence are presented later in Chapter 11. Here, we focus in particular on whether the AAI and CRI are related to a secure attachment experience in infancy.

Overall, our findings regarding infant attachment and the AAI at age 19 were not strong, with the exception of predictions from infant disorganization (Weinfield, Sroufe, & Egeland, 2000). Disorganized infant attachment was modestly predictive of a nonautonomous state of mind. In addition, and in accord with theoretical predictions, continuous ratings of disorganization in the infant attachment assessments related to unresolved abuse ($r = .48$; Weinfield, Whaley, & Egeland, 2004); that is, not only was disorganized attachment related to abuse in childhood, but also those abused children who were disorganized as infants more often showed a failure to integrate these experiences on the young adult AAI.

Despite these impressive findings for disorganization, we found that neither infant ABC attachment status nor the integrative early care variable were significantly related to the AAI at 19 years, either based on category analysis or with use of continuous scores for coherence of the AAI transcript (Weinfield et al., 2000, 2004). Quite strikingly, only 37% of our participants were classified as autonomous, and 8% were classed as preoccupied. The majority of our participants (55%), and even the majority of those who as infants had been secure, were *dismissing* on the AAI. They claimed perhaps no memory for childhood attachment experiences or derogated attachment experiences (e.g., trivialized their importance), or they may have idealized their parents, describing them in globally positive terms, but without being able to provide supporting examples. In some way, they kept attachment feelings at a distance. In any case, such a high proportion of dismissing cases guaranteed weak results from infancy, where only 22% had been avoidant (the category conceptually linked to dismissing).

Some studies have found a link between secure infant attachment and later AAI autonomy. Both Hamilton (2000) and Waters, Merrick, Treboux, Crowell, and Albersheim (2000) reported such a link using *low-risk* samples, in contrast to our findings with a high-risk sample. Main, Hesse, and Kaplan (2005) also reported significant associations between AAI autonomy and secure attachment assessed at age 6 and in infancy with a low-risk sample. They also reported interesting connections between specific scales from the infant assessment and AAI scales. However, the overall significant relation between infant security and AAI autonomy was found only when they included the infant disorganized category as insecure in infancy. Including disorganization with other insecure patterns did not lead to a significant overall finding for us.

Other studies failed to find a link between infant ABC measures and later attachment representation with low-risk samples (Becker-Stoll & Fremmer-Bombik, 1997; Lewis, Feiring, & Rosenthal, 2000; Zimmerman, 1994). None of these studies, however, used the AAI coding procedure. In addition, the Lewis and colleagues (2000) study used a truncated Strange Situation assessment that was not demonstrated to have validity as a measure of attachment.

Our own failure to link infant attachment security in general to the AAI is more complicated. Our assessments of attachment have been amply validated, throughout this book and in numerous publications. Moreover, our assessments were conducted primarily by the same people who did the coding in the successful Waters study. Likewise, our AAIs have some validity. They were predicted by family measures at 13 years, and they predicted quality romantic relationships 1–2 years later (Roisman, Madsen, Hennighausen, Sroufe, & Collins, 2001), as we discuss in more detail in Chapter 11. Finally, we showed that discontinuity between infant and early adult assessments was lawful (Weinfield et al., 2004). For example, those who changed from secure toddlers to nonautonomous young adults had experienced greater life stress throughout childhood and adolescence than those who remained secure. They also showed poorer parent–child relationships at age 13. Those who changed from insecure to autonomous had more supportive home lives at age 6 and less frequently experienced maltreatment than those who remained insecure. Thus, it seems unlikely that our nonsignificant findings are simply due to measurement error.

Given the total array of findings, we concluded at this point that the results had something to do with the nature of our high-risk sample. Even Waters and colleagues (2000) and Hamilton (2000) found evidence for some change between infancy and adulthood, and this change was related to major stresses (e.g., divorce). Clearly, the life stress and general instability of our sample was much greater than in either of their studies, so much so that "divorce" is not even a meaningful variable for us. Still, we have found infant attachment to be related to other early adult outcomes, so life instability cannot be all there is to it. Also, the large number of dismissing cases needs to be explained. We think this may have to do with level of development of the young people when this first AAI was administered. The AAI presumes that one has matured to the point of stepping outside of one's childhood experience, so that perspective taking and a reflective integration are possible. For young people, many from economically disadvantaged circumstances and still living at home, this may be challenging. Consider, for example, those who hold that negative experiences in the family had no impact on them (one manifestation of a dismissing state of mind). While in late adolescence, and still living at home, such a stance may be a prudent temporary adaptation. How can one face that it is a terrible situation and stay in it? Thus, the age of our participants and the nature of our sample may have reduced the validity of the AAI. The Becker-Stoll and Fremmer-Bombik (1997), Lewis and colleagues (2000), and Zimmerman (1994) studies, which also failed to find significant ties between infant attachment and attachment representation, used adolescents as well. Our longitudinal data allowed us to sort through some of these alternatives by repeating the AAI at a later age. We report on our somewhat more positive findings at 26 years in Chapter 14. There were notably fewer dismissing cases.

In contrast to the AAI, and in accord with our developmental construction theory, representation measures derived from the CRI were significantly related *both* to ABC attachment history and to later experiences (Roisman, Collins, Sroufe, & Egeland, 2005). Perhaps this is because the participants were slightly older, or perhaps it was due to discussion of a nonparental relationship. Still, it is a striking finding over a gap of 20 years. The CRI also was related to a variety of self-report measures of relationship closeness and satisfaction, and to directly observed quality of the interaction of the couple. Moreover, CRI responses added significantly to prediction of couple behavior, above and beyond the other self-report measures. At the same time, infant attachment security added to observed couple behavior in predicting the CRI. *Thus, how one represents a current relationship is based in part in early history and in part in current experience with the partner.* We say more about these kinds of complex relations in Chapter 11 on the developmental process.

EDUCATIONAL OUTCOMES

We examined three educational outcomes in early adulthood. First, we looked at those who had and had not dropped out of high school by age 19. Then, at age 23, we looked at the number of years of education completed, which could serve as a continuous measure. Finally, in subsequent years, we did a special analysis to determine predictors of returning to complete the high school degree for those who had earlier dropped out.

Predicting High School Dropout

Dropping out of school is a serious problem among youth, in terms of both personal and societal implications (Jimerson, Egeland, Sroufe, & Carlson, 2000). These literally millions of young people are ill-prepared for the modern workforce, and are consequently likely to face economic hardship, as well as pay less tax to support the general welfare. Moreover, they are disproportionately represented in criminal activities and incarceration statistics (Kirsch, Jungeblut, Jenkins, & Kolstad, 1993), with attendant personal and societal costs.

Dropping out, like many phenomena, is best viewed as a dynamic developmental process. It follows a course that can be described. At this point in time, dropping out no longer poses a mystery. It is well understood and largely predictable. Early studies of the problem pointed to achievement test scores or attendance and discipline problems in high school and junior high school as predictors. We wanted to elaborate and extend these findings, especially drawing upon our wide-ranging data from the early years.

As had so many others, we found that our achievement test measures from high school, middle school, and even early elementary school were related to later dropping out. However, in our project, we came to view such achievement problems not as causes, but as *markers* of the process late in its unfolding (Jimerson et al., 2000). In other words, many of the young people doing poorly in school, irregularly attending, and so forth, already are dropping out, at least psychologically. At some point, they are so far along the path that it stretches the term "prediction."

We were interested in finding out both how early the pathway to dropping out is initiated and what some of the key steps are along the way. As in traditional studies, we included IQ, SES, and achievement test performance in our analyses. We also looked at behavior problems, as others have done, although we included problems apparent at the beginning of school, as well as late elementary school problems. In addition to these traditional measures, however, we also looked at the history of early care and the early quality of the home environment, as measured by the Caldwell HOME Inventory, as well as parental involvement with school and successful relationships with peers.

Our comprehensive investigation led us to see both that the process begins quite early and that psychosocial factors play a critical role (Jimerson et al., 2000). The first finding was that all of the early psychosocial variables were significantly related to dropping out, the average correlation being around .30. This was comparable to the strength of the preschool WIPPSI and third-grade WISC-R IQ tests (r's = .29 and .27, respectively) and achievement test results across the school years. Only behavior problems and peer competence measures in elementary school predicted outcomes better (r range = .30 to .40).

Next, we used logistic regression to combine predictors. Logistic regression is similar to other regression techniques but can be used with categorical data, for example, dropping out or not dropping out of school. It allows one to say what percentage of cases may be predicted. We found that we were able to predict dropping out with 77% accuracy, *using only quality-of-care measures up to age 42 months*. Thus, by age 3½ years, dropping out was substantially predictable, even within our largely lower SES sample; that is, our findings in part control for the well-known influence of poverty on dropping out. Neither IQ nor achievement test data improved upon this prediction.

Finally, we used discriminant function analysis to test directly the relative power of the entire set of predictors up to grade 6 to discriminate dropping out from completing school. The most powerful variable was behavior problems in grade 6 (Wilkes lambda = .83). This is not surprising and probably reflects alienation from school, as well as difficulty getting along with peers and teachers. The next two significant variables were early quality of care (.77) and sixth-grade parental involvement (.74). Grade 1 problem behavior was next (.72), followed by gender (more boys; .71) and SES at grade 3 (.70). Neither IQ nor achievement test scores were significant when considered within this set of variables.

These findings strongly attest to the importance of psychosocial variables in the process of dropping out. Young people do not drop out of school because they are inherently incapable of doing the work. They do indeed become unable to do the work (later achievement tests predict better than earlier achievement tests), but this is in important ways influenced by psychosocial factors. By age 3½, well before the start of formal schooling, some children already are on a pathway that probabilistically leads to dropping out. Later, lack of parental involvement contributes to maintaining the child on the path. The other strong predictor of dropping out—earlier behavior problems—itself is predicted by a history of inadequate care, lack of support, and high stress (see Chapters 8 and 9).

Finally, in our interview at age 19, we asked all of the young people if they had ever had a teacher who was "special" for them, who took a particular interest in them, and whom they felt was "in their corner." A dramatically significant result was obtained. The vast majority of those who completed high school said "yes," and often were able to name more than one teacher. Most of those who dropped out said "no," and many of them looked at the interviewer as if an unfathomable question had been asked. Having such a special relationship with a teacher is, of course, another developmental outcome, predictable from earlier history. Nonetheless, relationships with teachers clearly are important, and we very much enjoyed sharing this information with the many remarkable teachers who participated in our study. Of more than 1,000 teachers that we asked to provide information over the years, only two declined.

Educational Attainment by Age 23

Educational attainment, like every other major outcome in our study, was based upon the young adult's cumulative history, beginning early in life (see Table 10.1). The 6- to 42-month early care composite, for example, correlated .32 with years of school completed by age 23, and the quality of the HOME environment at school entry correlated .30. As was the case with earlier educational outcomes, child behavior with the mother in our 42-month teaching tasks also was predictive of educational outcome at age 23, with the correlations for persistence, enthusiasm, and compliance all highly significant.

TABLE 10.1. Correlations between Child Experience and Adaptation across Time and Highest Educational Attainment (23 Years) ($N = 126$)

Variable	Highest educational attainment
Early caregiving experience (6–42 months)	.32***
Quality of home environment (30 months)	.30***
Child Persistence rating (42 months)	.30***
Child Enthusiasm rating (42 months)	.27**
Child Compliance rating (42 months)	.29***
Emotional health teacher ranking (grades 1–3, 6)	.46***
Peer competence teacher ranking (grades 1–3, 6)	.42***
TRF Behavior problem (grades 1–3, 6)	−.38***
WISCR IQ (grade 3)	.33***
Parental expectations of child achievement (grade 1)	.39***
Child–parent collaboration (13 years)	.48***
Overall adaptation (19 years)	.61***

$^*p < .05;$ $^{**}p < .01;$ $^{***}p < .001$

Again, not just the early years were important. In fact, predictions from psychosocial adjustment in the elementary period were notably stronger. Teacher emotional health/self-esteem rankings across the elementary years correlated with final educational outcome (.46), while the correlations for behavior problems and peer competence rankings were .38 and .42, respectively. *These were notably higher than the correlation for IQ (.33) and remained significant with IQ controlled.* The ongoing context of development in elementary school also was important, with both experienced family stress and social support being significant. Parental expectations for achievement at grade 1 correlated with future attainment (.39). This measure also was significant above and beyond measures of early care and IQ (Englund et al., 2005). Thus, both caring for and believing in the child are of great importance.

Early adolescent measures also were related to adult educational outcome. The correlations with scales for parental support (balance in the relationship) from our age 13 assessment were modest but significant. Recently, coders who were blind to all knowledge about the child rescored these tapes, this time focusing on child behavior and rating scales specifically designed to forecast educational outcomes (e.g., Englund et al., 2003). These scales included the teen's engagement with the tasks, enthusiasm, positive and negative affect, self-assurance, and collaborative attitude. The collaborative attitude scale reflects the child's desire to work together with the parent, based on the eager, receptive quality of cooperation, and on actively striving for joint understanding. Children who scored at the lowest level were distancing, or attempted to redefine joint tasks as individual ones. Each of these scales predicted number of years of education, with the collaborative attitude scale correlating the highest. The composite of all scales correlated (.46) with ultimate educational outcome. Not surprisingly, measures of adaptation in later adolescence correlated strongly with adult educational outcome, with correlations generally in the .40s. The global adjustment measure at age 19 correlated (.61) with this outcome 4 years later.

Combining measures through regression analysis allowed us to forecast ultimate educational attainment quite well. Thus, by school entry (combining early care and the grade 1 HOME), the multiple correlation was .35. Early care plus elementary peer competence or emotional health ranking yielded even stronger correlations (in the high .40s). This is a substantial predictive relationship across more than a decade.

All of these results were even stronger when we reanalyzed this database using our age 26 interview. With the educational story now more complete, even the composite early care variable was strongly predictive (.42).

As with our assessment of dropping out, ultimate level of educational attainment appears to be heavily influenced by psychosocial history. While causal conclusions cannot be derived from correlational data, it is noteworthy that measures of care, self-esteem, and supportiveness of surrounding context were consistently more powerful than child or maternal IQ in predicting this outcome. It is, on the one hand, discouraging that so many children face so much adversity in the school area; on the other hand, it is encouraging to consider that their problems often are not due to inherent limitations.

Finally, when we returned to the question of accounting for those who returned to finish high school or to get their GED after dropping out, we found that those who accomplished this task had more positive early care than those who did not. We continue to collect these data.

WORK OUTCOMES

Work Ethics and Work Competence

Our primary analyses of work attitudes and competence have been based on our interview of participants at age 23. Questions we asked were more extensive at this age, and it is obviously easier to gauge work-related competence after the participants have more experience. One key feature of these analyses was our a priori interest in middle childhood predictors. Following Erikson and others, we view middle childhood as the era in which children generally develop work habits, effectiveness, and a sense of the self as competent and hardworking (the sense of industry). We believed that measures of middle childhood competence in general, and measures of initiative and diligence in the school setting in particular, should be related to work ethic and work competence in early adulthood (Collins et al., in press-b; Hyson, 2002).

In addition to measures of achievement and peer competence in elementary school that we have already described, we also derived specific measures of "initiative" from teacher ratings on subscales of the Devereaux Elementary School Behavior Rating Scale (see Chapter 4). The subscales used for our initiative composite were level of organization, initiative in group discussions and activities, need for direction in completing work, and perseverance (Hyson, 2002). The outcome for our first analysis was "work ethic." This 5-point rating scale tapped both the importance of work in the young person's life and the level of responsibility shown regarding work during the past year. Again, as with the global adjustment scale, anchor descriptions were provided that fit various scale points to guide the rater. In addition to our initiative variable, other predictors included in this first analysis were achievement, IQ, and SES.

The strongest predictor of work ethic was, as predicted, the elementary school initiative measure ($r = .35$). Elementary achievement test scores also predicted work ethic significantly, but more modestly, and only initiative was significant when these two measures were combined in the same model, using path analysis (Hyson, 2002). Although in the expectable direction, neither IQ nor SES were significantly predictive.

In a subsequent analysis, another measure of work competence was used (Collins et al., in press-b). This composite of three scales tapped the degree to which our participants had explored possible career choices, evaluated their career goals, and formulated an overarching plan. Together, these were thought to capture work maturity. Predictors here included early care and peer competence in middle childhood. While both of these variables modestly predicted the work competence outcome, the middle childhood peer competence measure was the more powerful predictor (and, again, larger than IQ). Only it remained significant in regression analysis. Moreover, path analysis showed that it in part mediated the effect of early care, which became nonsignificant.

CONCLUSION

Age by age, at every point, negotiation of the salient issues of the era has been found to build upon foundations laid down in the previous phase, which, in turn, were supported by adaptations and supports in the previous phase, and so on, all the way back to the earliest years of life. In this sense, certainly, the early years are important. Beyond this, in certain arenas, and at certain times, early experiences in caregiving relationships seemed to be of notable importance, even in comparison with later experiences. When we discuss disturbance in Chapter 12, we encounter this again, for example, in describing the profound consequences of maltreatment. Nonetheless, virtually without exception, predictions to later outcomes were most powerful when early care was combined with later care, when measures of care were combined with measures of surrounding context, and when experiences with both parents and peers were considered.

We believe the cross-time associations we have described are compelling. To us, however, these data are only the starting point for the more intriguing developmental questions. These questions concern the processes underlying these connections, the principles that govern continuity and change, and the relations between normal and disturbed development. These are questions to which we turn our attention in Part III of this book.

PART III

Development and Psychopathology

CHAPTER 11

The Developmental Process

> In a sense, early experiences (especially with a primary
> caregiver) help to create a "grammar of emotion" that may
> be enduring, even though the language of emotion continues
> to unfold in the years to come.
> —THOMPSON (2003)

The motivation for our study always has been much more than
demonstrating the predictive significance of early experience or even that
each age forecasts behavior at the next. Primarily, we were interested in
understanding the developmental process; that is, how development
works. We wanted to know not just that there were connections between
salient experiences at one age and behavior at the next, but why and
how such connections happened. And we wanted to understand the
complexities of how prior history and current circumstances worked together, not just that both were important. Why do individuals show continuity of functioning across development? How is change accomplished? And what happens to prior adaptation or the history of
experience following developmental change?

We return again to discussion of the developmental principles that
have guided our work, trusting that these principles now will be more
readily understood, in light of the data presented in the preceding chapters. The first of these principles concerns the *unity of the organism*, that
is, the idea that the behaviors, thoughts and emotions of the person cannot be segregated. That the mind and the body are one has much to do
with the continuity of human development. "Mentalizing" about experi-

ence, to use Peter Fonagy's (1999) term, is part of what connects past to present. The second major principle has to do with *emerging complexity*. This is the idea that the child, as developed to any given point, transacts with current challenges and supports such that new complexity of organized functioning emerges. This new complexity is not foreordained by the prior functioning of the child, nor is it dictated by the new conditions. It is always a product of the interplay of both. Something qualitatively new is now present that embodies both continuity and change. The third principle concerns *children as active creators of their own development*. Experience creates the child but, at the same time, the child creates experience, through seeking, reacting to, and interpreting the world in individual ways.

These three principles lead to a dynamic view of the developmental process. It centers on the ongoing interplay of person and environment. Because humans participate actively in creating their own experience, what they experience and take forward from any given age frames their later experience to a notable degree. At the same time, salient experiences, especially experiences in important relationships, can have a transforming influence on the person. As we discuss later, this does not mean that the prior experience is then erased; rather, it simply means that there is a new level of complexity of the person. In keeping with the notion of hierarchical integration that we described in Chapter 2, we argue that the meaning of the prior experience is altered by virtue of its organization into a more complex personality structure. In light of transforming experience, prior experience now is part of a different framework for facing the future and interpreting the world. But it is "still there," and its relative salience depends on many complicated factors, such as particular circumstances, particular stresses that may arise, particular settings, and the nature of subsequent experience. In this chapter, we amplify upon these considerations, with special attention to continuity and change in development, the problem of resilience, and the interplay of representation, experience, and behavior.

CONTINUITY AND CHANGE

Continuity and change both are inherently part of any definition of development. Development means something emerging from what was there before. Continuity is the relationship between the two, whatever that may be. A simple kaleidoscope of forms would not be development. Likewise, development is change, although, to us, a particular kind of change—toward increasing complexity of organization. Without such change, there is no development. Thus, development always entails both continuity and change. This is no different when our focus becomes individual development. Asking whether individual development is most characterized by continuity or by change is not an apt question. In our view, past experienced and former patterns of adaptation are never erased; they are always part of an increasingly elaborated structure. At the same time, patterns of adaptation cannot remain exactly the same. Not only do changing contexts press for new ways of adapting, but emerging issues of life at different ages also make different requirements and call for greater complexity of organization. Thus, for continuity in competence, the adaptation of the individual *must* change. Important questions, thus, center not on the fact of continuity and change but on the nature of continuity and the nature of change, and how they are governed.

Several different supports for continuity of individual development may be put forward. The simplest, and most widely embraced, is that there is continuity in basic environmental assets, challenges, or general circumstances. For example, Alicia Lieberman (1977) years ago reported that parents of securely attached children also tended to promote encounters with peers (supporting visits, etc.). Thus, some of the tie between attachment and peer competence could be due to linking environmental supports. Similarly, we found some connection between early childhood support and later parental involvement at school. Moreover, we actually examined the continuity in the general quality of parental care. Such empirical study has been surprisingly rare given how much importance has been attributed to this proposition. As reported in earlier chapters, we found moderate correlations across periods, both from infancy to the preschool period, and from age 3½ to age 13 (Hiester, 1993; Pianta, Sroufe, & Egeland, 1989). Thus, continuity in the environment is one explanation for individual continuity, but not likely the only one.

The second explanation centers on early-established brain systems, especially those regulating arousal and emotion (Schore, 1994; Siegel, 1999). Related to this are dyadic patterns of emotional response that are reactivated in later social encounters. There is little direct human evidence for these positions, with the exception of early extreme circumstances of deprivation (e.g., Nelson et al., in press). However, increasing knowledge regarding early brain development and emotional development makes such a position plausible, especially in terms of lasting vulnerabilities. Also, many findings fit with such notions and are not easily explained without them. For example, the data we presented in Chapter 7 on empathy and peer victimization in preschool call for such an interpretation. Children who experienced parental mistreatment were not themselves reinforced for being mean, yet when seeing someone else in a condition of striking vulnerability, such a malevolent response seemed almost automatic. In contrast, children who were treated empathically responded with care or concern. Thus, prior dyadic patterns of emotional regulation appear to have been carried forward. We have more to say about this in Chapter 14. For now, keep in mind that, in our view, this explanation does not require immutability, just that different patterns may be more or less readily activated in individuals with different histories.

A third explanation for continuity, which ties together the above considerations, centers on the transactional developmental process. The nature and impact of new experiences are conditioned by history. For example, toddlers who have experienced inconsistency, chaotic care, and ultimately resistant attachment in infancy often have tantrums and are difficult. What they need as toddlers is clear, firm, consistent limits with support, and they need this more than do most toddlers. This, of course, is precisely what is difficult for their caregivers to provide, so the pattern of adaptation is deepened and carried forward. Kochanska and colleagues (2004) have described the converse case: Those with secure attachment histories are more responsive to parental socialization efforts when they are toddlers, which promotes emerging moral behavior in the preschool years. Understanding this process is critically important for understanding continuity and thinking about how to effect change.

Finally, continuity may be explained at a different level in terms of cognitive–motivational concepts such as representation (Bretherton & Munholland, 1999; Main et al., 1985), internal working models (Bowlby, 1973) or expectations (Sroufe & Fleeson, 1986, 1988). Such structures are viewed as being based upon experience and as guiding individuals in seeking and interpreting experience. People not only naturally behave in accord with their expectations about the world (i.e., generalize from their past experience) but also even seem to behave so as to confirm what they expect. There is security in what is known (Breger, 1974), so seeing the world in familiar ways is somehow comforting, even when this is ostensibly negative. Thus, even when circumstances change, speaking objectively, the individual may react to them as though they are the same, and also behave in ways that elicit familiar reactions from new people. This is how we interpreted our finding that preschool children who did not experience responsive care wound up neglected or disliked by other children. If, because of early experience, the preschooler doubts the interest and responsiveness of others, and isolates himself from the peer group or fails to initiate positive contacts, he removes himself further from positive social experiences (see also Ladd, 1983; Rubin et al., 1998). Dodge, Pettit, McCluskey, and Brown (1986) found that when accepted or rejected children were placed in new groups of peers, they soon had the same status with their new peers. Likewise, some children (those with histories of chronic rejection) behaved in ways that ultimately elicited controlling and even angry behavior from our teachers (see Chapter 7). A regulatory process in which familiar experience is recreated makes more sense than assuming that punishment is somehow rewarding for some children. No child really likes to be punished, but for some, it is what can be understood or is familiar.

A role for processes such as expectations is now prominent in most theories of behavior. About the same time as the "move to the level of representation" in attachment theory (Main et al., 1985), Dodge and Frame (1982), operating within a social learning theory, proposed that cognitive biases or deficits led aggressive boys to misinterpret ambiguous social behavior as entailing malevolent intent. Subsequently, this was reframed within attachment theory. Now, such interpretations are viewed not as deficits but as the result of normal generalization processes, founded upon historical experience in which ambiguous situations indeed were threatening. Confirmation of this idea came from a German study (Suess, Grossmann, & Sroufe, 1992), using similar procedures to those of Dodge. It was found that kindergartners with histories of avoidant attachment indeed made the kind of attributions of aggressive intent that Dodge described. We, too, found that measures of representation from preschool through adolescence are predictable from actual experience at earlier ages (Carlson et al., 2004). We say more about the role of representation in continuity in the later section of this chapter on the dynamics of development.

In summary, each of these explanations of continuity not only is plausible but is also supported by data from our study. We do not see them as in conflict, but as in simultaneous operation. Moreover, understanding the factors that promote continuity likewise points to critical factors underlying change in adaptation. Change would derive from changes in stresses and supports in the actual environment and transforming relationship experiences, which would result in altered interpretive frameworks. We have provided numerous examples in the preceding chapters of the impact of changing stressors and supports. Likewise, changes in the support available to caregivers, and especially the quality of their personal relationships, were among the most salient factors accounting for change in adaptation. We present more evidence for this when we discuss disturbance (Chapter 12). Finally, consider our findings regarding breaking the cycle of abuse across generations (Egeland et al., 1988; see Chapter 5). Alternative, supportive caregivers in childhood, long-term therapy experiences, and/or presence a supportive spouse were key factors. All of these are experiences that likely promoted changes in relationship expectations.

THE FATE OF EARLY EXPERIENCE
FOLLOWING DEVELOPMENTAL CHANGE

Questions concerning the fate of prior experience or prior adaptation following change are important for understanding continuity in development. Our view is that just as continuity requires change (for the evolved structure to apply in the new developmental context), change does not negate continuity. Change and continuity are not antagonists; both are always present (Sackett, Sameroff, Cairns, & Suomi, 1981). Even with notable change in adaptation, prior experience remains a part of the individual.

Given our comprehensive, age-by-age assessments, we were able to illustrate this in a way that had not been previously accomplished. In the initial analysis, we began by defining two groups of children (Sroufe, Egeland, & Kreutzer, 1990). Both groups showed consistently poor functioning across three assessments between 42 and 54 months. One of them had also shown consistently poor adaptation in three assessments between 12 and 24 months. The second group, however, had shown consistently positive adaptation during this early period. Note two essential points. First, based on the 42- to 54-month assessments, these two groups are the same. From one point of view (in which, with change, it is assumed that prior adaptation is erased), there is only one group—a group of children functioning poorly in the preschool period. They are only two groups if we take seriously the idea that prior history always remains part of the individual. The second point is that the consistency of functioning within each age period reduces the likelihood of measurement error (i.e., the possibility that the second group is still functioning well, but just was assessed poorly). Are they two groups, as our developmental view would suggest, or are they just one? Does the change, which apparently is real given the consistency of problems in preschool, mean that the earlier history is erased? These questions can be answered by looking at the functioning of these children in elementary school. We found that those children, functioning poorly as preschoolers but with positive early histories, as a group had significantly fewer problems than those with a continuous history of problems across the two earlier periods.

Subsequently, we did a similar analysis following up children into adolescence (Sroufe, Carlson, Levy, & Egeland, 1999). These children had shown notable behavior problems during the elementary school years. In this case, one group of children had histories of secure attachment and the other, histories of anxious attachment, but children in both groups showed comparable levels of problems in elementary school. When examined in adolescence, those with secure histories had, as a group, significantly fewer problems. Again, history was not erased despite clear evidence for change.

There are many other examples in the literature of early adaptation or early experience persisting after developmental change. Perhaps the most famous book on resilience is *Overcoming the Odds* by Werner and Smith (1992). As an interesting footnote to this study, Werner and Smith found that those who overcame early adversity and were successful as adults more often also had psychosomatic problems than those who did not have to overcome adversity. This accords with our view that one does not really erase early history; the children paid a price, even though the changes were real and profound. In another very interesting study, Suomi described a group of rhesus monkeys who had experienced early, extreme deprivation (Novak, O'Neill, Beckley, & Suomi, 1992). By living for years in well-functioning colonies, these animals had recovered adequate functioning and could not be discriminated from others by their social behavior. Nonetheless, when, as part of a learning study, the animals were put in test cages, the researchers noted something striking. Each engaged in disturbed, ritualistic behavior. Suomi referred to such behaviors as "signature stereotypies," because they were idiosyncratic and mimicked the very particular disturbed behavior each had shown as an infant. These patterns had not been erased; they were latent and always had potential for reactivation. Again, real change occurred: The young animals functioned normally in the colony under normal (not highly stressful) conditions. The last example we give is perhaps the most dramatic (Hinde & Bateson, 1984). When a caterpillar changes to a butterfly, the changes in structure and function are profound and unparalleled by anything in human development after the embryonic period. Still, remarkably, when that butterfly subsequently lays its eggs, it will do so on the type of vegetation that had nurtured the caterpillar. Something from early experience was retained across the developmental change.

RESILIENCE

The kind of data just described led us to a distinctive viewpoint on resilience (Egeland, Carlson, & Sroufe, 1993; Sroufe, Carlson, et al., 1999; Yates, Egeland, & Sroufe, 2003). Resilience has been an important topic in developmental psychology in recent decades, but it has on occasion carried some unfortunate connotations. Especially in some earlier writings, it was taken to imply some invulnerability or other magical qualities in the child; that is, certain inherent features in some children were seen as granting them a special capacity to overcome adversity or to rebound from periods of difficulty. It is easy to see how this came about.

There *is* great variation in how well children develop in the face of some known risk (e.g., poverty or high stress), and some children who are troubled for a period get better, while others do not. There is something to be explained here, and a label such as "resilient" seems apt. However, it was all too easy to go from the term as a mere description to using it as an explanation. Why do some children do well in the face of adversity (or recover functioning)? *Because* they are resilient. How do you know they are resilient? Because they did well. This was an unsatisfactory circularity.

One can see how such thinking might have evolved by looking at just one part of our 1990 study. Suppose the study had begun only in the preschool years? Among all of the children having problems at that time, some would later do better in elementary school. Without other data, such differences in recovery would have indeed been mysterious. One might have been drawn toward seeing these children as just somehow having "the right stuff" to overcome their problems. Again, this is not descriptively inaccurate. Some children are more able than others to overcome problems. However, given our antecedent data, we can see that a critical difference for this group of "resilient" children is that they had an early positive foundation that supported their recovery. "Even when floundering, some children may not lose the sense that they can affect the environment" (Sroufe, 1978, p. 56). This is so because it has been their experience previously that the environment will support them.

Similarly, as have others, we find great individual differences in children's reactions to high stress. As we reported in earlier chapters, stress is one of the predictors of problem behavior. At the same time, groups of children can be defined who are experiencing comparably high amounts of life stress, yet one group shows problems and the other does not. It seems appropriate to refer such children as "stress resistant" or "resilient." Indeed, they are. Again, however, it is not appropriate on the basis of such data to imply that some children are born inherently able to withstand stress, while others are inherently weak. As in the case of changing behavior problems, our study shows that if one has comprehensive developmental data, such resilience loses its mystery. As Masten (2001) has written, it is "ordinary magic." Children with histories of early positive care and early histories of competence are significantly less likely to evince problem behavior in the face of stress than those with unsupportive histories (Egeland & Kreutzer, 1991; Pianta, Egeland, et al., 1990). "If self-esteem and trust are established early, children may be more resilient in the face of environmental stress. They may show poor adaptation during an overwhelming crisis, but when the crisis has passed and the environment is again positive, they may respond more quickly." (Sroufe, 1978, p. 56).

Early support is not the only factor that promotes what has come to be called "resilience." Also important are changes in stress and support that occur at later times. Thus, when children change in positive ways following periods of difficulty, we often find either increased supports or decreased stress, or both. Likewise, children with and without serious levels of behavior problems in conditions of stress may be distinguished by the supports that are concurrently present. It is the balance of supports and challenges that must be considered, not simply the challenges alone (Sameroff, 2000). When this is done, resilience again loses its mystery.

Thus, both early support and contemporary changes in stresses and supports account for improvements (or declines) in functioning. When we considered both in the same analysis, we found that we accounted for 80% of what would have otherwise been simply referred to as resilience without explanation (Sroufe, 1999). Within the reliability of available measures, this left little to explain.

Many times when we have given oral presentations on our findings regarding the power of experience to predict behavior, one of the first questions is, "But what about these 'resilient' children?" The question implies that there are children who are not a product of their experience, but, rather, are impervious to it. A specific example used by critics is "earned security" on the AAI; that is, those individuals who describe negative experience with parents, yet are autonomous on the AAI. It turns out, however, than when one looks at prospectively gathered information, these people were not more likely to have been anxiously attached as infants, and the observed parental support available to them was comparable to that of others achieving autonomous status (Roisman, Padron, Sroufe, & Egeland, 2002). *Those who overcome adversity do so because of a positive platform or balancing supports available later.*

In the end, we came to view resilience as reflecting developmental process. While it becomes in time a defining feature of some individuals, it is better thought of as the product of the child's experiential history, and ongoing supports and stresses, not as an inherent, immutable characteristic. Resilience is undergirded by unwavering positive expectations regarding self and others (expecting positively even in tough times), flexible self-regulation, and an array of competencies that can be called upon as needed. Each of these is an outcome of development, built up over time within a context of adequate support. Moreover, resilience is not just based on characteristics of a freestanding person; it also depends on historical and ongoing supports. Thus, in our view, resilience is not an individual trait but a feature of the developmental system.

In previous writing we have contrasted our process view with a trait view (e.g., Yates, Egeland, et al., 2003). One telling example lies in the data showing that some children function well, have a period of trouble, then function well again. The interpretation that a history of positive adaptation reflects an underlying individual trait called "resilience" would have some paradoxical consequences. One would have to argue that some of these children were "resilient," then were not, and then were resilient again. Rather, our interpretation of these data is that the process underlying resilience is manifest in the entire developmental course. Children who were troubled and later rebounded drew upon an early history of supportive and consistent care. "Children who are competent are indeed more likely to manifest resilience at some point; however, competence is a characterization of functioning at a particular point in time, whereas resilience encompasses a developmental process over time" (pp. 251–252).

Our process view varies somewhat from those who have emphasized designated child factors, such as temperament and IQ. The primary study cited as evidence for a temperamental basis for resilience is that of Werner and Smith (1992) cited earlier. Close reading of this study, however, reveals that the single temperament variable that predicted resilience was the mother's rating of the child's "lovability" at age 2 years. We would submit that such a variable may be more reflective of the caregiver's positive perception of her child (which we would see as being of great importance) than an inherent child characteristic. In addition, this measure at age 2 and other temperament variables also may be viewed as developmental constructions.

Studies suggesting a prominent role for intelligence in resilience often have emphasized achievement and educational attainment in the outcomes. We, too, found IQ to be highly related to achievement test scores and, occasionally, preschool IQ and early cognitive ability were protective factors regarding later adversity (e.g., Pianta, Egeland, et al., 1990). But IQ turned out to be less powerful than we expected. It predicted far more modestly to social and behavioral outcomes, and recovery of functioning, than it predicted to achievement test performance. For example, recall that IQ did not add to our early experience predictors for dropping out of school. Moreover, even IQ is itself predicted in part by history of care and stimulation in the home (see Chapter 7) and is subject to change in the face of changing support (Chapter 8). Functional intelligence is no doubt even more strongly related to such variables.

IQ and temperament constructs certainly have an important place in a comprehensive picture of development. The relation of IQ to school achievement is important in that success in school is related to economic opportunity and other advantages. Moreover, as we discuss further in Chapter 12 on behavioral and emotional disturbance, temperament measures sometimes play a role in predicting outcomes as well, especially in interaction with other variables.

As a final word, it should be clear that we are distinguishing between the term "resilience," as used by developmental psychopathologists, and "ego resiliency," as used by personality theorists (e.g., Block, 2002). Ego resiliency is synonymous with "self-regulation" and has to do with flexibility in adjusting controls as permitted or required by circumstances (see Chapter 4). This personal characteristic, which is strongly related to secure attachment history (see Chapter 7), does become quite stable, as we reported in Chapter 8. It is a personality trait in that sense, and it is related to the capacity to cope with stressful circumstances. But it, too, is a developmental construction, and it is distinctive from resilience as used here, because only the latter refers to rebound following a period of difficulty. We have been interested in both of these developmental constructs.

THE DYNAMICS OF DEVELOPMENT

In accord with the biological principle of epigenesis (Sameroff & Chandler, 1975; Werner, 1948), we view the development of the person as a dynamic process, wherein self-regulatory structures and functions evolve from successive transactions between the developing child and the environment. The interplay between person and surround is total and complete, operating on every level. Environment and individual are mutually creating in an ongoing way. Thus, the person is constructed over time in a process in which history influences what is experienced, and experience alters history.

A developmental, transactional view of person and environment means much more than that both child and surround are important, or that one can predict behavior better by considering both. It even means more than considering person-by-environment interaction in a simple sense. It means that child and environment are mutually transforming. Thus, prior patterns of adaptation may be transformed by fundamental environmental changes and, at the same time, environmental features have different meaning and influence for different people. Psychologists speak of the "effective environment," that is, what we notice, ignore, seek out, or even bring about—what we take advantage of or use to our own disadvantage. We change what we can change ourselves.

Moreover, individual development is a recursive process characterized by progressive epicycles of transaction between person and environment. At the beginning of the child's life, an adaptation is formed. Such adaptations represent the confluence of the entire histories of parents, the infants they meet, and the circumstances within which they operate. At this early phase, we believe, they are best thought of as dyadic or systemic adaptations rather than adaptations of individual infants. Still, patterns of regulation are established, and these patterns become proto-expectations of infants regarding the interactive world. Thus, they become part of subsequent adaptations. Now, a new transaction is in operation, in which established patterns are part of the history that interfaces with new challenges and opportunities in the environment. Such new encounters now play their role in adaptive outcome, solidifying the previous pattern, or altering it, disrupting it, or transforming it. Given the probability of some continuity in the environment, discussed earlier, some degree of stability is the usual circumstance. Nonetheless, the new adaptation is formed. Expectations are deepened or modified, and this new adaptation is carried forward to ongoing encounters with the environment. With development, children become increasing forces in their own adaptations. This is both because they have more history to bring to bear and more deeply established and autonomous patterns of regulation. It is also because, with cognitive advances, expectations become beliefs, then attitudes and sophisticated frameworks for interpretation. Increasingly, therefore, children not only create their own unique environments but also interpret what is ostensibly the same environment. Capacities to tolerate challenges and draw upon available resources become more distinctive. Nonetheless, new environmental circumstances always play a role in adaptation as development continues to unfold.

Early supportive care promotes both positive self- and other-expectations and the capacity to regulate emotional arousal. Such capacities become especially important in conditions of high stress and emotional intensity, which are commonly encountered by high-risk children. External stress is challenging to adaptation but not uniformly so. How one views the stress and one's capacity to access personal and social resources is critical. Expecting positive outcomes, maintaining arousal regulation, and effectively utilizing available help all are important, because they support sustained and flexible coping efforts. For the child who does not expect that his or her efforts will be effective and cannot perceive available support, even a moderate amount of stress can be overwhelming. As a concrete example, a supportive mentoring relationship with an older individual is most readily achieved by those children who are able to trust and relate to such a person (Yates, Egeland, et al., 2003).

We have viewed this process as the progressive construction of experience (Carlson et al., 2004) or of the person. In this construction, a key role is played by expectations or representation. While experience over time creates expectations, expectations and behavior inspired by them, in turn, shape experience. Behavior and experience are therefore mutually creating through the medium of expectations. Put another way, expectations and representations are the "carriers" of experience. They are the connection between behavior–experience at one age and behavior–experience at the next. They are abstracted from experience and are the frames for ongoing encounters with the environment (see Chapter 8). At the same time, representations of the self in the social world continue to be modified by new experiences. Experience, representation, and ongoing adaptation are a nondissociable triad, inextricably linked together in a cyclical fashion.

Such a hypothesis is extraordinarily difficult to test, and we have been working on this problem for the last three decades. It involves trying to show that representation and behavior–experience have mutual influence in a progressive fashion. Both must not only be correlated at a given age, but each must also forecast the other. Thus, for example, representation must predict later behavior, with prior behavior controlled, and vice versa. And this must occur repeatedly, age by age.

While conceptually challenging, the task was especially difficult in practical, measurement terms. In addition to good behavioral measures, it involves having dependable measures of representation across ages from early childhood to adulthood. Given cognitive changes over this period, it is clear that such measures must be vastly different at different ages. Giving preschoolers sentence completion tests or formally interviewing them about important qualities of friendships is not very revealing. Likewise, one must have dependable measures of behavior–experience at the same ages—not quite as challenging, but important nonetheless. Any weak link in the chain damages the investigation. Furthermore, it is critical that measures of the two sets of constructs be completely independent. As just one example, if a child interview is used to measure both expectations regarding peers and competence with peers, a child's low expectations may color his or her description of peer acceptance, which conceivably may be objectively adequate. In such a case, both measures may be, at least in part, measures of representation. Thus, one cannot know whether the underlying conception is valid, whatever the results. This is a common problem in studies that rely on the same kind of instruments (or the same reporter) for all measures.

Design of the Study

Our plan called for us to begin with measures of early relationship experience and then assess representation and behavior from preschool through adolescence, with all the measures obtained at parallel times (Carlson et al., 2004). The early experience measures were attachment quality at 12 and 18 months, and relationship quality at 24 months. Specifically, we used a combination of Avoidance and Resistance scale scores from the Strange Situation (in order to achieve a continuous variable), and Experience in the Session from the tool problems.

Representation measures were diverse. All are described more fully in Chapter 4. At age 4½, we first derived three scales from the Preschool Interpersonal Problem-Solving Test, wherein the children are asked what they might do in certain interpersonal situations. The three scales were Mother–Child Relationship Quality (the child's expectation that the mother would accept an apology, offer affection, etc.), Peer Relationship Quality (cooperative solutions and/or expectations of empathy), and Cognitive Flexibility (e.g., seeing multiple alternative solutions). Each of these scales showed concurrent validity with relevant measures of care, social skill, or behavioral flexibility. These scales were composited to form the preschool measure of representation.

At age 8 years, representational measures were derived from family drawings. Ratings of Supportive Family Relationship and Security of Self were used. Criteria for the first scale were positive expectations regarding interactions and projected pride in the family (cf. Fury et al., 1997; Kaplan & Main, 1984). Some specific indicators were inclusion of all members, organized positioning of members, and positive indices of connection (e.g., figures holding hands, shared activity). Ratings of Security of Self were based on clarity of the child figure in the drawing, grounding, and proper proportion of the child figure (e.g., not very tiny, floating, or dismembered), and child expressions of positive affect. Again, these measures showed concurrent validity (Carlson et al., 2004).

At age 12, a sentence completion task, projective (TAT-type) stories, a moral fable interpretation, and a friendship interview were the basis for representation measures. The sentence completions included stems, such as "Other kids always. . . ." The story pictures depicted ambiguous social situations. The fable entailed a conflict of rights and needs between two parties (mice and a porcupine trying to live in a cave; see Johnston, 1988). Parts of the friendship interview also dealt with issues of conflict and closeness. (See Chapter 4 and Carlson et al., 2004, for details.) Ratings of two aspects of representation were made following study of the child's responses to each of these four procedures. The two scales were Peer Relationship Quality and Self-Coherence. High ratings on the peer scale reflected expectations of sustained positive emotional relationship connections; low ratings reflected expectations of isolation, lack of satisfaction, or aggression in relationships. High self-coherence was reflected in responses that were consistent across stimuli, yet plausibly and flexibly adapted to stimulus content. These scales again showed concurrent validity, for example, being related in the .50s to social competence and emotional health ratings in the summer camps (Carlson et al., 2004).

At age 16, a friendship interview, with similarities to that used at age 12, was the basis for representational measures. Friend Relationship Quality and Self-Coherence were again the scales derived from this material. At this age, there was somewhat more emphasis on the portrayed valuing of emotional closeness in the friendship rating than at age 12, and the coherence rating necessarily tapped more the young person's active efforts to integrate and organize relationship experiences. Good concurrent validity was demonstrated.

Finally, at age 19, we administered Main's AAI (see Chapters 4 and 10). Main has provided an elaborated Coherence of Transcript scale (Main & Goldwyn, 1998), which we used in our analyses. A high rating requires a "steady and developing flow of ideas regarding attachment," maintenance of a collaborative attitude, and adherence to the rules of discourse (succinctness, relevance, truthfulness, and understandability). This coherence rating was significantly correlated with coherence of the friendship or romantic relationship interview given at the same age (Carlson et al., 2004).

In kindergarten, grades 3 and 6, and at age 16, teacher rankings of peer competence and emotional health/self-esteem were used as parallel behavioral measures. As outlined in Part II of this book, these rankings had strong contemporary correlates (e.g., in the preschool, the summer camps, and the camp reunions) and were moderately stable from age to age. They were composited to form a single behavioral measure at each age. At age 19, the global adjustment and social support network measures (see Chapter 10) were combined and used as the measures of behavioral competence.

We argue that the two major sets of variables reflect at each age the representation and behavioral constructs of interest, and that they are valid measures. Moreover, it is important to note that the representational measures reflect the content and structural quality of the child's internal experience. All tap attitudes, expectations, and feelings. In contrast, the behavioral measures reflect the assessments of teachers and other external observers of the child's overt behavior. Thus, the measures have a large degree of independence, as is required for this analysis.

As a necessary control, we also used the intelligence estimate we had based on four subscales of the Wechsler Intelligence Scales for Children—Revised (WISC-R). Controlling for intelligence is especially important when using representational measures. We need to know that we are not simply measuring general verbal ability when we are trying to tap the content of the child's mind.

Findings

We used two general strategies for examining these data: a simple series of partial correlations and formal structural modeling. Both procedures begin with the array of correlations within and between the behavioral and representational measures. Several preliminary points may be made from these correlations (see Table 11.1). First, there is good stability of the representation measures from the preschool period to middle adolescence. The range of correlations between the preschool composite measure and the family drawing measure at grade 3, and the narrative measures at grade 6 and age 16 was .39–.46. The correlation with AAI Coherence at age 19 was not significant. Likewise, there was good stability for the behavioral measures (correlations in the .30s and .40s). Representation and behavior measures at the same age were always significantly related and usually were related across ages. The preschool representation measure, for example, related to all behavioral measures from ages 5–19 (correlations = .28–.41). In general, relations were stronger when the representation measure was a composite across domains and qualities of experience, or when there were multiple levels of assessment (e.g., the preschool scales of parent and peer expectations and cognitive flexibility; the grade 6 battery using multiple formats—stories, sentence completions, etc.). Likewise, the multifaceted age 19 behavioral measure was a strong outcome, being related to every measure of representation across ages. This likely is because it tapped broad domains of functioning. Controlling for IQ did not change the significance of any of the obtained relationships (Carlson et al., 2004).

In general, when we carried out partial correlations between adjacent ages, results were significant; that is, the behavioral–experiential measure predicted representation at the next age, with representation at the earlier age controlled, and representation predicted to behavior, with earlier behavior controlled. For example, the preschool representation composite predicted the combined grade 3 teacher ranking of peer competence and emotional health/self-esteem, with these same rankings in kindergarten statistically controlled. Put another way, change in behavioral adaptation between the two ages was forecast by representation at the earlier age. In turn, the middle childhood teacher rankings predicted representation from the grade 6 battery, with the grade 3 family drawing representation measure controlled. Back and forth, experience seemed to predict changes in representation, and representation provided the frame for subsequent experience.

Carlson and colleagues (2004) also carried out formal modeling, with the models varying in complexity and assumptions being made. These structural models were a format for considering the array of rela-

TABLE 11.1. Intercorrelations among and between Representational and Behavioral Measures

Variables	Representational measures					Behavioral measures				
	1	2	3	4	5	6	7	8	9	10
Representational measures										
1. Early childhood (4½ years)	—	.36*** (152)	.46*** (159)	.39** (145)	.13 (145)					
2. Middle childhood (8 years)		—	.25** (167)	.16*a (155)	.01 (152)					
3. Early adolescence (12 years)			—	.34*** (162)	.19* (160)					
4. Midadolescence (16 years)				—	.25** (152)					
5. Late adolescence (19 years)					—					
Behavioral measures										
6. Early childhood (5 years)	.28*** (155)	.21** (161)	.22*** (170)	.15 (155)	.10 (153)	—	.50*** (174)	.34*** (173)	.30*** (16)	.31*** (156)
7. Middle childhood (8 years)	.41*** (158)	.24** (168)	.28*** (175)	.22** (163)	.09 (160)		—	.49*** (180)	.41*** (172)	.27*** (163)
8. Early adolescence (12 years)	.30*** (159)	.27*** (169)	.31*** (179)	.17* (163)	.20**a (163)			—	.38*** (174)	.31*** (166)
9. Midadolescence (16 years)	.37*** (152)	.07 (161)	.22** (170)	.26** (161)	.18*a (161)				—	.31*** (165)
10. Late adolescence (19 years)	.31*** (145)	.24** (153)	.40*** (162)	.28** (156)	.30*** (163)					—

Note. From Carlson, Sroufe, and Egeland (2004). Copyright 2004 by Blackwell. Reprinted by permission. Coefficients represent zero-order correlations. Parentheses indicate sample size. Composite representational ratings: *Early childhood*: Mother–child relationship, peer relationship, cognitive flexibility; *Middle childhood*: Family relationship, security of self; *Early adolescence*: Peer relationship, self-coherence; *Midadolescence*: Friend relationship, coherence; *Late adolescence*: AAI coherence. Composite behavioral rankings/ratings: *Early childhood through midadolescence*: Peer competence and emotional health; *Late adolescence*: Socioemotional functioning and social support.

aPartial correlations controlling for IQ were not significant. Remaining partial correlations did not lead to meaningful reductions in significance levels.

*p < .05; **p < .01; ***p < .001.

tions across ages in single analyses. Most pertinent here, it was possible to compare the fit to the overall data array of interactive versus noninteractive models; that is, models allowing for mutual influence between representation and behavior–experience, and models that did not. In each case, interactive models yielded substantially and significantly better fit than noninteractive models. One of these models is depicted graphically in Figure 11.1.

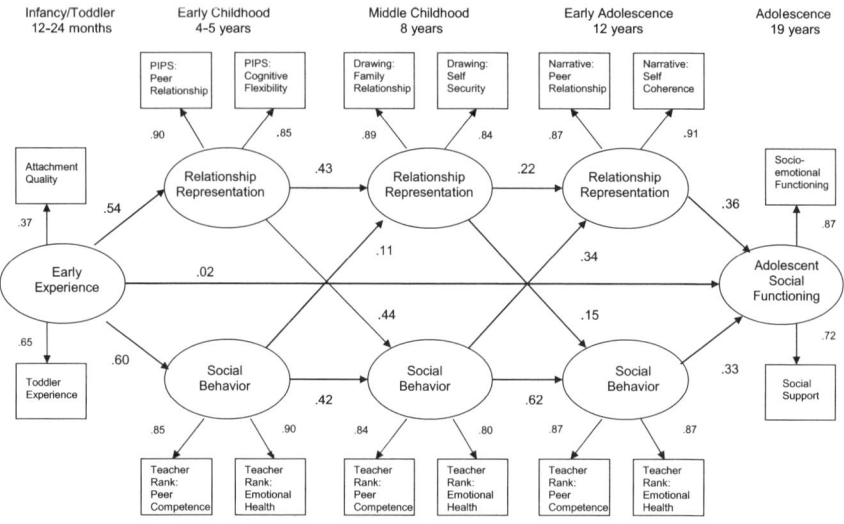

FIGURE 11.1. From Carlson, Sroufe, and Egeland (2004). Copyright 2004 by Blackwell. Reprinted by permission. Model standardized coefficients $\chi^2[92]$ = 116.51; χ^2/df = 1.29; goodness-of-fit index = .92; root mean square error of approximation = .04. Path coefficients are significant at $p < .05$, with the exceptions of paths from Early Experience to Adolescent Social Functioning and from early childhood Behavior to middle childhood Representation.

We have begun to extend these findings into early adulthood (Roisman et al., 2002). We reported in Chapter 10 that an effective parent–child relationship process at age 13 predicted a similar effective process in romantic relationships when our participants were in their early 20s. It is also the case that this link between a family behavioral predictor and the later behavioral outcome is mediated by the young person's representation of parental attachments at age 19, which is significantly related to both of the other measures.

We take these findings as confirming in general our epigenetic, organizational model of development, in which psychic structure is formed in a dynamic process. More specifically, the findings support the particular hypothesis that representation is a carrier of experience. "It is noteworthy that representational measures were related to earlier experience with earlier representation controlled and, at the same time, to later experience with prior experience controlled" (Carlson et al., 2004, p. 78).

CONCLUSION

In this section of the book, we present findings on disturbance and the clinical implications of our work. Yet we begin with this discussion of the process of development. This is no accident. We believe the same principles and processes that govern normal development also govern abnormal development. Years ago, the biologist Paul Weiss said: "Pathology and developmental biology must be reintegrated so that our understanding of the 'abnormal' will become but an extension of our insight into the 'normal,' while ... the study of the 'abnormal' will contribute to the deepening of that very insight" (Weiss, 1961, p. 150; see also Cicchetti & Cohen, 1995).

The capacity to function well in school, the capacity for intimate relationships, and the capacity for resilience are developmental outcomes. Personality itself is a developmental outcomes. In the same way, we view psychopathology as an outcome of development (Sroufe, 1997). Disturbance is the result of the progressive transactions between person and environment, the recursive, mutual influence of experience and expectations. This view holds whatever role one assigns to genes or other endogenous factors. The developmental process is the same whether one is investigating normal development or disturbance.

The developmental–transactional view of psychopathology has been affirmed even in studies of serious adult disorders, such as depression and schizophrenia. While some have argued that these problems are caused by endogenous pathogens, developmental studies show that such a position is oversimplified. For example, Cadoret, Troughton, Merchant, and Whitters (1990) carried out an adoption study, in which offspring of depressed and nondepressed mothers were compared for adult outcome. As have many others, they found a small effect for biological inheritance. However, they also examined early environmental risks, namely, number of placements before final placement, or age at final placement. Such variables also predicted depression, even with genetic risk controlled. More importantly, they found that the interaction term for the psychosocial and biological risk factors was dramatically more powerful than either risk factor alone. In an equally important and parallel study, Tienari and colleagues (1990) found the standard genetic risk for schizophrenia in adopted away children (5% for the offspring of schizophrenic mothers, 1% for those of nondiagnosed mothers). However, what was unique about this study was their assessment of the quality of the adoptive home. In brief, they found that it was the combination of being in a disturbed home and genetic risk that accounted for all of the psychosis. There was no increment in schizophrenia for those at genetic risk who grew up in healthy homes; nor was there schizophrenia in unhealthy homes in the absence of biological risk. They concluded that it would be no more appropriate to say that having a biological mother with schizophrenia *causes* schizophrenia than to say that growing up in an unhealthy home causes schizophrenia. Rather, even schizophrenia is the product of transactions between organism and environment over time. Disturbance is always the result of development.

In Chapter 12, we turn our attention to the behavioral and emotional problems of children and adolescents. Not surprisingly, we find that a developmental approach to such problems is most revealing. In contrast to explaining disturbance as something some children just have, we describe a probabilistic, epigenetic conception in which complex, interacting factors are considered that place children on pathways to disorder and maintain them on, or deflect them from, such pathways.

CHAPTER 12

Behavioral and Emotional Disturbance

> The process of development constitutes the crucial link
> between genetic . . . and environmental variables, between
> sociology and individual psychology, and between physiogenic
> and psychogenic causes.
>
> —RUTTER (1980)

$\mathbf{W}$e embrace a developmental view of disturbance. As discussed in the preceding chapters, we hold that emotional problems are developmental outcomes; that is, they derive from a process of successive transactions of the child and the environment (e.g., Sroufe, 1997). Thus, disturbance is created by the interplay of multiple factors operating over time, and links between antecedent conditions and disturbance are probabilistic and nonlinear. Stated another way, disturbance is the outgrowth of patterns of maladaptation interacting with ongoing challenging circumstances in the absence of adequate support. In general, we argue, the same processes that govern continuity and change in normal adaptation govern the development of disturbance. Before discussing our abundant data on behavioral and emotional problems, we first outline our developmental position in more detail.

A DEVELOPMENTAL MODEL OF DISTURBANCE

Our developmental viewpoint has been inspired by Bowlby's (1973) elaboration of Waddington's (1957) developmental pathways model (see Chapter 2). While Bowlby described this model in terms of diverging and converging tracks in a railway yard, we have preferred a more biological depiction of a tree with its branches. In either case, serious disturbance would be represented by branches at the far outside of the tree, or away from the center of the train yard, and such a condition would be the result of a series of branchings that progressively take the individual to the outside. There are four other implications of the model:

1. There are multiple pathways to the same or similar outcomes. Thus, there would be various developmental courses leading to the same "final common pathway." (Two individuals could begin on different major branches but, because of subsequent branching, wind up in a very similar place.)
2. The same initial pathway, because of divergent patterns of branching, can lead to multiple outcomes (Cicchetti & Rogosch, 1996). Physical abuse, for example, is associated with later conduct problems, alcoholism, depression, or other problems. Understanding which outcome arises requires consideration of not only initiating conditions but also subsequent conditions.
3. Change is possible at many (any) points in development. The nodes in the tree may be thought of as points of developmental transition, which provide both new challenges and new opportunities and thus, perhaps, special opportunities for fundamental change.
4. Change is constrained by prior development. Change becomes more difficult the longer a pathway has been pursued, and certain outcomes may become very unlikely over time.

Several noteworthy ideas are embodied in this set of assumptions. First, one can see that early experience is not destiny. With subsequent experience, different individuals who began on the same path may diverge into various patterns of adaptive or maladaptive functioning. Ongoing circumstances may support pursuance of potentially deviating developmental pathways or deflect the individual back toward more normal adaptation. At the same time, as "initiating conditions" (see Chapter 2), early beginnings constrain to some extent later possibilities and are *probabilistically* related to certain classes of outcomes. Final outcome cannot be specified from knowing the initial condition, but neither is it the case that development is simply chaotic and random. The degree and nature of likely change is conditioned by history.

Second, this model has implications for intervention. Clearly, because of implications 3 and 4, early intervention is encouraged. Change is easier before a pathway has become entrenched. At any point, a strategy for intervention would be to identify and alter factors maintaining the person on a maladaptive pathway or to identify interventions that would encourage a return to a more serviceable pathway. The strength of this approach is that patterns of maladaptive functioning, probabilistically leading to disturbance, may be corrected even before there is diagnosable pathology.

Finally, despite similar manifest behaviors at outcome, different interventions may be more or less effective for different individuals, depending on the developmental course they are following. Classification in terms of developmental trajectory may ultimately prove to be more valuable than classification of behaviors. We return to this point when we discuss particular disturbances in later sections.

This probabilistic, systemic approach to the development of disturbance is congruent with modern transactional models of risk and protection (e.g., Sameroff, 2000). In fact, early compromised experience and early maladaptation may be seen as risk factors for disturbance. Like any other risk factor (biological parent with disturbance, low SES, harsh living conditions), being at risk does not mean being destined for disorder. In fact, the majority of the people in the population of individuals having any of the risk factors just mentioned will *not* be disordered in current psychiatric terms. As mentioned in Chapter 3, a striking example is genetic risk for schizophrenia. Having one parent with the disorder only raises the probability of developing schizophrenia to about 10% from the population base rate of 1%, even when the child grows up with that parent (Sameroff, 2000). When the children are adopted away the probability is only 4% (Faraone & Tsuang, 1988). Thus, well more than 90% of such individuals will not develop schizophrenia. Similarly, anxious attachment in infancy, even disorganized attachment, does not make later pathology certain or even highly likely; it merely increments the probability of such an outcome. This is why we describe attachment as an "organizational construct" rather than as a causal trait (see Chapter 2). Variations in early attachment lead individuals to frame subsequent experiences differently, and for this reason, insecure attachment does compromise development. But if circumstances change enough, experience changes and so, too, do the inner frames that guide subsequent functioning. Note that in predicting competent outcomes, age by age, we always found that it was not early care or attachment alone that was most predictive, but the cumulative history of the individual (Egeland et al., 1990; Erickson et al., 1985; Sroufe, Egeland, et al., 1999). We find the same thing when it comes to the prediction of psychopathology, as we describe in later sections.

IMPLICATIONS OF A DEVELOPMENTAL MODEL

The uniqueness of a developmental approach can be seen in contrasting it to what may be called a "deficit model." Within such a model (Lazare, 1973), it is assumed that an inherent (perhaps inborn) deficit of the child leads directly to disturbance. This assumption may be explicit or implicit, but in any case, it leads to statements suggesting linear cause; for example, "AD/HD is largely the *result* of neurological dysfunction" (Frick & Lahey, 1991, p. 169; emphasis added). The widespread and growing use of medication with children also may be seen as an implicit endorsement of a deficit model. In our developmental–transactional view, child characteristics are only one feature of the developmental process, and they cannot be viewed as independent of the context of development. Disturbance is a reflection of a dynamic developmental process, not a condition a child *has*. Saying that a child *has* attention deficit disorder or conduct disorder has very different meaning than saying that a child *is* distressed or troubled or angry, or that a child *is* having great difficulty controlling impulses or paying attention in school. The former language implies immutability.

As with all development, given the immature status of the human at birth, early care, and the context of early care, play prominent roles in early adaptations and thus in initiating a cumulative developmental process that may lead to disturbance. Still, multiple factors, at times including organic disturbances, enter into the process over time. When some clear organic condition plays a role in disturbance, developmental processes must nonetheless be considered (Grossman et al., 2003). The impact of any organic feature depends on the total developmental context. For most childhood problems, organic features cannot be dissociated from history of care. A high-energy child (setting aside the complexities of the emergence of such a characteristic) may or may not ultimately fit criteria for attention-deficit/hyperactivity disorder (ADHD), depending on the pattern of supports and challenges experienced. (See Suomi, 2002, for a discussion of experimental studies with monkeys.) High activity level has a different meaning when a child is empathic, cooperative, and sociable than when the child is socially oblivious, dysregulated, and/or oppositional. Only the latter child will likely end up with a diagnosis of ADHD.

A disorder such as autism, in which disturbance seems to result despite a wide variety of caregiving contexts, is the exception, not the rule. Such children are qualitatively different from other children, even other children with problems. Such profound impairment is notably rare. There was not a single case of autism in the first-generation participants of our study, yet dozens of children fit criteria for ADHD, conduct disorder, or depression. We are arguing that the problems of these many children are best thought of as developmental outcomes, deflections from normal developmental pathways.

Adopting a developmental model has implications for viewing standard problems and findings in the field. As one example, neurophysiological or biochemical correlates of disturbance would be interpreted as "markers" of a developmental process and not necessarily as evidence of initial cause. Of course the electroencephalographic patterns of children with serious attention problems would be distinctive compared to those of children without such problems as they engage in a laboratory task. How could they not be, since their patterns of attention are different? But were distinctive organic differences present at or near birth? No one knows. Of course, in the midst of serious depression (or anorexia), altered brain chemistry may be apparent. But how do we know which is cause and which is effect? When young monkeys are permanently separated from their parents, they subsequently show the same brain biochemical anomalies as severely depressed patients (McKinney, 1977). Starving concentration camp victims show the same chemical imbalances as self-starving teenagers, and when persons manifesting anorexia eat again, chemical balance returns to normal (Steinhausen, 1994).

A second example concerns the relative intractability of certain problems, such as conduct disturbance. We again take a systemic view of intractability, calling attention to the way in which particular patterns of adaptation call forth exacerbating reactions from the environment. So, for example, the child with disordered conduct pushes away other children, infuriates teachers, and, in general, elicits great negativity from the environment. Such reactions deepen the child's alienation and curtail mastery of necessary social skills, and the process continues. Intractability need not imply deficit, as we discuss further later.

Finally, consider the issue of overlapping categories of disturbance. Every researcher and clinician is familiar with the fact that children qualifying for one diagnostic label (e.g., ADHD) often qualify for another (e.g., conduct disorder). Fully half of the children given one of these two labels also are given the other. Moreover, there is substantial overlap between both of these and depression, and so forth. In fact, such multiple possible diagnoses are the rule, not the exception. From a developmental point of view, this is an understandable state of affairs given the common core of arousal- and emotion-regulation issues underlying these common childhood problems. From a deficit model, however, this is a confusing state of affairs. Just what is the deficit that would lead to so many different disorders? It is no solution to simply say there is *comorbidity*. Like resilience, which we discussed in Chapter 11, this term is merely a description of the current state of affairs, not an explanation.

A developmental approach may ultimately shed light on this issue by uncovering the core developmental processes that currently utilized categories share, and it may provide insight into the heterogeneity within categories as well.

We believe that a crucial way to evaluate the merits of a developmental position on disturbance is to examine the results from prospective longitudinal studies such as ours. We first outline some of our findings on early experience and later disturbance, because such data have not been previously available; then we present our more complex analyses of the development of a variety of child problems.

EARLY EXPERIENCE AND LATER DISTURBANCE

For the sake of communication, we feel that it is important to relate our work to the standard DSM psychiatric classification system. Scholars and professionals have been interested for both theoretical and practical reasons in the possible ties between our early measures of attachment and maltreatment, and particular child and adult problems. Whatever its limitations, the current DSM system serves the very useful purpose of providing a common nomenclature for discussion. When we refer to young people who fit criteria for ADHD, or anxiety disorders, or conduct disorders, we have some shared idea of what we are discussing. In this section, we present an overview of our findings regarding predictions from our early assessments to formal clinical classifications. In later sections, we describe how our total body of information sheds light on some common disturbances of young people. At that point, we discuss ADHD, conduct disorders, depression, and anxiety.

The measures of disturbance to be discussed in the remainder of this chapter derive from four sources: (1) behavior problem checklist data from teachers, parents, and young people; (2) the Children's Depression Rating Scale (CDRS); (3) a formal diagnostic clinical interview administered at age 17½—the Schedule for Affective Disorders and Schizophrenia for School-Age Children (K-SADS); and (4) a self-report Dissociative Experiences Scale (DES; see Chapter 4 for a description). The K-SADS provides both symptom scores and formal DSM-III-R diagnoses. We used these to generate both specific diagnoses and a global pathology index, based on the number and severity of diagnoses.

A complete discussion of the reasons why anxious attachment in infancy would be related (probabilistically) to later psychiatric disturbance would be lengthy. We have discussed this in several papers (e.g., Carlson & Sroufe, 1995; Egeland & Carlson, 2004; Sroufe, Carlson, et al., 1999). This brief overview, centers on the problem of regulation. As discussed in earlier chapters, variations in attachment may be thought of as variations in dyadic regulation of emotion and behavior. Such patterns of regulation promote *to the extent possible* closeness with a particular caregiver and in that sense are the best adaptations possible. For children with secure histories, based in responsive care, ample proximity may be maintained through a flexible balance of exploration and direct signaling when in need. Sustained periods of alert organization and cycles of brief upset followed by relaxation are repeatedly experienced, supported by the infant's confidence in the caregiver's availability. Through such experience, there is a tuning of the central nervous system (see also Schore, 1994).

Children with anxious histories also establish patterns in their dyadic regulation efforts. By minimizing signals of need that may further alienate rejecting caregivers, or by heightening and chronically emitting signals of need toward an only intermittently responsive caregiver, those with avoidant and resistant attachments promote proximity to the extent they can. Even disorganized attachment behavior (simultaneous approach–avoidance; freezing, etc.) enables a degree of proximity in the face of a frightening or unfathomable parent.

For children in each group, these patterns become prototypes for subsequent regulation, even when apart from the caregiver. While in an important way serviceable early on, patterns of regulation of the anxiously attached groups seriously compromise later functioning (e.g., Kobak, Ruckdeschel, & Hazan, 1994). Blunting one's feelings so as not to express needs, isolating oneself, feeling alienated from others, and failing to turn to them when stressed, make life very difficult, especially in the social arena. Chronic vigilance, apprehension, and worry about needs being met take a toll. And being disorganized and disoriented cuts one off from vital experiences originating inside and outside of the self. As we have stated elsewhere:

> For children with avoidant and resistant histories, emotions that would have facilitated affective communication and exchange are defensively modified or cut off. . . . As a result, when experiencing distress the child may fail to signal directly a need for support, become embroiled in negative emotion, and be unable to draw from potentially supportive relationships. Moreover, . . . working defensive strategies of avoidance or resistance may themselves be vulnerable to breaking down under stress. . . . This is evident in low ratings of ego resiliency, inability to cope with frustration, and pervasive presence of negative affect of insecure children. . . . For individuals with (disorganized attachment relationships), the process of regulation, the consolidation or integration of self across behavioral states and acquisition of control over states, may be disrupted. (Sroufe, Carlson, et al., 1999, p. 10)

Given the centrality of emotional regulation and regulation of social re-lationships in all major psychiatric diagnoses, it therefore was plausible to expect a relation between adolescent disturbance and early attach-ment (Cole et al., 1994; Sroufe et al., 2000).

The results were clear and confirming. We begin with the global pa-thology index at 17½, based on number and severity of diagnoses. The strongest single predictor of this outcome from the first 6 years of life was disorganized attachment. The rating of disorganization from in-fancy correlated .34 with global pathology. Thus, severe dysregulation in the caregiver–infant dyad is associated with more extreme disturbance at the end of adolescence (Carlson, 1998). Avoidant attachment also was significantly correlated (.25), but resistant attachment was not.

Despite these impressive findings, it was also the case that predic-tion of pathology was increased when other measures were added to at-tachment history. For example, we found that cumulative early care and our parent–child measures at 13 years (especially boundary violation and support for autonomy) added to avoidant and disorganized attach-ment in accounting for pathology, as did assessments of the quality of peer relationships in elementary school (Carlson, 1998). One example regression, in which substantial variance is accounted for, is shown in Table 12.1. Attachment history, later parenting, and behavior problem history all were predictive, in a cumulative way. When middle childhood peer competence was substituted for elementary behavior problems in this analysis, the result was very similar.

Results for specific disorders were quite interesting. Resistant at-tachment in infancy was uniquely and specifically associated with anxi-ety disorders at age 17½ (Warren et al., 1997). By this, we mean that this pattern of attachment, and only this pattern, predicted anxiety problems, and anxious resistant attachment was not related to externalizing-type problems. These are remarkable findings, given the obvious connection to the chronic vigilance and heightened apprehension of the resistant group in infancy.

While avoidant attachment was *not* associated with anxiety disor-ders, it was related to pathology in general (discussed earlier) and to externalizing problems and later conduct disorders (Aguilar et al., 2000; Renken et al., 1989). This is in keeping with the viewpoint that chronic rejection is associated with interpersonal alienation and per-haps also with an abiding anger taken forward from infancy, as we discuss further in the section on conduct problems (Egeland, Yates, Appleyard, & van Dulmen, 2001). It is also consistent with the previ-ously discussed idea (see Chapter 7) that relationship qualities (here, hostility) are internalized and carried forward. Disorganized attach-ment also was associated with conduct disorders, we believe, because

TABLE 12.1. Summary of Hierarchical Regression Analysis Predicting Psychopathology Ratings (K-SADS, 17.5 years) from Avoidance and Disorganization (12–18 months), Behavior Problem Index (TRF, Grades 1–6), and Family Relationship Quality (13 years) ($n = 120$)

Variable	Model 1			Model 2			Model 3			Model 4		
	B	SE	β	B	SE	β	B	SE	β	B	SE	β
Avoidant attachment	.74	.25	.27**	.51	.25	.18*	.38	.23	.14	.38	.24	.14
Attachment disorganization				.20	.08	.25**	.17	.07	.21*	.19	.07	.23**
Behavior problems							.09	.02	.40***	.08	.02	.38***
Family relationship quality										.19	.09	.16*
R^2 change	.07			.06			.16			.03		
F for change in R^2	8.98**			7.36**			25.17***			4.23*		
R	.27**			.35***			.53***			.55***		

Note. From Carlson (1998). Copyright 1998 by University of Chicago Press. Reprinted by permission.
*$p < .05$; **$p < .01$; ***$p < .001$.

of the lack of self-integration and the impulse control problems associated with this disorder.

Anxious attachment in general, with no distinction between avoidance and resistance, was associated with depression (Duggal, Carlson, Sroufe, & Egeland, 2001). We believe that avoidance and resistance represent the initiations of two different pathways to depression, one based in alienation and the other based in helplessness and anxiety. Different factors likely would be required for perpetuating these two pathways, and different "comorbid" problems would be associated with the two types (e.g., conduct problems vs. anxiety). Limitation of our sample size has not allowed us to confirm this speculation, and it remains a problem for further research.

We predicted specifically that disorganized attachment would be linked to dissociative problems. Indeed, as others have written (e.g., Liotti, 1992; Main & Hesse, 1990), infants experiencing the conflict associated with a frightening or unfathomable parent have no choice but to engage in infantile versions of disrupted mental states (see Chapters 3 and 5). The situation posed by the simultaneous strong urge to flee from the source of fear (parent) and flee to the attachment figure (same parent) is not possible to resolve. And infants can only leave the situation psychologically, that is, with breakdowns in organized behavior and gaps in awareness (i.e., "protodissociative" experiences). Such a response then becomes a prototype for later adaptation. In fact, disorganized attachment was impressively related to DES scores (E. B. Carlson & Putnam, 1993) at age 19 years (.36) and modestly related to a composite of dissociation items on the behavior problem checklist at age 16 (Carlson, 1998). As have many others, we also found that dissociation was predicted by early maltreatment (Ogawa, Sroufe, Weinfield, Carlson, & Egeland, 1997). Moreover, there was a synergistic relation between disorganization and abuse with regard to dissociation. Children with histories of disorganized attachment, a "fragmented self," as we described it, were far more likely to show dissociative problems in the face of abuse than those with secure histories who experienced abuse. It has been frequently noted that not all who are abused dissociate. Reminiscent of our discussion of resilience in the preceding chapter, we argue that differential outcomes of abuse rest in part on prior history, certainly including disorganized attachment. Finally, in a structural model, we found that an early care factor (intrusiveness, low caregiving skill, and abuse) was strongly related to disorganized attachment, and that the link between early negative care and later pathology was mediated through disorganization (Carlson, 1998). We believe this is because of the disorganizing consequences of early malevolent care.

We conclude our discussion in this section with a presentation of

TABLE 12.2. Percentage of K-SADS Diagnoses in Adolescence by Preschool Maltreatment and Control Groups (*n* = 172)

Maltreatment	Depressed/ other mood disorders	Anxiety/phobia/ obsessive– compulsive disorder	Conduct disorder/ oppositional defiant disorder	Posttraumatic stress disorder	Comorbidity
Physical abuse	40	47	67	13	60
Unavailability	40	53	53	27	73
Neglect	31	62	38	15	54
Sexual abuse	64	64	55	27	73
Control	31	34	19	12	30

Note. From Egeland (1997). Copyright 1987 by University of Rochester Press. Reprinted by permission.

our overall findings concerning child maltreatment and later pathology (Egeland, 1997). Maltreatment represents such a distortion in the attachment relationship that it seems apt to include it here. These results are summarized in Table 12.2. Several points are clear. First, even though the nonmaltreated participants in our sample often qualified for some psychiatric diagnosis, such diagnoses were much more common when there was a history of maltreatment. For example, conduct disorder and oppositional defiant disorder (grouped together because of their close relation) are more than tripled in children with a history of physical abuse. Anxiety disorders are doubled in the face of neglect or sexual abuse. Posttraumatic stress disorder (PTSD) is doubled when there is a history of psychological unavailability or sexual abuse. Finally, the results on "comorbidity" are quite striking. This is the percentage of cases that qualified for at least two diagnoses of any kind. This characterized 30% of our nonmaltreated participants, thus confirming the general risk of being born into poverty. But the rate was 54% for neglect, 60% for physical abuse, and 73% for both sexual abuse and psychological unavailability. These straightforward outcome findings are dramatic. We provide an example of the place of maltreatment in a developmental process analysis in the later section on conduct disturbances.

DEVELOPMENTAL PATHWAYS TO SOME PROMINENT CHILD DISTURBANCES

Our research strategy, like our conceptualization of disturbance, is distinctive. In much research, one begins with children already diagnosed with the disorder in question and seeks to distinguish them from those with other problems or, more typically, children without problems. Such a strategy has clear advantages. It is an efficient way to ensure a sizable number of children with certain kinds of problems, and it has generated many important correlates. One disadvantage, however, is that it is difficult with such work to determine whether correlates obtained are antecedents or consequences. Even more important, it can reveal nothing about the developmental process. What are the precursor or insipient forms of the disturbance (i.e., what do the children look like before the diagnosable problem is manifest)? What are the steps in the emergence of the problem? What factors promote or interfere with movement along these steps? To answer these kinds of questions requires prospective longitudinal data. Longitudinal data also yield insights into antecedent–outcome chains. It is for these reasons that we used this approach.

Our approach, of course, has disadvantages as well. Gathering comprehensive data age by age means that sample size is constrained. This means that there are at times a rather small number of clinical cases. It also means that often our children had not been formally diagnosed until we did our own formal assessments at age 17½. This is because many troubled children do not get professional help. Therefore, before age 17, we relied on item summaries and scales from behavior problem checklists that had been validated against clinical groups. Still, we believe our data provided a start toward answering vital questions about the development of disturbance.

Attention-Deficit/Hyperactivity Disorder

ADHD has been the subject of a voluminous literature, with thousands of articles on neurophysiological correlates and drug treatment alone (see, e.g., Campbell, 2000, and Mash & Wolfe, 2002, for reviews). Every model and perspective on psychopathology, from genetic and biochemical models to sociocultural models, has been brought to bear on this set of problems, and it may well derive from numerous different pathways.

We begin with this set of problems specifically because it does *not* relate very well to attachment history. The occasional significant correlation with attachment history that was obtained probably derives from the fact that ADHD, like most disturbances, is very heterogeneous. Some of these children, for example, are very anxious, and attachment problems may contribute to this anxiety. Some are angry and thereby impulsive, and this anger may have attachment roots. However, it seems that for many children who qualify for this label, there is not a core secure-base problem or chronic emotional unavailability of the parent. Attachment is not related to everything and not everything is well related to attachment.

It is for this reason that we assessed multiple aspects of parenting. Certain of these aspects were specifically hypothesized to be influential in the development of ADHD problems. Given our developmental–organizational perspective, we expected attention, hyperactivity, and self-control problems to develop and thus to be related to experience, certainly including the nature of the care experienced. This would be true regardless of whether and how neurophysiological features contribute to pathways leading to these disturbances.

In our approach to ADHD, as with any disturbance, we began by asking why most children do not have these problems. For example, how do most children develop the capacities to sustain and flexibly deploy attention, to modulate their arousal (i.e., avoid extreme highs or lows, and settle themselves if too aroused), and to regulate impulses? What are the steps in such a normative developmental process? What kinds of supports are needed, and when are they needed? When such questions are answered, we can then ask how the process can go awry and begin our developmental analysis, which includes examining the role of caregiving across time.

We have previously described the developmental sequence underlying emergence of attention- and arousal-modulation capacities (e.g., Sroufe, 1989, 1997; see also Chapter 2, this volume). In the first months, such capacities are rather crude in the infant, and smooth, flexible deployment of attention and well-modulated arousal depends on the quality and timing of stimulation provided by caregivers and on caregivers' reading and appropriately responding to infant needs. As we discussed earlier, it is more a matter of caregiver regulation than infant regulation. Young infant control of state is primitive. The infant can turn on or shut down, but to sustain moderate arousal often requires appropriately trained stimulation at the hands of the caregiver. Caregivers learn to read infant signals and to provide care that keeps distress and arousal within reasonable limits. By effectively engaging the infant and encouraging ever-longer bouts of emotionally charged but organized behavior, they provide the infant with critical training in regulation.

Within the secure "holding" framework of the relationship (Brazelton et al., 1974), infants learn something vital about "holding" themselves, containing behavior, and focusing attention (Sroufe et al., 2000). When caregivers perceive that infants are becoming too aroused, they reduce or alter stimulation to keep arousal within manageable limits, thus entraining infants' nervous systems. In time, infants play a more active role by explicitly signaling needs and through increasing capacities to sustain attention and maintain moderate arousal. "If the caregiver misreads a signal, the older infant will adjust the behavior, often until the desired response is received" (Sroufe et al., 2000, p. 84). In the second and third years, the toddler's arousal modulation activities become more purposeful but still depend heavily on the caregiver to anticipate overly arousing situations and to step in when the child's capacities have been exceeded. There are many steps to the process that cannot be detailed here. "Basically, a process unfolds wherein what begins as caregiver-orchestrated regulation becomes dyadic regulation, with increasingly active participation by the infant. Then, progressively, transfer of the regulatory responsibility to the child occurs over the course of early childhood through a series of phases" (Sroufe, 1997, p. 258).

Given this analysis, it can be seen that this process can be derailed in various ways at different points in development. What we have described as intrusive or "uncooperative" care (see Chapters 3 and 5) would have serious effects in the first half-year. When unpredictable, sudden stimulation is frequent, with no preparation of the infant, the infant repeatedly experiences arousal jags with insufficient modulation, sensitizing certain brain systems toward overreactivity. Similarly, at a later point, when children typically are mastering some degree of self-modulation, if too much is required from the child at certain precise times, this can distort development. In particular, if time and time again caregivers further stimulate the child just as the child is at the edge of his tolerance, such that he is pushed over the edge into overarousal and disorganization, both arousal regulation and cognitive supports will be compromised. Inhibitory and excitatory brain systems will not be tuned, and the child will have the expectation that, when highly aroused, he will surely lose control. We developed our parent–child boundary dissolution measure at age 42 months with precisely these considerations in mind. For high scores on this scale, the parent teases, taunts, giggles with, or otherwise provokes the child precisely at the point when tension is elevated and the child is beginning to lose control. This could be viewed as promoting the development of ADHD-type problems, and it was the basis for our strongest hypothesis, formulated before any of our children entered school (Jacobvitz & Sroufe, 1987).

It should be clear from all of our earlier discussions that we do not view such aspects of parenting as inevitably causal in a simple, linear way. Rather, our hypothesis is that such patterns of care initiate and serve to maintain the child on a pathway probabilistically associated with later disturbance, along with a variety of other factors. Moreover, we know that parents are heavily influenced by their own histories and their current circumstances. And some children pose more challenge for some parents. Therefore, in our analyses, we examined child factors and aspects of the caregiving ecology, as well as these early parenting variables.

In our first analysis (Jacobvitz & Sroufe, 1987), we showed that both the intrusive care measure at 6 months and the overstimulation (boundary violation) measure at 42 months predicted activity and attention problems in kindergarten, based on a scale consisting of 11 pertinent items from the Achenbach and Edelbrock (1986) Child Behavior Checklist (e.g., easily distracted; can't concentrate; can't sit still, restless; talks out of turn). This scale strongly discriminated between clinical and nonclinical cases in Achenbach's large sample. While no temperament measures, including infant activity level, were predictive, one measure of newborn neurological status was predictive: the Brazelton motor maturity score on the NBAS. Even though we had no specific prediction for this variable, and other Brazelton variables with perhaps greater plausibility were not significant, it is nonetheless interesting to note that there was little overlap between cases captured by motor maturity and those captured by the caregiving variables (Jacobson & Sroufe, 1987). This is in accord with the possibility of multiple routes to these kinds of problems. We confirmed the distinctiveness of these pathways in later analyses during the elementary years (unpublished data).

Aside from the newborn motor maturity score, no measure of child behavior up through age 2½ predicted kindergarten activity and attention problems. However, distractibility of the child, when working with the mother in the teaching tasks at 42 months was predictive. Thus, by age 42 months, a pattern of child behavior becomes stable enough to predict the later outcome. It should be noted that distractibility itself was predicted by caregiver intrusiveness at 6 months (.31).

In a later analysis of attention and activity problems in first grade, we focused specifically on the 6-month intrusiveness variable (Egeland, Pianta, et al., 1993). Again, intrusiveness was strongly related to attention problems. Moreover, a key finding in this study was that this relation held even after statistically controlling for measures of positive parent–child interaction; that is, with regard to the development of attention problems, intrusive care is more than just the absence of positive care. There is specificity to many of our findings on disturbance; that is, we claim to do more than simply show that good things predict good things and bad things predict bad things (see the discussion of anxiety below).

Finally, we carried out a systematic and comprehensive analysis of attention and activity problems from early childhood through the elementary school years (Carlson et al., 1995). There were four phases of the project. First, we determined whether caregiver intrusiveness was related to early temperament, newborn neurological status, or any aspect of medical history. It was not. It was, however, related to prior measures of parental anxiety and to a key contextual variable; namely, the mother being single at the time of the child's birth. These analyses supported the contention that intrusiveness and overstimulation are caregiving variables and not simply caregiver reactions to temperamental infants. At the same time, we trust that readers are dissuaded from blaming caregivers given the contextual bases for these difficulties (see also below).

Next, we looked at links between early infant variables, caregiving, contextual variables, and child distractibility at age 42 months. Newborn motor maturity, caregiver intrusiveness, and relationship support for the mother all were significant. Only the correlation with intrusiveness was in the .20s (.27). No later measure of activity level or other aspect of infant temperament predicted distractibility.

In the third phase, we predicted to attention and activity problems in grades 1–3. No infant behavior variables, including numerous ratings of activity level and irritability, were related to this outcome. In contrast, both caregiver intrusiveness at 6 months and our boundary violation (overstimulation) variable at 42 months were predictive. So too were all three context measures included in the assessment (single status at birth and the mother's relationship support at 30 months and in grades 1–3). Single status at birth was the largest single predictor (.30). In hierarchical regression, the caregiving and contextual variables accounted for 17% of the variance in attention problems at this age. The child distractibility measure at 42 months accounted for a significant 3%. Overall, these are clear findings concerning the role for exogenous factors in the development of attention problems. When we arrayed our exogenous variables in chronological order, they were significant step-by-step. Single status predicted attention problems, then intrusiveness added, then relationship support at 30 months, overstimulation at 42 months, and current support in early elementary school added to them. We would argue that ADHD is a developmental outcome.

Moreover, the latter contextual variables also may be seen as accounting for change in the trajectory of the attention problem pathway from one age to the next, since they were significant after taking early care and 42-month distractibility into account. Each age represents the possibility of deflection away from attention and activity problems or of consolidating the tendency toward attention problems.

In predicting attention and activity problems at age 11, we found that the dominant predictor was prior attention problems. The correlation between grades 1–3 and grade 6 attention problems was .54. In regression analyses with prior attention problems entered first, overstimulation at age 42 months was still a significant predictor, but no other variable was. While this affirms the power of an early caregiving variable, it also supports the premise that the longer a pathway is pursued, the more difficult change becomes. (However, in a separate analysis, we found that our measures of parent–child boundary dissolution from the assessment at age 13 also were related to ADHD-type problems and predicted change in behavior problems from ages 11 to 16; see Hiester, 1993; Nelson, 1994.)

The preceding analysis was a harsh test of the influence of context, since context already was a part of attention problems in grades 1–3. Indeed, when entered prior to attention problem scores in grades 1–3, context variables (single status at birth, the mother's relationship support) did account for significant variation in attention problems at age 11. Moreover, when we looked at grades individually, rather than compositing across grades 1–3, we found context effects at each age. For example, relationship support for the mother accounted for change in attention–activity problems between grades 1 and 3, and relationship support at age 11 accounted for change between grades 3 and 6. And this is without specific intervention to bolster the context of parenting. We remain optimistic that supports for parents could alter the course of attention problems in some cases, even at this late age.

In the preceding analyses, we referred to these children as exhibiting attention and activity problems, since they, for the most part, had not been formally diagnosed as fitting criteria for ADHD. As a follow-up, we specifically compared children likely to meet clinical criteria for ADHD in early and late elementary school. This was done using T scores on the Achenbach Child Behavior Checklist of 67.5 or greater on an average of the "inattentive" and "nervous/overactive" factors. (Scores in this range have been clinically validated). This resulted in 22 cases for grades 1–3 and 19 for grade 6. Controls had T scores of less than 55. Single relationship status at birth, intrusive care at 6 months, and overstimulating care at 42 months distinguished these groups at both ages. Relationship support also distinguished the groups in grades 1–3. No infant measure or medical history variable distinguished the groups at either age. Thus, the importance of caregiving and contextual factors in the above analyses is not likely due to our use of non-clinical cases.

Conduct Problems

Conduct problems of children have been the focus of a great deal of research in the last two decades, and some important developmental hypotheses have emerged (e.g., Egeland et al., 1996, 2001; Moffitt, 1993; Rutter, 1997; Shaw, Owens, Vondra, Keenan, & Winslow, 1996; Stouthamer-Loeber et al., 1993). The profound consequences of early emergence of such problems and the related notion that there may be at least two groups of children with conduct problems, based on age of onset, have been especially important ideas. We sought to bring our long-term, prospective longitudinal data to bear on these issues.

For example, Moffitt (1993), presenting results from the Dunedin Longitudinal Study, made the distinction between what she referred to as life-course-persistent and adolescent-limited conduct disorders. She considered only the first group pathological, partly because of the persistence of the problems. These children showed early beginning and very persistent aggression and other conduct problems in childhood and adolescence, and on in to adulthood. Problems in the second group emerged first in adolescence, perhaps as a striving for autonomy, a desire to be popular, or mimicry of deviant peers. She did not see these children as truly troubled, although they were similar (though somewhat less severe) with regard to level of problem behaviors during the teen years. She expected them to account largely for the normative drop-off in antisocial behavior that occurs between adolescence and adulthood, although this has not yet been confirmed by her or by others (Roisman, Aguilar, & Egeland, 2004). Moffitt also argued that these two groups are distinctive in that the problems of the persistent group derive from an inherent neuropsychological deficit.

We found the first part of Moffitt's (1993) hypothesis exciting and compelling. The idea that young people with manifestly similar problems in adolescence could represent two distinctive pathways, with different potential outcomes, was seminal for developmental psychopathology—a first demonstration of the importance of pathway over "syndrome." This part of the thesis seems well supported and marks this as one of the most important papers of the previous decade.

We were more skeptical, however, concerning the conclusion that there was a neurological foundation for persistent conduct problems. There are compelling psychogenic alternatives that would explain the persistence of such problems as well, as we introduced earlier. Attachment theory, for example, began with Bowlby's observation in the 1940s that juvenile thieves routinely had backgrounds of parental abandonment and profound early privation. A very large number of studies have found an association between parental neglect or harsh treatment and later conduct problems (Elder, Nguyen, & Caspi, 1985; Eron & Huesman, 1990; Farrington, Ohlin, & Wilson, 1986; Patterson, Capaldi, & Bank, 1991; Patterson & Dishion, 1988), as have we (e.g., Egeland et al., 2001). The studies by Patterson and colleagues are perhaps most compelling, because they provide data on a cumulative, back-and-forth developmental process between parent and child, and demonstrate the impact of family intervention.

Persistence of early conduct problems would be explained by psychogenic theories based on the nature of this adaptation. Because harsh, chaotic treatment leads to interpersonal alienation and anger, a lack of internalized empathy, and impulse control problems due to early dysregulation, these children engage in disruptive, oppositional, and aggressive behaviors. Such behavior prompts further anger in, and harsh treatment from, parents, and alienates teachers and peers, leading to further rejection all around. Part of what is meant by *mal*adaptation is a pattern of behavior that elicits conditions that perpetuate the problem. Moreover, within a psychogenic position, comorbidity of conduct problems with ADHD is not paradoxical but expectable, due to the common core of dysregulation. Comorbidity with depression may derive from alienation underlying both conditions.

Our concerns with a neurological interpretation of the Moffitt data (1993) were both empirical and conceptual. Her empirical support for this supposition was that the persistent group had lower verbal abilities than the adolescent-onset group, based on psychological tests given in middle childhood. This is a good example of a finding in which one cannot conclude whether the neuropsychological measure represents a cause or a consequence; yet the Moffitt study is widely cited as demonstrating a neurological basis for conduct problems. The Dunedin study, impressive and important as it is, has no information on early temperament or direct signs of early compromised neurophysiology. In fact, the study begins with children at age 3, quite late in terms of development of temperamental and neurophysiological differences. Moreover, it does not have strong measures of parenting, and no observational measures of parenting at all.

We were able to test Moffitt's (1993) hypothesis more completely, because we had very early data on newborn neurological status, birth complications, and other medical problems, as well as temperament. Likewise, we had observational measures of early care and a variety of contextual measures. Finally, we had extensive measures of conduct problems and verbal ability outcomes.

We examined 15 temperament measures, and none showed the persistent group to be at a disadvantage compared to an adolescent-onset group (Aguilar et al., 2000). Likewise, we examined 10 early "neuropsychological variables," including delivery complications, nonoptimal newborn status on the Brazelton NBAS, infant anomalies, Bayley Scales of Infant Development, early language comprehension, and scales from the WIPPSI IQ test. Again, there were no significant differences. Even a neurological risk composite and a temperament risk composite failed to differentiate groups. Thus, no measures of language or cognitive functioning *in the preschool years* distinguished between those who would develop conduct disorders and those who would not.

In contrast, early psychosocial variables were predictive. We wanted a challenging test of our own hypothesis, in order to avoid capitalizing on chance. Therefore, we began with an overall psychosocial risk index made up of 15 variables. We required that this be significant before we examined specific variables. As in analyses throughout this book, we included parental care (e.g., intrusiveness, avoidant attachment, physical abuse, and neglect) and contextual variables (e.g., SES, life stress). This risk index was significantly higher for the early-onset group than for the adolescent-onset group (see Aguilar et al., 2000, for details). Moreover, groups differed significantly on numerous individual psychosocial risk variables. These included intrusiveness at 6 months, avoidant attachment, a parental involvement/support factor at 42 months, physical abuse, psychological unavailability, mother single at child's birth, and early family life stress. Abuse and neglect in the later elementary school years also were strongly discriminating but are best interpreted as signs of the ongoing process rather than as initiators of the pathway.

What about the differences in verbal ability reported by Moffitt (1993) in the elementary years? Such measures indeed revealed differences in our data, supporting the replicability of her results for such late measures of cognitive functioning. Specifically, we found lower performance among the early-onset cases compared to the adolescent-onset conduct problem group on both the Peabody Individual Achievement Test in elementary school and the Woodcock–Johnson Psychoeducational Battery in high school. However, such ability differences may be best interpreted as consequences of being on this pathway beginning early in life. Rather than being viewed as underlying causes of conduct problems, they might be better viewed as factors serving to maintain individuals on this pathway. To repeat, there were no differences on verbal measures in the early years.

For the most part, our data were in accord with the idea that adolescent-onset cases of conduct problems were similar to our participants without conduct problems in many ways. For example, social support and life stress experienced by the family in middle childhood were not distinctive, nor did parental reports indicate greater stress in adolescence. Thus, we had difficulty accounting for individual reasons for why conduct problems emerged in these young people. However, members of the adolescent-onset group did report experiencing greater stress and distress in adolescence. Therefore, while such a pathway may not represent the same degree of disturbance as that for the early-onset group, the condition also may not be entirely benign.

We believe that the most important work to be done on conduct problems in the future concerns the process by which risk factors lead to these problems (Egeland et al., 2001). Where we firmly agree with Moffitt (1993) and others is on the importance of early onset of conduct problems (Gilliom & Shaw, 2004). If this pathway is enjoined early and followed even up to age 7 or 8, later negative outcomes are quite likely.

Thus, a priority in our work has been to understand the complex processes supporting this pathway early in life. In one model that we tested, we found that early physical abuse represented an initiation of the pathway, and that its impact in part was mediated through subsequent alienation from the parent (Egeland et al., 2001). Thus, a latent alienation factor was created from noncompliance, negative affectivity, and avoidance of the mother at age 42 months, and this accounted for a significant portion of the link between abuse and externalizing problems in the first 3 years of elementary school. This work on our project is ongoing.

Depression

Our primary work on the development of depression, like our study of conduct problems, was a guided by prevailing hypotheses concerning two distinctive conditions. In this case, however, the key idea was that childhood depression and adult depression may represent different problems (e.g., Harrington, Rutter, & Fombonne, 1996). There have been many reasons for suspecting this distinction. Childhood depression is more rare than adult depression, and there is a striking difference in gender makeup at the two age periods. In childhood, the ratio is even, or perhaps there are slightly more boys; beginning in adolescence, there are dramatically more females. Not surprisingly, given these demographics, there is rather little stability from childhood to adulthood. In fact, one study found that child conduct problems were a better predictor of adult depression than was childhood depression (Robins & Price, 1991). We found a correlation of only .22 between levels of childhood and adolescent depression, well less than half of the stability coefficient that we obtained for conduct problems. Based on all of this, as well as cross-sectional data on correlates at the two ages, Harrington and colleagues (1996) argued that adolescent onset depression more often was an early onset of adult depression and perhaps had a genetic base, whereas childhood depression was more associated with psychosocial adversity and not necessarily a precursor to adult depression. But they called for longitudinal studies to clarify the matter.

Our study again offered several advantages for approaching these questions. Not only did we have longitudinal data on depression, with multiple measures of depression in both childhood and adolescence, but we also had data on all of the pertinent predictors. Our measures of child depression included the CDRS, and our measures of adolescent depression included the K-SADS, with behavior problem checklist data at both age periods from multiple reporters (see Chapter 4). We also had measures on mothers' depression (the Beck Depression Inventory), and all of the measures of parental care and family adversity discussed previously. Direct observational measures of parenting are extremely important in this case. Studies that rely on interview or self-report measures of parenting are subject to bias, because it is well known that one consequence of depression is negative perceptions (Chi & Hinshaw, 2002). Therefore, if depressed parents (or children) describe parenting in negative terms, then this could be a consequence of depression and not point to a cause. Our measures were completely independent.

There was already a substantial literature suggesting that inadequate care, especially neglect and physical or sexual abuse, was associated with depression in children (e.g., Cicchetti & Toth, 2000; Toth, Manly, & Cicchetti, 1992; Trickett & Putnam, 1993). Such a connection was viewed as likely mediated by low self-esteem, negative expectations concerning relationships, and emotional dysregulation associated with inadequate care. As Toth and colleagues (1992) concluded, "Disruption in or the unavailability of adequate care provides a unifying framework for understanding the occurrence of depression" (p. 98). We sought to add to this literature by comparing the caregiving and contextual antecedents of child- and adolescent-onset depression (Duggal et al., 2001).

In the case of childhood depression, we found that the single strongest predictor was some form of early abuse (.30), and an early supportive care composite, an early life stress measure, and a measure of relationship support for mother all were significant as well. Mother's depression also was related to childhood depression (.24), but each of our four adversity variables predicted above and beyond maternal depression. In regression analysis, there was a significant interaction of maternal depression with gender, which revealed that a mother's depression had a greater impact for boys than for girls in childhood (accounting for 5% of the variance). Even after maternal depression and this interaction were included, the four psychosocial variables still explained an additional 13% of the variance.

In the case of adolescent depression, maternal depression (.29), early care (.31), and abuse (.18) were the significant predictors. In regression, there was again a large maternal depression–child gender interaction, accounting for 10% of the variance. In this case, however, the impact was dramatically greater for *girls*. Even after taking this effect into account, supportive early care and family stress still contributed significantly to adolescent depression.

There is some support in these data for the greater involvement of adversity in producing childhood depression and a greater role for the mother's depression (a possible surrogate for a genetic factor) in adolescent-onset depression. This was even more clear when we looked at clinical groups; that is, young persons who had depression scores high enough to be clinically significant. Both abuse and early family stress were significantly higher for child cases than for adolescent-onset cases. Within adolescence, the depressed clinical group was distinguished from control cases only by maternal depression.

Considering gender as well yields a richer picture. For boys, quality of early care predicted depression not only in childhood (.27) but also in adolescence (.40). In fact, *early* care was more strongly predictive of the adolescent outcome than was later parental care. Care was not significant for girls at either age. Maternal depression, on the other hand, was significant only for girls in adolescence (.41), not for boys (.15). Thus, with our data, the case for depression as two distinctive conditions may fit better for girls than it does for boys or, alternatively, childhood depression in boys and adolescent depression in girls may be distinctive problems. In fact, for boys, maternal depression was more strongly related to childhood depression (.26) than to adolescent depression (.15), perhaps through its consequences for maternal behavior.

One interpretation of these data, of course, is that females are more vulnerable to early-onset adult depression, with a genetic vulnerability being an additional risk. However, there are alternative explanations for the impact of our genetic surrogate, maternal depression. Numerous investigators have demonstrated that parental depression has an impact on parenting. Downey and Coyne (1990), following an extensive review, concluded that the parenting of depressed mothers is characterized by constricted affect and expressiveness, flat speech, less attentiveness, and less positive responsiveness to their children. They also "show heightened levels of child-directed hostility and negativity, and . . . coercion rather than negotiation" (p. 63). Embry and Dawson (2002) have shown that atypical brain functioning in infants and preschoolers whose mothers are depressed is mediated by insensitive interactions by these caregivers. When insensitivity is controlled, significant differences between these children and controls disappear. Moreover, children of mothers whose depression remitted by age 3 years no longer showed brain patterns different from normal. Finally, Crockenberg and Covey (1991) have shown that when children of depressed mothers interact with nondepressed fathers, the patterns of interaction are not different than those of control children. Thus, the atypical behavior and emotional expression of these children are early on based in the relationship with their mothers.

Studies also have found evidence that the link between parental depression and later offspring depression may be mediated by parental behavior (Bifulco et al., 2002; Johnson, Cohen, Kasen, Smailes, & Brook, 2001). Once parental behavior was taken into account, parent depression was no longer a significant predictor. Since these studies relied on single reporters for measures, the mediation effect may be overestimated.

We recently conducted a similar path-analytic study and supported the same conclusion to a lesser degree, and only for boys (Burt et al., in press). Nonetheless, this remains an important consideration.

In our data set, we have found with a variety of outcomes that characteristics of the mother consistently are more predictive for girls, while maternal care, life stress, and family disruptions have been more predictive for boys (Sroufe & Egeland, 1991). Why this should be so, and why it should be especially true in adolescence, can be explained by "gender intensification theory" (Hill & Lynch, 1983). Differential role expectations increase following puberty, and as identity issues become salient, girls are influenced by the identity of their same-sex parent. Mothers confide more in their daughters, and depressed mothers more often use daughters for comforting (Radke-Yarrow, Richters, & Wilson, 1988). Reciprocally, daughters may become overly involved with them and worry about them. This greater burden could play a large role in the differences in depression of adolescent females versus males. Studies with two-parent families are needed to explore whether a similar process would occur with fathers and sons.

Anxiety

In our studies of anxiety problems, we have focused on models of developmental process and on the way in which newborn neurophysiological status and early temperament combine with experience. We reported earlier that anxious–resistant attachment history predicted anxiety disorders at age 17 (Warren et al., 1997). In that study, it was also the case that one measure of newborn functioning, habituation to startle on the Brazelton Neonatal Behavioral Assessment Scale, showed a significant relation with that same outcome. Resistant attachment was still significant when controlling for this variable. However, the key finding was that resistant attachment and the temperament variable showed a notable interaction effect; that is, the combination of the two had an effect on later anxiety, above and beyond either variable considered alone.

In a more recent paper, we explored in more detail a developmental pathways analysis of anxiety problems (Bosquet & Egeland, in press). Here, we found support for a model in which anxious attachment and nonoptimal temperament (a combination of nurses' ratings of newborns and Brazelton NBAS state and habituation factors) predicted first to problems of emotional regulation in our Barrier Box situation at age 3½ and, partly through that, to childhood anxiety problems, and on to anxiety in adolescence. A central finding was that this model showed discriminant validity vis à vis depression and other disturbances. This important demonstration is not simply a case of good things predicting good things and bad things predicting bad things. That the model predicted anxiety and not depression was a stringent test, because these two sets of problems have proven especially difficult to distinguish in research.

CONCLUSION

With each pattern of disturbance we examined, the validity of the developmental–construction viewpoint was supported. Generally, pathways to disturbance appear to be initiated early in life. Given the time span covered, early care measures were at times remarkably predictive, as in the .40 correlation of early care with adolescent depression in boys, and the .36 correlation between disorganized attachment and dissociation tendencies at age 19. However, even given this demonstrable role for early care and experience, we do not view links with later problems as direct or inevitable. Always, cumulative measures of care and adversity were stronger, and pursuing the pathway to ultimate psychiatric classification entailed maintenance or deflection by ongoing quality of experience and the surrounding context.

We did not often find evidence that early temperamental variation was strongly predictive of later psychiatric problems. It is noteworthy that in those cases in which we found temperament to be predictive, it was largely in interaction with experiential factors. Such interactions between biological and experiential factors are getting increasingly more attention in the field (e.g., Caspi et al., 2002; Gilliom & Shaw, 2004; Kochanska et al., 2004). Perhaps in time, studies using stronger measures of temperament than were available to us will find even more compelling results. Until such prospective, longitudinal data on objectively measured early temperament are available, however, we would urge caution in interpreting claims of simple endogenous etiology, especially when couched in terms of linear causal models.

Our work has clear implications for the research agenda in psychopathology. When disturbances are viewed in developmental perspective, process questions are central. When developmental pathways rather than inherent deficits are emphasized, prevention and alterations of course, rather than treatment, come to the fore. Rather than simply seeking singular roots and correlates of disorder, researchers would focus instead on complex factors that initiate pathways and the array of factors that keep individuals on, or deflect them from, such pathways.

Our promotion of a developmental perspective certainly does not disallow consideration of biological and neurophysiological factors in the study of disturbance. Central nervous system and hormonal functioning are always part of the ongoing context of development (e.g., Cicchetti & Cannon, 1999). A place for such considerations is clear and obvious, even in our data. For example, we find huge gender differences in both rates and development of disorder, and further differences before and after puberty. While we, of course, take a complex, interactive view of gender and experience, gender and puberty are nonetheless biological markers that command attention. Other biological and physiological markers likewise will have important roles to play in differentiating pathways that may manifest in similar behaviors at certain times. In the end, converging psychological and neurophysiological data will be the greatest assurance that we, as scientists, are on the right path in seeking to understand behavioral and emotional disturbance.

CHAPTER 13

Clinical Implications

> Once the [therapeutic] process has started he begins to see the old images (models) for what they are, the not unreasonable products of his past experiences or of what he has been repeatedly told, and thus to feel free to imagine alternatives better fitted to his current life.
>
> —BOWLBY (1988)

The findings reported in the previous chapters, and the perspective on development that they support, have implications for conceptualizing child disturbance, for etiology and classification of child problems, and for prevention and intervention efforts. Indeed, not only other developmental researchers (e.g., NICHD, 1997) but also clinical investigators have drawn upon our research findings, concepts, and methods. We briefly overview the implications of our research for clinical work in this chapter.

Since we began our research within Bowlby's attachment theory, we begin our discussion with his ideas regarding psychopathology and clinical practice, and later bring in the work of more contemporary clinical investigators. In the end, our work strongly supports some widely held propositions, including the idea that the early years have special importance in the formation of the personality, that emotional life is central in human functioning, and that malevolent experience can lead to distortions in cognition and feeling, the causes of which may lie outside of awareness.

These ideas may be viewed as broadly psychoanalytic. But the content and the nature of Bowlby's explanation of the origins of psychopathology took psychoanalytic theory in a distinctive direction. Bowlby followed a branch early abandoned by Freud, which emphasized the child's actual experiences rather than the child's inherent conflicts and fantasies (Breger, 1974; Loevinger, 1976). Contemporary workers have now integrated the emphasis on experience with a concern about the child's interior world as well (e.g., Slade, 1999; see section on intervention below).

CONCEPTUALIZING DISTURBANCE

Following Bowlby, we view the actual experiences of the child as central in the etiology of disturbance. In our study, caregiver psychological unavailability, physical abuse, sexual abuse, and serious distortions in the infant–caregiver relationship (disorganized attachment) were strong predictors of later psychopathology (see Chapter 12). Without such experience, psychopathology was not nearly as common. Of course, all children experience the entire gamut of emotions with some frequency. But it is not normal to have strong and pervasive feelings of hatred or suspiciousness toward one's parents. As Bowlby (1988) suggested, when children do feel pervasively angry or guilty, or are chronically frightened about being abandoned, they have come by such feelings honestly, that is, because of experience. When, for example, children fear abandonment, it is not in counterreaction to their intrinsic homicidal urges; rather, it is more likely because they *have been* abandoned physically or psychologically, or have been repeatedly threatened with abandonment. When children are pervasively filled with rage, it is due to rejection or harsh treatment. When children experience intense inner conflict regarding their angry feelings, this likely is because expressing them may be forbidden or even dangerous (see also Jacobvitz, Hazen, Curran, & Hitchens, 2004). "Irrational" fears and worries, too, generally are rooted in experience.

Bowlby (1988) described one case in which a child was terrified that pieces of furniture would become animate and hurl themselves at her. He argued that this was not in response to inner conflict regarding the child's own destructive urges. Rather, as it turned out, the child's father, in blind rages, had actually thrown pieces of furniture and hit her with them. In general, Bowlby argued that thoughts or feelings that now seem distorted or out of place were at one time reasonable responses to actual circumstances.

In his essay, "On Knowing What You Are Not Supposed to Know and Feeling What You Are Not Supposed to Feel," Bowlby (1988) pointed to the importance of both explicit and implicit messages that are contained in the parents' actions. By being told repeatedly that something does not hurt and that big boys do not cry, for example, children learn to not recognize such feelings. A girl repeatedly told by mother that father died in a car accident, when the child found him hanging, can lead her not to access the memory of the witnessed death and to have no place to put the attendant feelings. In addition, of course, this child would add emotional abandonment by mother to death of the father in her experienced losses.

Beyond being explicitly told not to remember things, there are three other explanations for failures to access experience. First, Bowlby pointed out the problems that occur when the child's inner working models of self and other, based upon direct experience, are contradicted by what the child explicitly is told is the case ("You are lucky to be treated so well"). Children have no choice but to believe, at a conscious level, what parents tell them is the truth. When the representation of actual experience is contradictory to what they have been told, this must remain outside of awareness, engendering various kinds of distortions of thinking and feeling. The child thus has inner conflict, but this is because two powerful sources of information are in contradiction. When children must disown powerful experiences they have had, problems created include "chronic distrust of other people, inhibition of their curiosity, distrust of their own senses, and a tendency to find everything unreal" (Bowlby, 1988, p. 103).

A second reason for shutting off memories is that parents have treated children in ways that are too unbearable to think about. A child cannot easily face recognizing that a parent (his protector and guardian) has malevolence toward him. For example, Bowlby reports a case in which a mother locked herself away from her young child when he was crying and frequently left him alone, screaming in terror. He later was for a time unable to recall such scenes. Similarly, the child with the fear of flying furniture for a long time had no memory of the causal events. Equally important, there also is "exclusion from consciousness of the thoughts, feelings, and impulses to action that are the natural responses to such events" (p. 113). Thus, a particular child may well have pervasive angry feelings and strike out in an apparently random fashion, but these are consequences of particular malevolent experiences. Repeated rejection of the child across the early years, especially when combined with contempt for the child's desire for care and comforting, was argued to be the foundation for personality disorders, ranging from a false sense of self to fugue and multiple personality.

The final reason for shutting off memories, the one embraced more generally by psychoanalysts, is that the child did or thought something about which he or she feels guilty or ashamed. Even here, the intensity of such feelings and the failure to resolve them, likely have to do with the treatment the child experienced. It is parents that first engage in unacceptable practices or that find the child's natural behavior to be shameful. The child with a pervasive sense of shame has somehow *been* shamed.

Support for the Role of Negative Experience and Atypical Representations

In addition to his clear and compelling logic, Bowlby used three sorts of evidence to bolster his theory about the experience-based etiology of dissociation and disturbance. First were developments in cognitive science, in which processes and mechanisms had been revealed that demystified the process of shutting off experiences from memory. There are multiple levels of information processing. External perceptions (and, presumably, internal perceptions as well) are screened for relevance at a preconscious level. Only some of the many possible matters that we could consciously entertain do we in fact attend to consciously. One need merely assume that certain kinds of experience can lead to distortions in what gets marked as "not relevant." Excluding information per se is a normal process (Carlson, Yates, & Sroufe, in press). The second source of evidence was certain kinds of experimental data, studies demonstrating both nonconscious processing of information and concordances between parental exclusion or denial of certain kinds of information and their children's exclusion of the same kind of material (see Bowlby, 1988). Finally, Bowlby drew upon many clinical case studies, wherein recounted histories or uncovered memories seemed to confirm the role of negative experience. Such cases, of course, have been criticized because of their retrospective nature and the possibility that "memories" were created in therapy and did not reflect actual events.

What was needed, and what Bowlby explicitly called for, were longitudinal studies that could confirm the origins of inner working models (the child's particular way of seeing him- or herself and others), the link between malevolent experience and later disturbance, and, especially, the relevance of distortions in early caregiving relationships and later tendencies to dissociation. This is where our work and the work of other longitudinal researchers came into play. Bowlby was an avid supporter of such work.

In general, our study strongly supported the predictive power of childhood experience. Observed experiences of sensitive, responsive care; consistent availability of parents for comforting, support, and nurturance; and later encouragement and guidance predicted measures of competence at every age. Likewise, intrusive care, chronic rejection and rebuff, hostility and boundary violations, physical and sexual abuse, *all documented at the time of occurrence*, were predictive of a host of problems, including serious disturbance. More specifically, we were able to document that early distortions in the caregiver–infant relationship (disorganized attachment), accompanied by documented maltreatment of the child, were strongly predictive of dissociative problems at 19 years of age (Carlson, 1998; Ogawa et al., 1997). Thus, in accord with Bowlby's theorizing, a profound inability to remain conscious of one's salient experience and to integrate diverse aspects of experience seems to be a legacy of early malevolent experience. Such incapacities are acquired.

A Case of Recovered Memory

Oftentimes we found that early frightening or otherwise threatening experiences (abuse, witnessing parental violence, multiple family disruptions) were more strongly predictive of later problems than were similar negative experiences in middle childhood. This was perhaps because, at an early phase of differentiation, the developmental structure is more broadly impacted by a disorganizing influence or because, as Bowlby suggested, young children are more vulnerable to following implicit or explicit proscriptions not to remember, and therefore to experiencing the distortions in emotional life that follow.

In this regard, we recount a case of memory loss and recovered memory that we have published (Duggal & Sroufe, 1998). In comparison to retrospective reports that previously were cited as testimony to recovered memory, our case had several strengths. First, the presence of sexual abuse at the hands of the father during the preschool period was authenticated at that time. Child Protection intervened, and visitation with father was temporarily terminated; there was a police investigation, and the child entered therapy. Therapy notes made at the time later were, with consent, made available to the project. Moreover, this child was in our nursery school during this period, and observations of her difficulties at that time made by her teachers (who were unaware of the abuse) corroborated the therapist's impressions. Finally, the experiences were described by the child's mother during our yearly interviews. Thus, the abuse in this case was documented at the time, not based upon recall.

Second, project data also confirm that for a time the child talked about the abuse (e.g., as noted in interviews with early elementary school teachers). Thus, the experiences did register and were represented.

Third, a period of "forgetting" was documented. No mention of the abuse was in the later records of interviews with teachers. Moreover, in two of our adolescent interviews, young people were asked, with probing, if they had ever experienced abuse. (Our interviewers were, of course, always blind to history.) This child said explicitly that nothing "like that" had ever happened to her. This is important, because if events were always consciously remembered but just not talked about, this is not the kind of shutting off Bowlby was suggesting. And in this case, it is not likely that the child was merely withholding from the interviewer. For example, she had no hesitance to share information about her own sexual activity.

Finally, the child recovered a partial memory of the abuse, and not in the context of therapy; that is, there is no way that it was suggested by a therapist. As it turned out, our interviewer, again, having no knowledge of the 19-year-old's history, was partly involved. This time, when a question about sexual abuse was raised, the child said that it was very interesting, because she recently had experienced a vague sense of something. When talking to a girlfriend about earliest memories, she had the sense that there was something that she could not quite remember, but it was frightening. As she talked to the interviewer, more came back. She had an image of being in a particular room on a bed and seeing her father approaching her. He was naked above the waist (she could "see" no more) and he bent down toward her, and it was very frightening. Recovering this fragment left her very upset and avoidant of her father, who would not acknowledge his behavior.

She could not, and still cannot, remember more, but the sleeping situation when she was 4 years old was as she described from her memory. She stated that she previously had absolutely no memory of this. Her mother was surprised, due to all of the talking about it that was done in early childhood. However, we think the memory disappeared at around age 7 or 8, when custody arrangements changed and the child was again staying with her father. It would have been too overwhelming to be conscious of the prior abuse in that context. Moreover, the father had never admitted to her or anyone else that he had been abusive, and she would have experienced pressure to conform to this viewpoint. We believe that this longitudinal case supports the numerous retrospective cases of traumatic exclusion of experience cited by Bowlby.

Representations Outside of Verbal Awareness

Our work also supports the contention that negative experience will be represented in the child's mind, regardless of whether it is consciously accessible. We find many cases in our study in which young people state on the Adult Attachment Interview that they have no memories whatsoever of early maltreatment, even though we have documented that it occurred (Huston, 2001). In some cases, this may not be due to lack of memory, but simply to not seeing parental mistreatment as abuse. Some cite examples of obvious maltreatment as though they confirm the parent's love. Here in Minnesota, we believe that being shut out of the house, barefoot, on a winter night, is cruel and prosecutable, but such things have been described by some of our participants as "caring," for example, "because it showed how much she wanted me to be a better person." Still, despite shutting off such memories *or* feelings from awareness, they do show up it certain forms of representation. Projective stories, for example, of children being pursued by malevolent people or dangerous animals, in fact more often are told by children who experienced maltreatment at home (McCrone et al., 1994). Children whose drawings depict ominous signs significantly more often have histories of disorganized attachment relationships (Carlson & Levy, 1999; Fury et al., 1997). Preschoolers whose play is absent of people more often have experienced chronic emotional unavailability (Rosenberg, 1984). Those whose play is filled with unresolved conflict more often have histories in which anxiety about relationships has been prevalent. Time and again, the content of children's minds, as well as their expectations and interpretations of others, reflect their lived history (see also Chapters 7 and 11).

One telling example is the dream of RN, a preschooler. Over the course of the term, RN was developing a great fondness for Jane, one of our teachers. Indeed, Jane had been extraordinarily nurturing of her, despite RN's emotional lability and explosive temper. Midway through the semester, RN told of a dream she had, in which Jane had hurled her against a wall. Jane told RN that she would never do that, to which RN responded, "Why not?" "Because I love you," said Jane, to which RN responded, "Why?" To this child, such statements of genuine caring and affection were perplexing. As one might expect, RN had received harsh, unpredictable treatment from her emotionally unstable mother. Her internal world reflected the external world she had known. Her feelings of intense anger were especially aroused in response to those who drew near to her. While she only rarely overtly expressed anger at Jane, their developing closeness intensified her feelings of vulnerability regarding rejection. RN's sense of the terrible things that can happen when one entertains longings for closeness, and her intense anxiety about rejection, are reflected in her dream (see also Kalsched, 1996).

Continuing Questions

We by no means would claim to have completely demonstrated the validity of the theoretical propositions outlined earlier. Our work represents only a beginning. We have shown only in a coarse way that adverse experience is internalized and is associated with later problems. There is a very long way to go in linking the particular problems, and patterns of problems, shown by children and youth, the *particular* experiences they have had, and the representations that mediate them.

One example of this need for further research comes from our study of children in nursery school and elementary school. In this work, we established a broad association between a history of seductive care and a predefined class of problems (Sroufe & Jacobvitz, 1989). Some of these children who had experienced earlier seductive care were later victimized by other children. Others were impulsive, inattentive, and hyperactive. Still others were highly anxious and tense, or very coy, eliciting a great deal of attention and affection from adults and older children. There were various combinations of these problems, and sometimes the manifestation changed over time. For example, one boy who was impulsive and victimized as a preschooler was seen as primarily nurtured and protected by older girls in early elementary school. He was highly anxious at both ages. As a young adult, he sexually exploits women. While such links are quite interesting and confirm the importance of thinking in terms of branching pathways (see Chapter 12), our point here is that we cannot at present account for why one child showed one pattern or another, or why the manifestation may change as it does from one age to another. Moreover, the number of cases involved was not sufficient to link this up with individual patterns of representation. Perhaps this level of understanding could be reached with a larger study, and with more detailed and comprehensive information regarding early and changing experience. In general, much more work is needed on how particular combinations of experience at different ages work together to impact the development of problems.

CLASSIFICATION AND ETIOLOGY

Our developmental study and the foregoing theoretical considerations regarding etiology lead to some distinctive ways of thinking about classification of children's problems. Our study has implications for evaluating the current approach to the classification of children's problems and perhaps for setting a direction for a fundamentally new approach. The boldest interpretation of our work would lead to a system based on classifying patterns of adaptation and developmental trajectories, rather than manifest problems alone.

Approaches to classification are always intertwined with thinking about etiology, even when this is not explicit, or when classification principles are not consistent. For example, in a deficit model, there is an assumption of a specific pathogen and a specific disorder (Sameroff, 2000). Discrete causal influences and discrete resulting categories are presumed, with clear distinctions among resulting taxa. As we discussed in Chapter 12, this is no longer accepted even in medicine, because in modern medicine multiple interacting factors of various kinds can lead to disorders such as heart disease. Nonetheless, in psychiatry and psychology, all too often the single pathogen–discrete entity connection is assumed, even though this is challenged by the rampant problem of comorbidity (see Chapter 12).

In contrast, in the developmental–organizational approach that we advocate, cause is complex. Early patterns of maladaptation, or extreme adversity, such as a history of physical abuse, are seen as creating vulnerabilities that in interaction with later factors are probabilistically linked to a range of various manifestations. Thus, a history of physical abuse is associated with both externalizing problems, such as conduct disturbance, and internalizing problems, such as depression. This is actually consistent with the reality that externalizing and internalizing problems routinely are found to correlate, including in our study, in the .50s or above. Groups of children with certain commonalities of history may be defined by common core issues, but these are looser groups than implied by the standard approach, with great individual variation in patterning of particular problems.

Evaluating the *Diagnostic and Statistical Manual of Mental Disorders*

The current approach to classification, as represented by the *Diagnostic and Statistical Manual of Mental Disorders* (DSM) of the American Psychiatric Association (1994), certainly has a number of strengths. First, it is widely known and accepted, and therefore aids communication among professionals and compilation of research findings. Second, it is comprehensive. It is difficult to find a seriously troubled child whose problems do not fit into the scheme at one or more places. Third, the multiaxial system allows consideration of contextual factors, such as stress, and certain aspects of history. Fourth, subcategories defined for many problems are an acknowledgment of the heterogeneity of most disorders, as is the fact that different combinations of problems can lead to the same diagnosis. As one example, in DSM-III, there was a distinction between "socialized" and "nonsocialized" conduct disorder, which allowed for the possibility that some conduct disturbed young people were simply adhering to peer norms. This important idea anticipated the later work on early-onset and adolescent-onset conduct disorder (see Chapter 12). Unfortunately, this distinction was dropped in later versions of the

DSM. Finally, there are some other developmental ideas imbedded in the DSM. Age of onset of symptoms is given notable attention. Antisocial personality disorder, for example, cannot be given as a diagnosis in the absence of a history of childhood problems. Sudden onset of violent behavior in adulthood, in the absence of child conduct problems, likely suggests a serious, organically based problem. Often, diagnosis of children requires greater frequency of particular problems than are usually manifested by children at that same age. This is another developmental feature. Moreover, there are descriptions in a number of categories of how the problem profile may change between childhood and adolescence. In general, description of the categories has become more concise and clear in the DSM.

Despite these strengths, the DSM system is also plagued by a number of problems. There have been numerous critiques in the literature (e.g., Cantwell, 1996). Some have expressed concerns regarding its structure (e.g., the range of categories from quite broad to exceedingly specific) or the lack of unifying theory. Others have expressed concern about its overinclusiveness, in which every manner of problem is encompassed (e.g., implying that difficulties with math or reading are psychiatric disorders). Still others have called attention to the ubiquitous problem of comorbidity (e.g., Caron & Rutter, 1991). To date, research has shown that "comorbid" children have a worse prognosis, but no one has shown that this is not simply a function of having more problems, regardless of number of categories represented. Comorbidity is just assumed to have some kind of meaning, because the children's problems span multiple, preconceived categories.

Beyond these problems, we are concerned primarily with the relative lack of developmental thinking in the DSM, even acknowledging the few examples provided above. At one time, child categories essentially included psychosis, retardation, and "adjustment reaction to childhood." These categories were at first proliferated as downward extensions of adult disorders, rather than considering childhood in its own right. Subsequently, committees of clinicians met and defined new categories. But there was no discernible attempt to start with normal development and define deviations from there. Among the developmental concepts not present is differentiation; this would include the possibility that there are rather fewer, more general child categories that ultimately branch into a larger number of categories. Rather, more and more child categories have been added with each version of the DSM. Likewise, there was insufficient attention to transformation. Thus, researchers had to discover, as they now have, that oppositional defiant disorder and conduct disorder really are not two distinctive problems (see Rutter & Sroufe, 2000, for comment and references). More typically, oppositional defiant disorder is a developmental precursor of conduct disorder or a "stepping-stone" toward conduct disorder (e.g., Farrington, 1995). In general, we believe that these conceptual problems derive primarily from embracing a deficit model, with diseases rather than problems of development as the focus.

Posttraumatic Stress Disorder and Attachment Disorders

Some colleagues have asked whether categories such as PTSD and attachment disorders are not encouraging signs that this system is becoming more inclusive of psychogenic factors and developmental considerations. At first glance, it may appear that way. Indeed, it is important that there is recognition that trauma, if severe enough, leads to attention, cognitive, and affective problems that are hallmarks of disturbance. However, it is unfortunate that the consequences of trauma, and harsh experience more generally, are sequestered into such a category. The link between trauma and other problems, such as anxiety, depression, or ADHD, is not considered. Thus, if one fails to meet specific criteria for PTSD (including identifying a specific trauma), we risk a presumption of organic etiology. Trauma, or a generally threatening environment, likely is one of the foundations for many of the problems of childhood.

The category of attachment disorders has similar problems. It is to the good that the particular problems specified have been included and that the experiential base is required. There has been some very good thinking about the nature and variety of attachment disturbances (e.g., Zeanah, Boris, & Lieberman, 2000). Moreover, it has been very important to recognize the plight of institutionalized and other extremely deprived infants. One could think of this as an appropriate start toward inclusion of attachment issues in the DSM. But there is again a sequestering of attachment problems into a few very specific syndromes, as well as an absence of developmental thinking. According to this system, if one is not excessively inhibited, hypervigilant, or ambivalent toward caregivers, or indiscriminately friendly or totally unable to form a relationship, one does not have an attachment problem. Only 2 or 3 of the 180 children we studied would have truly fit these categories; yet attachment problems, at times severe, were common. The vast majority of children, even those who are both avoidant and disorganized as infants, do not fit this diagnosis, even though they are dramatically more likely to have a range of serious problems later (and fit numerous DSM categories). Those with avoidant histories can be atypically forward in new social situations, and they rarely formed close friendships in our summer camps, but they do not meet criteria. Even many of the East European orphans, whose relational abilities are seriously compromised, do not meet diagnostic criteria. Finally, this categorization of attachment problems may shift the focus from relationship to individual diagnosis and treatment.

We are not advocating a broadening of the attachment disorders categories. To the contrary, we do not think avoidant or disorganized attachment should be thought of as *disorders*. Rather, as we have argued in earlier chapters, patterns of anxious attachment should be thought of as initiating pathways, which over time can terminate in a variety of forms represented in the DSM. Thus, as with the earlier discussion of trauma, it should be recognized that attachment issues are prominent foundations of many childhood disturbances, ranging from anxiety problems and other internalizing disorders to oppositional defiant disorder, conduct disorder, and other externalizing problems. Having an "attachment disorder" category has the potential of drawing attention away from the broader role of attachment (for further discussion, see Carlson, Sampson, & Sroufe, 2003).

A Task for the Future

The DSM system has been in ascendance for the last 25 years. It is our hope that the next 25 years will witness at the least a parallel effort to evolve a developmental approach to the classification of children's problems. This will require starting "at the other end"; that is, instead of beginning with adult disorders and extending the system down into childhood, we would urge beginning with the study of development. Patterns of adaptation in early childhood would be defined and progressively refined. We suggest that those appraising children begin first with a broad assessment of core emotional issues and problems of arousal regulation; that is, to what extent do the manifest problems derive from feelings of rejection, fears of abandonment, or anxiety with regard to meeting emotional needs? How does the world look through this child's eyes? How seriously, and in what way, is the child's capacity to regulate arousal compromised? And to what extent are such disabilities the result of current emotional states, and to what extent are the patterns of dysregulation more deeply established and intractable? A very promising line of work in this regard has been done by the "Zero to Three" group (e.g., Greenspan & Wieder, 1994). This work should be elaborated and extended into the middle childhood and adolescent years.

We believe that adaptational problems first begin as disturbed patterns of relationships, characterized by distinctive forms of dyadic dysregulation (Sameroff & Emde, 1989). Maladaptive patterns may entail overregulation, underregulation, and various particular forms of dysregulation. Such patterns are internalized as the child plays an increasingly active role in regulation over the first few years. Once defined, these general patterns could then be traced as they are differentiated and transformed in subsequent phases. Ultimately, maps of associated outcomes, some appropriately characterized as disordered, would be constructed. Clinicians would have to discern the trajectory, as well as the manifest problems, because the decision to intervene and the type of intervention would follow from that. This is a huge, complex undertaking, but it would be worthwhile both in terms of what would be learned about development and what it could do for the well-being of children.

INTERVENTION

We see our work as supporting certain kinds of approaches to individual therapy with adults and with children, and to working with families. Even more so, the work suggests the value of early intervention into developmental systems, before manifest child disturbance emerges and, especially, the importance of prevention. We believe the data confirm (1) that pathways to disturbance often begin early, and (2) that the longer a pathway is pursued, the more difficult change becomes. Thus, for example, intrusive care in infancy, anxious (and, especially, disorganized) attachment, and other aspects of early developmental problems predicted late adolescent disturbance with some power. Adding externalizing problems in early elementary school led to even more substantial prediction. By age 7 or 8, a history of enjoining and pursuing a conduct problems pathway reflects an adaptation that is very difficult to change (see also Dodge, 2000; Farrington et al., 1986). Therefore, early identification of relationship disturbances and other developmental problems, and of risk factors for such problems, is critical. So too is putting in place supports that are required by such families to promote the child's development. We take up these levels of intervention in turn, beginning with implications for treatment of children and adults who show disturbance.

Treatment of Infants and Children

Attachment theory and research, certainly including our own, have guided the development of treatment strategies in infancy and toddlerhood (Lieberman, 1993; Lojkasek, Cohen, & Muir, 1994; Muir, 1992), middle childhood (Minde & Hesse, 1996; J. Sroufe, 2003), and adolescence and adulthood (Fonagy, 1999; Slade, 1999). The rise of "infant psychotherapy" in particular was a direct consequence of attachment work. The work of the Muirs (Lieberman, 1991; Lojkasek et al., 1994; Muir, 1992) is prototypical, attachment-based work, focusing as it does on working with parent and infant together toward the goal of greater parental awareness of the child's attachment needs and feelings.

Clinical researchers have drawn upon longitudinal data such as ours to provide conceptual frameworks (e.g., Lieberman & Zeanah, 1999), to make linkages between early experience and later adaptation (e.g., Lojkasek et al., 1994), and to design evaluation methodology (e.g., Zeanah et al., 1997). For example, our measures of parent and child behavior (e.g., Matas et al., 1978), and the maladaptive behavioral patterns we defined in early childhood (e.g., Sroufe, 1983), have provided direction for intervention and evaluation studies of the toddler and preschool years (e.g., Egeland & Erickson, 2004; Erickson & Egeland, 1999; Lieberman & Zeanah, 1999; Zeanah et al., 1997).

One excellent example of the kind work being done with young children is Alicia Lieberman's (1992, 1993) work with toddlers. Lieberman draws on concepts closely related to ours to elaborate on the emotional life of the toddler. Her work suggests the same steps that we described in Chapters 5–7, as the child moves from confidence in support to guided regulation, to internalized confidence. She notes that while "impetus to explore propels the toddler forward, the ability to rely on a supportive relationship is still at the core of the child's capacity to learn" (Lieberman, 1993, p. 24). While the infant may be preoccupied with the actual whereabouts of the caregiver, and fear of separation and loss, the older toddler may contend more with subtle threats of parents' disapproval (i.e., loss of love, abandonment) and competing desires toward dependence and independence (cf. Breger, 1974). Autonomy assertions in the context of supportive care and firm limits deepen the child's trust in the relationship and in the self, and restoring closeness after conflict helps the child to acquire more behavioral control, facilitating the long-term goal of constructing a stable internal world.

As Lieberman (1992, 1993) describes it, maladaptive patterns in toddlerhood often take the form of persistent deviations in the balance between the attachment and exploratory systems, leading to inflexible behavioral styles (e.g., inhibition, recklessness, and precocious competence in self-protection). Underlying these deviations, there remains a core anxiety regarding caregiver availability that begins earlier in infancy but becomes more complex in the second year. Throughout development, the growth of competence requires that children can rely on feeling safe and protected. In a responsive home environment, or in the environment that is created in a therapeutic setting, the toddler begins to experience him- or herself freely exploring the world of objects. However, it is not the manipulation of objects or play alone, but the manipulation of objects during engagement with another that creates the child's sense of him- or herself. The mother, or therapist, affectively shapes the child's experience, giving it meaning. Through ongoing support, guidance, and acceptance, the intimacy of the first year survives and "is woven into the new order of things" (Lieberman, 1993, p. 37).

Intervention strategies in early childhood have varied in focus or "port of entry" into the relationship system (i.e., caregiver representation, parent behavior, child behavior). They have in common, however, the goal of providing a holding environment in which the child can explore unmet attachment and exploratory needs, and the caregiver can explore feelings stirred through infant activity (Lojkasek et al., 1994, McDonough, 2000; Muir, 1992; Stern, 1985). They share the goals of facilitating more authentic experience in the caregiving relationship, regulating emotion (e.g., emotional expression and containment), and addressing lapses or breakdowns in coping strategies.

Therapy with Adults

Work with adults that derives from attachment theory and research bears many similarities to the work with children just discussed. With adults, of course, there can be more cognitive engagement, and a less exclusive focus on engaging the individual at an emotional level.

Bowlby (1988) himself proposed a list of five "therapeutic tasks" in clinical work with individuals. These tasks followed directly from his proposal that disturbances derive from salient childhood relationships in which distortions in thinking and feeling were required for adaptation. The vital nature of these distortions, and the fright or pain that required them, makes it impossible for the individual to see their source and to recognize that they may not be appropriate in present circumstances. The first task, then, is for the therapist to provide "a secure base" from which the person can explore painful aspects of past and current experience. Second, the person is encouraged to examine expectations concerning self and others in current relationships, and to see what unknown biases are being brought forward. Third, since these expectations inevitably also apply to the relationship between the therapist and the client, this relationship too is to be examined. Fourth, the person may now be ready to examine how current expectations and perceptions may be the product of childhood experiences—what was done by parents, or what they said or implied must be believed. This step, of course, can be very difficult given the painful nature of some of the things to be remembered and thought about. Finally, the person may be enabled to see that these images and expectations may not be appropriate to the present. (This step is summarized in the introductory quotation for this chapter.) While in some ways similar to other psychoanalytic therapies, here there is less emphasis on therapist interpretations. Much more, it is a matter of supported exploration.

Bowlby's ideas regarding therapy have been extended in recent years by a number of clinical investigators, with an increased integration of the individual's inner world and consideration of likely actual experience (e.g., Cortina & Marrone, 2003; Eagle, 1995; Sable, 1992; Shane, Shane, & Gale, 1997; Slade, 1999). Arietta Slade provides an excellent synthesis of much of the current thinking. She draws heavily on Main's (1995) ideas regarding coherence of narrative and "metacognitive monitoring" and her adult attachment classification system, as well as Fonagy's concepts of "mentalizing" and "reflection" (Fonagy et al., 1995).

These concepts are closely interrelated. They refer to the capacity to monitor, attend to, and reflect upon thought and internal emotional experience in a dynamic and complex way. The broader term, "mentalizing," refers to the capacity to see, think about, and understand one's self and others in terms of inner states. Such capacities are acquired, as our work on empathy confirmed (Chapter 7), through relationship experiences in which caregivers are emotionally attuned to young children.

Embracing these ideas leads to a new form of "clinical listening," as the therapist focuses on gaps and inconsistencies in discourse. Such gaps reveal acquired styles of coping with attachment feelings in response to failures to be understood in an emotional, intersubjective way. Without such experiences of another engaging one's inner experience, the person is now unable to make his own or another's experience understandable. Fonagy ties insensitive parenting to such a history of failed shared experience, and thus explains the intergenerational process. This parent cannot now engage and contemplate in a coherent manner the child's inner states, which undercuts the child's experience of the self "as real, known, and intentional (which is) central to security" (Slade, 1999, p. 581).

This clinical work is closely tied to research with the Adult Attachment Interview (e.g., Hesse, 1999; Main, 1995). Two common results of histories with insufficient emotional responsiveness are dismissing inner experience or being overwhelmed by feelings. These two patterns present different issues to therapists (Holmes, 1998; Slade, 1999). On the one hand, those with dismissing tendencies may deny the need for help or attempt to divert attention away from emotional issues (Dozier, 1990). On the other hand, those showing the preoccupied adult attachment pattern can overwhelm a therapist to the degree they are overwhelmed by, and unable to reflect upon, their feelings. In a very interesting study, Mary Dozier documented that therapists who themselves were autonomous on the Adult Attachment Interview were more responsive to clients, without themselves becoming overwhelmed (Dozier, Cue, & Barnett, 1994).

Whether with adults or children, the approaches just discussed require some time to carry out, because they hinge on establishment of a trusting relationship between practitioner and clients. As is the case with attachments (either in infants or in romantic partnerships), such relationships cannot be formed quickly. It requires time to establish trust. Certain aspects of our findings support this point of view. First, we documented the negative expectations that children with histories of anxious attachment and/or maltreatment bring to their new relationships with peers and teachers (e.g., Sroufe & Fleeson, 1988; Suess et al., 1992). Moreover, anecdotally, we saw the time required for teachers to penetrate and alter the negative expectations the children brought to them. Finally, in our study on breaking the cycle of abuse, it was therapy of some duration (6 months or longer) that had a significant effect (Egeland et al., 1988).

In our understanding of the development of children's problems, the formation of expectations and patterns of adaptation is constructed over time. The longer such organization has been established, the longer it likely will take to alter it. This makes us doubtful concerning "quick fixes" for attachment-based problems. Many brief procedures, which at times have been referred to as "attachment therapies," have developed independent of attachment research, and have not been demonstrated to be effective. One should be especially cautious concerning those premised on physical intrusion with a child (forced-holding therapy). These would run the risk of confirming and deepening inner models of the self as flawed and of attachment figures as malevolent. Likewise, we cannot offer any support for "rebirthing" therapy. All of the cognitions and feelings from the past are represented in some way currently and can be accessed in the here and now. Again, any claim that long-standing, relationship-based problems can be treated quickly should be considered with caution (see also Slade, 1999).

Nothing in this model implies, however, that work must be individual, or that targeted work with particular problems is not useful. With children, especially, given our data on the way ongoing circumstances maintain trajectories, work with parents and with the entire family would seem very important, if not absolutely essential. Changing the way parents relate to the child would be more important than any relationship the child could have with a therapist. Reducing family chaos could greatly help a child with arousal regulation problems.

Moreover, many children need specific help with learning to self-regulate. Certainly, there is a role for working on the anxiety that contributes to such problems, but if problems are long-standing, changed self-expectations may not be enough. Cognitive-behavioral approaches to such problems may therefore also be useful. Targeted work on self-control, peer relationships, or academic progress also makes sense based on our data. We obtained clear evidence for a back-and-forth interweaving of behavior problems, peer competence, and school achievement, with each predicting the others across time (see Chapters 8 and 9). Therefore, helping the child in one of these arenas might well produce a cascade of positive effects. Where early care was at least marginally adequate and trauma was not prevalent, such intervention may be enough.

Specific, problem-oriented treatment may work best with persons with secure attachment histories, though, at present, there is only clinical evidence to support this proposition (e.g., Korfmacher, Adam, Ogawa, & Egeland, 1997; J. Sroufe, 2003). We expect that for those with seriously malevolent histories, transforming relationship experiences, and not just targeted help, will be required.

It also bears repeating that neither attachment theory nor Bowlby's (1988) suggestions for treatment should be taken to imply blaming of parents. As Bowlby states, "The misguided behaviour of parents is more often than not the product of their own difficult and unhappy childhoods" (p. 145). In Chapter 14, we present our very recent data confirming the continuity in treatment of young children from one generation to the next. Persons providing inadequate support were indeed themselves inadequately supported. Therefore, helping parents free themselves from their own negative expectations and distortions can also be an important part of helping the child, as we discuss further below.

Prevention and Early Intervention

One key part of early intervention and prevention efforts is enhancing sensitive responsiveness of caregivers to infants. Our research supports this proposition in two ways. First, our measures of sensitivity and cooperation at 6 months were consistent predictors of outcomes throughout the juvenile years. Second, sensitive, harmonious care has proven to be a robust predictor of attachment security in both our study and a number of other studies (e.g., de Wolff & van IJzendoorn, 1997; NICHD, 1997; Pederson et al., 1998; Posada et al., 1999). Given the important role for attachment that we have demonstrated, promoting attachment security would also seem to be important, and altering caregiver sensitivity is an important way to do that.

An important question, therefore, concerns how to go about changing caregiver sensitivity or responsiveness. Probably only in the least complex cases will a focus solely on training parents to alter interaction patterns have significant effects, as was the case in one study in the Netherlands (van den Boom, 1989, 1995). With multiproblem families, a much broader, comprehensive approach to prevention or intervention

TABLE 13.1. Steps toward Effective, Enjoyable Parenting (STEEP) Intervention Goals

1. Promote healthy, realistic attitudes, beliefs, and expectations about pregnancy, childbirth, child rearing, and the parent–child relationship.
2. Promote understanding of child development and form realistic expectations for child behavior.
3. Encourage a sensitive, predictable response to the baby's cues and signals.
4. Enhance parents' ability to see things from the child's point of view.
5. Facilitate the creation of a home environment that is safe, predictable, and conducive to optimal development.
6. Help parents identify and strengthen support networks for themselves and their child.
7. Build and support life management skills and effective use of resources.
8. Help parents recognize options, claim power, and make healthy choices.

Note. From Egeland and Erickson (2004). Copyright 2004 by The Guilford Press. Reprinted by permission.

likely would be required (Egeland, Weinfield, Bosquet, & Cheng, 2000; Lieberman, 1992, 1993). Our research has consistently revealed the effects of life stress and available social support on the quality of parenting. Likewise, parents' own history of treatment, their understanding of this treatment, and their subsequent ways of viewing their infant all were shown to be important (Egeland, Bosquet, & Levy-Chung, 2002; see also Chapter 5). Thus, while the infant is only impacted by how it is treated and the quality of stimulation provided, these factors are dramatically influenced by the surrounding context. When this context provides few supports and poses many challenges, it is unlikely that parents will be able to respond easily to training efforts. Thus, most of the programs in the literature that have proven to be successful have been comprehensive (Egeland et al., 2000). Sometimes these interventions have targeted families of infants previously assessed to be anxiously attached. Others, like the program we evolved, work with high-risk families even before attachment problems have developed.

Based on our research findings, we developed, implemented, and evaluated STEEP (Steps toward Effective Enjoyable Parenting), a preventive intervention program for high-risk mothers and infants. The goals of the intervention, which begin at birth, are described in Table 13.1 (from Egeland & Erickson, 2004). In general, in addition to striving directly to enhance the sensitivity of caregiver interactions, we worked at every level of context that was germane to promoting such interactions.

Some of the work was directed at the *intra*personal level, especially the models and expectations concerning self and others that might interfere with parenting. For example, expectations of rejection could interfere with developing the necessary relationship with the project facilitator or even lead to misinterpreting needy infant behavior as hostile (Korfmacher et al., 1997; see also Chapter 7). Failure to integrate past malevolent experiences could lead to blind spots with regard to properly interpreting the infant. Recall that those parents who tended to be high on dissociating experience were most likely to perpetuate the abuse they had experienced in the next generation (Egeland & Sussman-Stillman, 1996; see also Chapter 5). Thus, helping parents to recognize and to integrate their own past experiences was deemed important.

Work was also directed at the *inter*personal level, in terms of both developing realistic appraisals and decisions concerning partners, and evolving a broader social support network. The same facilitator was with the parent throughout our yearlong intervention for individual contacts, for home visits, and for group meetings. The parent group meetings themselves promoted a sense of belongingness, as well as an opportunity to learn from other parents. Finally, other efforts were made to develop mutual support between mothers in the project. For example, a home visitor might on one occasion take a mother and infant to the home of another participant, and the next week reverse the procedure. In this way, friendships were supported in what were sometimes isolated parents. All of this followed from our finding that the most potent predictor of change in quality of parent–child relationships was changing the level of social support (see Chapters 7–10). There also were efforts directed at the broader context surrounding the family. For example, mothers were helped to locate available community resources and to gain access to them.

Finally, there were direct efforts to help the parents be more responsive to infant signals and more harmonious in their stimulation and care. Videotapes of the mother interacting with her infant were utilized for this purpose. This work was not viewed as teaching the mother a set of tricks, but rather as helping develop her understanding of the infant—to see the world from the infant's point of view. We had found that one of the major predictors of poor-quality parenting was a lack of understanding of the "psychological complexity" of the infant (see Chapter 5), that is, recognizing that the infant is an autonomous being, with its own agenda, yet highly dependent on the parent for its well-being. Therefore, as the facilitator reviewed videotapes with the mother, she would ask questions about what the baby was indicating that he or she wanted, or did not want, what was liked and not liked, in the ongoing interaction. It was a gentle, nonconfrontational process, in which the parent (1) gradually learned that the baby had a "language," and (2) learned to understand the meaningfulness and meanings of the various messages. Increased sensitivity to signals and less strident care seemed to follow naturally from this learning. These taped sessions also afforded excellent opportunities for the parent to recognize her own feelings and, at times, to explore their connections with her own treatment as a child (Erickson & Egeland, 1999).

We do not claim that these ideas are unique. They have much in common with other workers in the field, such as the work of Marvin, Cooper, Hoffman, and Powell (2002) on the "circle of security," Fraiberg, Adelson, and Shapiro's (1975) writing on "ghosts in the nursery," and the interpretive play therapy utilized by the Hinck's Institute in Toronto (e.g., Lojkasek et al., 1994; Muir, 1992). What we do claim is that our rationale, and these practices, sprang from specific findings in our research, as well as from attachment theory.

CONCLUSION

The findings from our study have implications both for understanding behavioral and emotional disturbance and for clinical work. Three of these findings are (1) that the describable, lived experience of children predicts the presence of later disturbance; (2) that individual pathways can be described and are probabilistically associated with various forms of disturbance; and (3) that disturbance, in most cases, develops step-by-step over time. Moreover, the earliest robust markers of pathogenic experience or of maladaptive developmental pathways lie in infant–caregiver relationships. As has been noted previously, disturbance in early childhood is best characterized as relationship disturbance, not disturbance in the infant or toddler (Sameroff & Emde, 1989; Sroufe, 1989).

Our results have implications for all aspects of clinical work. For classification, they suggest greater attention to developmental trajectories as a way of approaching problems of "comorbidity" and within-class heterogeneity. One goal would be to predict and to understand which children will have problems that cut across current categories. "Comorbidity" should be predictable, not a mystery. Another goal would be to understand likely differential outcomes for children manifesting similar problems at a given time, in order to tailor interventions for different children within categories. Implications for treatment follow. When we better understand pathways, we will better know how to adjust intervention at different developmental points. Proper timing and appropriate kinds of interventions could achieve maximum leverage. Finally, it is clear from our work that early prevention would be best achieved by establishing comprehensive programs to support parents (or reestablishing those supports that have been dismantled). While difficult, we believe that helping parents overcome the legacy of their own malevolent experiences is especially important.

In this book, we have been concerned primarily with the implications of our work for conceptualizing development and for promoting further research. We recognize that in this chapter we have only begun to outline the clinical implications of our study. We look forward to expanding these ideas in the future in collaboration with those engaged in more clinical work.

It is more than obvious that much work remains to be done in this developmental field. In Chapter 14, we describe some of the directions in which our current work is taking us. We are giving particular attention to intergenerational transmission of patterns of behavior and to processes governing continuity and change in patterns of adaptation.

CHAPTER 14

The Tasks Ahead

Serena, age 2, works hard on the lever problem, following her mother's leads until, finally, she gets the candy out of the box by weighting down the board. Her mother Jessica smiles and says in an animated voice: "There, now you've got the candy out! You got it!" Two decades later, Serena watches Dustin, her own 2-year-old, as he works hard to solve the same problem. At last he solves the problem and smiles brightly. "There you go. Good job!" she says, and smiles warmly at him.

When Ellis seeks help from his mother as he struggles with the problem, she rolls her eyes at the ceiling and laughs. When he finally does manage to solve the problem, his mother says, "Now see how stubborn you were." Two decades later, as Ellis watches his son Carl struggle with the same problem, he leans away from the child, laughing and shaking his head. Later, he taunts the child by pretending to raise the candy out of the box, then dropping it as the child rushes to try to get it. In the end he has to solve the problem for Carl and says, "You didn't do that, I did. You're not as smart as me."

When we started this project, our goals were to learn something about the origins of parental care, including maltreatment, and to document the consequences of variations in care. We learned that the way parents treat their children is a complex product of their histories, and the resultant understandings they have about childrearing, as well as their current supports and stresses. We are continuing to document this in the second generation.

287

.ng consequences of care, we have established to our satis-
: nothing is more important in children's development than
.re treated by their parents, beginning in the early years of life.
)rehensive study, in which both care and other influences were
.sured, makes this clear. At the same time as we conclude that
psychosocial factors, including family experiences, are incredibly powerful influences on children, we also conclude that parents ought not be
blamed. Yes, patterns of care, stimulation, and parental involvement are
strong predictors of behavior problems and school success and failure,
even in competition with intelligence. Some children have little chance at
school, even before they begin. Others early on begin pathways to problems with peers and/or psychopathology. Still, patterns of care that children experience are conditioned by the stresses and supports available to
parents. For there to be "no child left behind," we will have to do a
better job in leaving no family behind.

As important as these questions and findings about conditions and
outcomes are, what has occupied us most throughout this study is the
more basic question of how development works, that is, the complex
process through which we become who we are. In fact, we now look at
the importance of early experience in terms of this process. Early experience may have a lasting impact not primarily because of its immediate
impact on brain structures and emotional regulation, but because it
leads to short-term consequences that themselves become risks for later
development (see also Sanchez, Ladd, & Plotsky, 2003). We used the example in Chapter 6 of parenting difficulties in infancy leading to difficulties between parents and toddlers. More generally, one may look at early
secure relationships between parents and children not as a permanent
protective coating, but as a foundation for later positive relationships
with parents, peers, and others. As Eleanor Maccoby (1992) describes it,
it is "money in the bank" for parents and children. This is why we view
all the time parents spend building the early relationship with the child
as crucial, not just for that time, but for their relationships throughout
childhood and adolescence.

Attention to process, of course, takes one beyond a consideration of
early relationship experiences. Our abundant findings on change in individual adaptation, as well as our findings on the myriad ways in which
multiple influences work together, make it clear that old ways of posing
developmental questions are inappropriate. The question is not whether
early experience or later experience is more important. Important as it is,
early experience does not *cause* later outcomes in a direct way. Just as
you were not born to be who you are, neither did you become who you
are when you were 2 years old. Rather, early experience initiates a process and thereby frames subsequent encounters with the environment.

Such later encounters, however much guided by past experience, none-theless have the potential for transforming prior experience—not in its fact, but in its meaning relative to functioning and subsequent develop-ment. We are indeed *prone* to live out our early histories, as the vignettes we have cited and our broader findings suggest, but as some other cases show, we are not *destined* to do so. Our way of being is always a prod-uct of our cumulative history of experience, our resources and the chal-lenges we have faced, and our current circumstances.

The concern with process, and with understanding both continuity and change in development, continues in our present work. In this final chapter, we describe some of the current work we are doing and some of the questions that guide us in our continuing research. As was the case in the beginning, we continue to see the importance of studying both nor-mal and abnormal development concurrently. Likewise, the same three prongs of activity continue to this date. We are studying social relation-ships, behavioral and emotional disturbance, and development of the self, in terms of both the negotiation of life tasks and the representa-tional world of the person. In the social domain, our current foci are adult partnerships and parenting, although we track broader social net-works as well. In the realm of disturbance, we focus on the nature and development of characteristically adult disturbances and on changing trajectories of problems. In the realm of self-development, we have a special interest in the capacity to integrate past experiences and the on-going interplay among representation, social behavior, and relationship experience. In all cases, our attention is increasingly devoted to ques-tions of developmental process.

ONGOING ISSUES IN SOCIAL RELATIONSHIPS

Our position is that the capacities for social relatedness and effectiveness in social relationships are developmental constructions; that is, the per-son draws upon all previous, salient social experience to engage profit-ably in current social relationships. In relating to peers, for example, early experience with parents, later parenting, and prior experiences with peers and siblings all are important. Adult romantic relationships build upon these, as well as upon prior experiences with intimate friend-ships and earlier romantic relationships. Moreover, all of these experi-ences within and outside of the family, plus the current network of sup-portive relationships, are expected to undergird the capacities needed to be an adequate parent. Thus, not only childhood experiences with par-ents and peers but also current adult relationship supports provide sup-port for parenting.

As discussed in previous chapters, the process is not simply a quantitative, additive one. The critical issue is certainly not the number of relationships in which the person has participated. In fact, we have found, for example, that having a large number of prior sexual partners is a negative indicator regarding quality of romantic partnerships. Nor is it the case that "all relationships are equal." The timing, content, and quality of particular relationship experiences are central to any later influence. One illustration of this presented in Chapter 10 was that experiences with parents and peers were primarily associated with different facets of later romantic relationships (e.g., trust vs. negotiating conflict). We expect this to continue to be the case as we follow our participants through the early adult years.

Current Issues in Romantic Partnerships

Effectiveness in romantic relationships, like competence with peers and the quality of friendships in childhood and adolescence, stems from experiences in multiple earlier relationships. Because we assess diverse aspects of people's relationships with their current romantic partners, we are able to identify the distinctive ways in which particular earlier relationships, occurring in particular developmental periods, play a role in functioning with romantic partners. Two examples that illustrate these distinctive patterns follow.

One example comes from our repeated finding that the quality of caregiving up to 42 months of age significantly contributes to predicting *quality* of romantic relationships in early adulthood but is not a significant predictor of whether individuals are currently involved in a romantic relationship in this age period (Collins & Madsen, in press; Hennighausen, 1999). Another example is our finding that relationship involvement—whether an individual is in a romantic relationship at ages 23 and 26—is especially well predicted by teacher-rated peer competence in middle childhood. To the surprise of many, the quality of an individual's friendships over time in childhood and adolescence has little bearing on whether an individual has a romantic partner at ages 23 and 26. But *for those who do*, trajectories of friendship quality in childhood and adolescence strongly predict the *quality* of those relationships (Collins, Hayden, & van Dulmen, 2005; Collins & van Dulmen, in press-a).

These findings support our position that competence in romantic relationships represents an integration of competencies drawn from diverse relationship experiences in earlier life. By implication, lack of competence in this key arena of adult functioning almost certainly reflects developmental trajectories in which there were earlier relationship dysfunctions of various kinds. In an initial study, we have found that the qualities of relationships with both parents and friends contribute to a likelihood of violence in early adult romantic relationships. Controlling for history of childhood physical abuse and exposure to parental partner violence, intrusive or overly familiar behavior (boundary violations) in our videotaped parent–child collaborations at age 13 consistently predicted perpetration and victimization toward romantic partners in early adulthood. In addition, friendship quality assessed at age 16 contributed over and above familial predictors (Linder & Collins, in press). Our prospective data on a wide range of relational experience variables give us unique opportunities to examine the processes by which positive and negative experiences in familial and peer relationships comprise trajectories toward effective or dysfunctional adult relationships with romantic partners.

Continuity and Change in Parenting across Generations

We have a keen interest in the quality of parenting our participants are now providing for their children in the next generation. We are well positioned to investigate continuity across generations. Having prospective, observational data, we do not have to rely on retrospective reports by either first- or second-generation parents. Parenting in the early years is an especially important area for study, because one's own experiences from that time cannot be verbally recalled. Thus, if these experiences are carried forward and impact upon one's own practices, then this must be due to nonverbal representation in some form. We believe that an especially promising hypothesis is that in relating to the emotional needs of one's own child, early established patterns of parent–child dyadic regulation are activated. Of course, demonstrating the validity of this hypothesis requires many steps. Among other things, one must take into account the consequences of later experiences with one's parents and even contemporary influences. Potential explanations based on shared genetics must be dealt with, and so forth. This will be an involved process, and we are still in somewhat early phases of this part of our project. Nonetheless, preliminary results are quite interesting.

At this point, we have completed several analyses based on our assessments at age 2 (Kovan, Kempner, & Carlson, 2004; Levy, 1998). This is an early enough age to preclude any verbal memory in adulthood, yet we have continuous variables available at this time. Data on continuity and change in infant attachment await a larger number of participants, due to the categorical nature of this data.

Since only 34 toddlers were available for these first analyses, we had to be restrained and strategic in the analyses carried out. As a first question, we simply asked: What is the correlation between the overall

TABLE 14.1. Correlations between First- and Second-Generation Parenting Construct ($n = 34$)

First generation	Second generation				
	1	2	3	4	5
Supportive presence	.50**	.54**	−.42*	−.52**	−.50**
Quality of assistance	.45**	.53**	−.30	−.50**	−.47**
Hostility	−.27	−.33	.42*	.65**	.44**
Nonresponsive physical intimacy	.07	−.07	.04	.15	.39*
Generational boundary dissolution	−.19	−.42*	−.34*	.50**	.37*

*$p < .05$; **$p < .01$; ***$p < .001$.

global quality-of-parenting rating for the two generations? As always, coding of these two measures was carried out with complete independence. (Indeed, some of the coders of the second generation were not born, or were toddlers, when the first-generation parenting was coded.) The obtained correlation was an impressive .52. The matrix of correlations for more specific scales is presented in Table 14.1. In general, the same scale correlates most highly with the same or closely related scales across the two time periods; for example, quality of assistance in the second generation was predicted by quality of assistance (.53) and supportive presence (.54) in the first generation. Thus, the correlations implied in our opening vignettes were indeed supported using group data.

For regression analyses, quality of assistance and supportive presence were averaged to form a positive parenting composite. Hostility, nonresponsive physical intimacy, and generational boundary dissolution were used to form a negative parenting composite. Positive parenting in the first generation correlated .56 with positive parenting in the second; negative parenting correlated .54 with later negative parenting. Such correlations, of course, could result from a number of mediating factors. IQ, SES, or education level of first- and second-generation parents could be concordant and could conceivably account for similarity in parenting, as could age of parents, psychiatric status, or common amounts of life stress. Only the first three variables were significantly related to first-generation positive parenting (r's from .17 for level of education to .28 for the Wechsler Adult Intelligence Scale). Therefore, only these three variables were used in the regression analyses as control variables. When these three variables were all entered in the first step of a hierarchical regression, none was significant in predicting second-generation parenting. Moreover, when positive parenting in the first generation was subsequently entered, it accounted for an additional 30% of the variance, a highly significant finding. For the second-generation negative parenting composite, none of the control variables showed even significant simple correlations. However, both positive and negative parenting in the first generation were predictive (overall R^2 = .48). These findings reveal that the impressive continuity in parenting across generations cannot be explained as being due to common intelligence or to generally similar circumstances.

We also examined the specificity of the predictors at age 2 by analyzing prediction from first-generation parenting quality at age 13 (the balance scale composite; see Chapter 9). While these variables were related to parenting at age 2 in the first generation, they did not predict second-generation parenting at age 2 nearly as strongly as when we used first generation measures from age 2. Moreover, when we statistically controlled the measure at age 13, the measure at age 2 still predicted. The two age periods together accounted for 37% of the variance in second-generation positive parenting.

We take this array of findings as initial support for our theorizing about intergenerational continuity in parenting, especially the role of internalized early relationship experiences. That age 2 predicts to age 2 better than does age 13 is in accord with this, and at a later time, this might be bolstered by showing that age 13 in the second generation is likewise best predicted by age 13 parenting in the first generation. Moreover, it seems unlikely that our findings can be explained by shared genetics. We have no direct information on this, but the fact that experience of parenting predicts one's own parenting, with IQ, level of education, and SES controlled, rules out the pervasive influence of some putative genetic mediators. We are currently coding certain discrete, behavioral measures, such as amount of talking to the toddler, amount of touching and physical proximity, and amount of smiling. Such variables might be thought a priori to be more influenced by genetic variation; yet in accord with the work of Bornstein (2002), we do not predict such variables to show the same level of continuity across generations as our more psychological constructs. Support can be shown in various ways.

At this time, we are training a new team of coders to rate our age 42 month variables. This, in addition to the arrival of more children in Generation 2, will allow us to expand our analyses in a number of ways. In time, we hope to have a sufficient sample size to carry out more sophisticated analyses and, especially, to account for change as well as continuity. Considerable variance remains to be explained, and we believe that there are promising candidates for explaining change. Notable among these would be the quality of current supportive relationships with parents or partners and/or Adult Attachment Interview status, that is, the openness and coherence with which the individual can process attachment related information. As described earlier, current partnership quality and Adult Attachment Interview status are related. This finding was not surprising. All close relationship experiences, not just those with a therapist, can have transforming influences on inner models of self and others. For these reasons, we predict that even with a history of poor early care, parents with supportive current partnerships have a better chance to parent adequately than those with poor histories and poor current support. The ultimate question concerns how early care experiences; later experiences with parents, peers, and adult partner relationships; and current stresses and supports all converge in support of adequate or inadequate parenting.

CURRENT WORK ON BEHAVIORAL AND EMOTIONAL DISTURBANCE

Three tasks currently occupy us in our study of disturbance. The first is tracing out trajectories of problem behavior from childhood and adolescence into the adult years. The example we discuss is conduct problems. In particular, we discuss the fate of the adolescent-onset cases in comparison to the early-onset–persistent cases described in Chapter 12. A specific interest is in factors associated with desistance in either of these patterns. Given the cost to individuals and society of this behavior, any leads for successful intervention are invaluable.

The second focus of our current work is continued developmental analysis of targeted problems, especially those that may be prevalent in a sample such as ours. The example we use is self-injurious behavior (SIB), which begs explanation. Why would teens or young adults deliberately harm themselves? Perhaps SIB is analogous to anorexia, which, in contrast, is prominent in middle-class samples. Perhaps both represent modern replacements for "hysteria," as suggested in a paper by one of our former graduate students (Bergmann, 1986). SIB also is interesting in that it shows the flexible applicability of a comprehensive longitudinal data set. It was not even on the horizon when our study began; now it is a widespread problem, and our prospective data shed light on its origins.

Finally, we are interested in characteristically adult disorders, especially those such as personality disorders that are exclusive to adulthood. Uncovering the antecedents and course of such problems, which have strong conceptual links to early childhood relationships, is a high priority. Personality disorders should be well represented in our sample, unlike rare disorders such as schizophrenia.

Pathways of Conduct Problems from Childhood into Adulthood

Adolescent-onset conduct problems have been distinguished from early-onset problems, which are more persistent and have much stronger associations with early psychosocial adversity (see Chapter 12). The former group at times has been referred to as "adolescent limited" (Moffitt, 1993), with the plausible suggestion that their problems may wane in adulthood. However, this has not yet been firmly established, and it is one of the questions we are pursuing. Beyond this, we also seek to identify factors associated with change; that is, can we distinguish between those who will desist and those who will continue to show problems? And will factors associated with desistance be different or the same for adolescent-onset and early-onset cases? To date, we have done preliminary analyses based on our self-report data at ages 23 and 26 years (Roisman et al., 2004).

At both ages 23 and 26, the early-onset group continued to have more externalizing problems, anxiety and depression, and drug problems than those individuals without a history of childhood problems, and at these ages, they also had significantly more externalizing problems and drug problems than did the adolescent-onset group. Moreover, only the early-onset group was distinguished by other problems in early adulthood, such as problems in the work and education arenas. Adolescent-onset cases, however, also had more externalizing problems and drug problems than did controls; that is, they were intermediate to the early-onset and not previously disturbed groups. This suggests that, at least at these ages, the term "adolescent-limited" should still be withheld, at least as a general characterization. It is noteworthy, however, that the adolescent-onset cases, as a group, had no more problems in work, educational attainment, or romantic relationships than controls. Thus, it is correct that this pattern reflects a less pernicious pathway.

Our next key finding was that successful involvement in work and successful involvement in romantic relationships predicted a decrease in externalizing problems at both ages 23 and 26. The latter is especially important, because the work and relationship measures were obtained at age 23 and are therefore independent of the self-reports of problems at age 26. It is noteworthy that these effects held especially for the *early*-onset group. We were unable to specify what led to the decline in problems for the adolescent-onset group. But for the early onset group, these "turning point" opportunities in work and relationships were specifically associated with change. For those having both successful work experiences *and* successful romantic relationships at age 23, the level of externalizing problems at age 26 was no different than that shown by those without a history of childhood or adolescent problems. This is a remarkable finding. We, of course, are now keenly interested in understanding how these individuals were able to attain such positive experiences, and whether they are, in fact, causal in the observed desistance.

Self-Injurious Behavior

We sought to take advantage of our unique data set to illustrate the potential of a developmental approach to certain targeted problems. One of these is SIB, such as self-hitting, cutting, or burning. SIB is drawing increasing attention from mental health professionals, because its prevalence is increasing, and because of the obvious distress of these individuals.

In our sample, 21% of the participants engaged in some degree of SIB by age 26, with 8% showing clinically significant, severe SIB (Yates, 2004). In contrast to observed patterns in clinical samples, where SIB is overrepresented among females, rates of SIB did not differ between males and females in our community sample. As we have observed with other forms of psychopathology (e.g., antisocial behavior), younger ages of onset were significantly related to more severe, recurrent patterns of SIB.

Contemporaneous correlates of SIB included higher levels of reported risk-taking behavior and more frequent endorsement of finding pain pleasurable. SIB cases were more than twice as likely than noninjurers to report having friends who engage in SIB. Suicide attempts were significantly more common among severe self-injurers, but examination of self-reported motivations for SIB indicated that suicidal behavior was distinct from SIB, in that "wishing to die" was among the *least* frequently endorsed reasons for SIB. In contrast to popular notions of SIB as a suicidal or manipulative gesture, the vast majority of injurers, and especially the recurrent, clinically significant SIB cases, endorsed *intrapsychic* motivations for SIB. These reasons included to release anger, anxiety, or depression; to punish oneself; and to escape bad feelings. These findings generally are in accord with the broader literature on SIB, particularly in community samples.

What our study allowed us to do uniquely was to examine prospectively potential antecedents of this behavior and to test certain prespecified developmental models. SIB would seem to require the convergence of at least two major antecedents: malevolent care and distortions in the development of the self. In accordance with broader theories of emotional development, we hypothesized that traumatic caregiving undermines the child's emerging capacities for affective–cognitive integration; symbolic processing, particularly through language; and self- and other-reflective capacities (see also Kalsched, 1996). Trauma-induced deficits in affect regulation and reflection may contribute to distortions in key self-processes. Thus, our collaborator, Yates (2004), tested whether early adversity in the caregiving environment (disorganized attachment and child maltreatment) contribute to SIB via dissociation and somatization, as assessed in adolescence using our clinical interview (the Schedule for Affective Disorders and Schizophrenia for School-Age Children).

Univariate analyses confirmed that disorganized attachment and child maltreatment, particularly sexual abuse, contribute to clinically significant SIB. Subsequent multivariate analyses demonstrated that child sexual abuse, physical neglect, dissociation, and somatization significantly predicted severe SIB, particularly for females. Moreover, these relations remained significant even when several associated risk factors were added to the model. SIB cases did not differ from noninjurers on measures such as infant temperament, child cognitive ability, or maternal life stress. Our data suggest that maltreatment, dissociation, and somatization make unique contributions to the development of SIB. Efforts to construct further and test developmental process models of SIB are ongoing. There seem to be two pathways, with child sexual abuse and distortion in self-processes leading to severe SIB, and physical abuse leading to mild SIB. With those who are clearly mild injurers (7 boys and 6 girls), physical abuse emerges as the only predictor of membership.

Ongoing Work on Disturbance

We have begun carrying out another major clinical interview with our participants at age 28, which will allow us to address a new set of issues. Our focus will be on those questions that take advantage of our unique, longitudinal data set. Thus, we have a particular interest in understanding linkages between childhood and adult disturbances, as well as distinctive developmental processes that may underlie them. Questions include the following: How are child problems transformed in their adult expressions? What kinds of adult problems arise in the absence of child disturbance? What are the differential antecedents of child and adult problems that are manifestly similar? When we identify a link between child and adult disturbance, exceptions become the subject of great interest. What factors promote disruption of this linkage, allowing some individuals to desist? Likewise, what factors lead to the emergence of disturbance in adulthood, when childhood experience was benign? In general, of course, the major question is, as always, how do history of experience and current circumstances combine in promoting the particular pattern of adaptation?

Within standard adult disorders, as listed in the DSM, we have a special interest in exploring the question of which disorders do, and which do not, seem to have some degree of origin in childhood relationship experience. As stated in the introduction to this section, this is one reason we are particularly interested in personality disorders, which should arise in sufficient numbers in our sample for systematic study. It was these adult disorders that Bowlby specifically hypothesized would be linked to early relationship experiences. Many of them have as primary characteristics profound relationship disturbances, such as instability in relationships (borderline personality disorder). Again, our goal is not only to uncover antecedents, both early and later, but also to shed light on the developmental processes underlying these disorders.

DEVELOPMENT OF THE SELF: ADULT STATE OF MIND REGARDING ATTACHMENT

In Chapter 10, we reported that while there was a significant relationship for infant disorganized attachment, there was no significant relationship between our infant Strange Situation classifications of secure, avoidant, and resistant attachment, and status on the Adult Attachment Interview (AAI) at age 19. We also pointed to several possible explanations for this, beyond the possibility of systematic change. Among these was the possibility that our participants, at least in this particular sample, were too young to do the kind of reflective abstraction required by the AAI. Another related possibility was that the transcripts were too difficult to score for this high-risk group at this age. We knew that both assessments had some reliability and validity, because of the array of meaningful correlates associated with each of them. All of this prompted us to carry out another AAI assessment at age 26. The results of this effort are just coming to light as we write this chapter.

While 12-month infant ABC classifications did not predict to the 26-year AAI, the 18-month classifications did (Sampson, 2004). The 3×3 matrix (from A, B, and C to dismissing, autonomous, and preoccupied) yielded a significant chi-square (12.95, $p = .012$). This modest stability was due entirely to the secure group. Those who had been secure as infants were more likely to be autonomous at age 26 (group F) than were those who had been resistant or avoidant as infants (53.2% vs. 35.1%). Moreover, disorganized infant attachment was even more strongly related to nonautonomous AAI status than it had been at age 19 ($\chi^2 = 10.35$, $p < .001$) and was also related to unresolved status. There was not predictability to specific classifications, from A to dismissing or C to preoccupied (see Chapter 4 for descriptions of these categories). The failure of the 12-month assessments to predict is not so surprising with our sample, since 38% of our cases changed classification between 12 and 18 months. Based on the data here, one possibility is that attachment had become somewhat more stable by 18 months.

The modest stability, even based on 18-month classifications, is in part due to the fact that only a minority of cases (45.4%) was autonomous at age 26 (compared to 62% secure at 18 months). While this is more autonomous cases than at age 19 years (35.5%), it still puts a boundary on the continuity possible. There may still be even more autonomous cases at a later age.

Critics no doubt will point out that we have not found a great deal of evidence for stability. However, any stability across 25 years, from infancy to adulthood, is impressive to us given the complexity of these constructs and how difficult they are to measure. Moreover, other aspects of early care also were related to the 26-year AAI outcome. A history of child maltreatment, for example, was predictive of non-autonomous AAI status, and it was so, above and beyond attachment classifications. Our cumulative early care variable (measures from 6 to 42 months) also was significantly related to "Coherence of Transcript" on the AAI, which is the continuous measure most related to autonomous classification.

For us, this evidence of stability is not the end of the story, but the beginning. Our primary interest was, and remains, the developmental process. The concordance in classification even to this degree provides the backdrop for examining those who changed from secure to insecure status, or from insecure to secure. It bears repeating that the AAI is not a measure of early history, but of *current* state of mind regarding attachment issues. Thus, it is theoretically a product of the entire history, including recent circumstances. We underscore this in the following paragraphs.

In addition to maltreatment, two other prespecified variables accounted for change in status from infancy to adulthood. First was family life stress, cumulated across the years of childhood and adolescence. For males in the sample, there was significantly more intervening life stress in the families where the participant changed from secure in infancy to insecure at age 26, compared to those who were secure at both ages. Second, quality of parenting at age 13 also distinguished participants that changed status. For the entire sample, those who changed from secure to insecure had lower family support scores (the combination of the three balance scales used in previously described analyses) than those who were secure as infants and remained secure (autonomous) as adults. In this case, there was no gender difference in how this variable worked.

Likewise, we were interested in stability and change between the age 19 and age 26 measures of adult state of mind. First, there was significant stability (Sampson, 2004). The greatest percentage of dismissing cases at age 26 had been dismissing at age 19, and so on, with *each* of the three categories. The overall 3×3 contingency table chi-square was 14.27 ($p = .006$). Still, there was substantial change as well. Such change is expectable, in part, because of the pronounced change in the distribution across the two ages. For example, there were 57.2% dismissing cases at age 19, but only 38% at age 26. We were again interested in accounting for changing state of mind status in general, and change in dismissing status in particular.

Since inner working models of relationships are thought to reflect cumulative experience, there was an obvious area within our data set in which to look for mediators of change in adult state of mind regarding attachment, namely, intimate relationship experiences in the intervening years. Two primary assessments were pertinent, our observational measures of couples made at age 20–21, and our interview-based assessment of romantic relationship quality at age 23 (Sampson, 2004). Two composites of observational variables were used: (1) relationship process, a combination of the security, support (Balance I and II), conflict resolution, secure base, and positive affect scales for the couples (Roisman et al., 2001); and (2) a negative affectivity composite. Both of these composite scales differentiated between male subjects who changed from insecure to secure AAIs and those who stayed insecure; that is, those showing positive change had more supportive and less affectively negative relationships with adult partners in the intervening years. This was not significant for females. Positive romantic relationship quality, based on the interview at 23 years of age, was strongly related to coherence on the AAI (.40) and again was significant in accounting for change from an insecure AAI at 19 to a secure AAI at age 26. In this case, the variable worked equally well for males and females.

We also were interested in how infant attachment and 19-year AAI, as well as romantic relationship experience, combined to predict the state of mind measure at age 26. For this analysis, we used either quality of relationship at age 20–21 or at age 23 for participants who had only one of these measures. Where participants had both measures, we combined them. We found that these three predictors together accounted for 18% of the variance in the outcome at age 26, a highly significant finding.

Having now looked at continuity and change in adult representations of relationships, and some of the factors that govern these processes, we plan to explore the ongoing role of representation in social and emotional behavior. As numbers permit, we can examine the place of representation in later romantic relationships and in parenting. Just as adult relationship experiences appear to impact on relationship representations, we also expect that changes in representation will then promote changing functioning in relationships. A major challenge for the field will be to more fully understand the interplay of actual experience (both early and late), and how that experience is integrated and represented.

LOOKING BACK AND LOOKING FORWARD

When Byron Egeland and Amos Deinard set out to explore the origins and early consequences of child maltreatment, they never realized the gigantic task they were starting. In the early years, none of us knew how far we would be able to take this project, or how challenging the task would be. We knew, of course, that development was complicated, but it has proven to be complex beyond our imaginations. Nor did we know how exhilarating the journey would be—all that we would see, discover, and come to understand in a deeper way. We were able to demonstrate some things that had not been previously established with appropriate controls, and this was very gratifying. At the same time, this work has been humbling, because we know that we have simply made a beginning in unraveling the processes of individual development.

There were, of course, surprises, and there certainly are things we would do differently were we to begin our study now. Perhaps the biggest surprise was the dramatic range of outcomes. On the one hand, we detected more child maltreatment than the earlier literature would have led us to believe, and more psychopathology than we had expected. On the other hand, a substantial number of the children we followed have done remarkably well in terms of every index of functioning.

Within the area of child maltreatment specifically, a finding that we could not have anticipated based on the previous literature was the devastating consequences of "psychological" maltreatment. The pattern of parental psychological unavailability had wide-ranging consequences from early childhood on into adulthood.

Another surprise was how patterns of influences and outcomes were so different for boys and girls. It was as though we actually conducted two studies. This might seem obvious now, but no one was talking about the genders as two distinct subcultures in the early 1970s (but see Block, 1979). Finally, before we began, we did not know the extent to which different aspects of parenting, and parenting and peer experiences, would have different outcomes. It is clear that in addition to the secure base function served by parents, there are many other ways that social relationships serve the child's development. Modulated stimulation and maintenance of boundaries are two constructs that proved to be quite powerful. Again, in retrospect, this seems obvious given the important place of emotional regulation in development.

Among things that we might do differently, we first suggest that we tried to do too much. Since assessments were always spread out over 20 months, and until age 8, we did them at least yearly, we were not finished with one when the next began. We were always behind, which inevitably compromised planning and forethought. Our constant assessments of children swamped us at times. Had we been more judicious, we would have been able to have at least one more parent–child observation somewhere in middle childhood. This was an important gap in our data. We would recommend not only larger studies with more control variables, but also studies with fewer participants and much more detailed information on process. Our study was coarse, and the field needs much more information on the daily parent–child transactions as the child develops the capacity for emotional regulation.

One of the clear hazards of longitudinal research is that one always knows better at the end of the project how the study could have been conducted in the first place. There is a built-in obsolescence to long-term studies. There are measures that we would have liked to have done, and there certainly are things we would measure were we starting now, given the state of the field. Among these would be neurophysiology measures and other biological markers of functioning, perhaps especially those having to do with stress reactivity (e.g., Gunnar, 2001). This is not because such measures are more valid or more real, or more important than social, emotional, or cognitive measures, but because they too are an important part of the complex field of influence. They equally reflect the developmental process. We view such measures not as singular causes but as critically important for their interaction with other variables and, perhaps especially, as a means of carrying forward the impact of experience. They likely will be of great help in tracking and clarifying processes of pathway initiation, and continuity and change.

In this book, we have emphasized the role of experience in shaping development. We did this both because our research revealed to us that experience is indeed critically important, and because at times there has been a risk in psychology of neglecting experience in a rush to embrace biological determinants of behavior. Our argument has been that whatever the role of child characteristics in determining the child's reaction to the social and physical world, and in determining reactions of others to the child, it is nonetheless what the child experiences that ultimately matters. One could, of course, say at the same time that what the child experiences can have impact only in that it shapes the child's emotions and cognitions, and the brain structures that underlie these. We would agree with that as well.

At present, many scholars are calling for interdisciplinary, "big tent," multilevel approaches to developmental psychopathology (e.g., Cicchetti & Dawson, 2002; Masten, in press), including the use of animal models and a broad array of measurement approaches (e.g., Sanchez et al., 2003). We would add our voices to theirs. The future tasks that we laid out in this chapter are daunting. Most of these represent tasks that go beyond the capabilities of our project by itself or any single investigation. They will require the concerted effort of many investigators and many teams of researchers.

CONCLUSION: IN THE END . . . WE COME TO THE BEGINNING

One way that we can sum up is to return to the two cases we introduced in Chapter 1, Serena and Thomas. You may recall that, in infancy, Serena was in a very stable situation. The quality of care she received was sensitive and responsive, consistent routines were established, and her parents were surrounded by a solid network of support. Serena herself was thriving. The situation for Thomas could not have been more different. The living situation was chaotic and ever-changing; his mother had no support, and the care she provided was haphazard at best, harsh at worst. Thomas was struggling then and had problems throughout childhood and adolescence. His adult adjustment is marginal; his partnership is very unstable, and his parenting poor. Serena, by contrast, is doing well on all fronts. She is an excellent mother; her marriage relationship quality received very high ratings, and she did well in college. These two cases are consistent with our group data. But lest we allow things to appear too simple, we hasten to point out that Thomas actually has some notable strengths (e.g., he works on his relationships, and he has had some educational success), and that Serena had a period of notable difficulty as an adolescent, which included substantial conflict with her parents. Peer relationships usually went very well for her, but not always. Each life has its twists and turns. Experience with a therapist, in Thomas's case, and experiences with caring teachers for both of these young people, seemed to be influential. While our group data were compelling, at every age there were children doing both better and worse than we would have predicted from our prior data. Still, often, intermediate experiences shed light on these changes. In the end, we are firmer in our conclusion that development is lawful, but we are only beginning, as a field, to describe adequately this lawfulness.

We are looking forward to the next phase of our study, during which we will assess our participants in adulthood (age 32). We will focus on the personal integration that has evolved from the cumulative experience in relationships and in life more broadly. We expect individuals to have developed relatively stable patterns of functioning within and across the domains of relationships, work and career, personality organization, and psychological health. We will examine how relationship experiences and life events that we have studied throughout the years have become organized into patterns of competencies and vulnerabilities. Moreover, from the participants themselves, we will learn how they understand their own development, and the experiences and relationships they viewed as influential.

LONGITUDINAL STUDY ASSESSMENTS

Assessment	Variable measured	Developed by
Last trimester assessment		
Shipley–Hartford Vocabulary Test	Intelligence	Shipley & Hartford

Personality Research Form
  Aggression
  Defendence
  Impulsivity
  Succorance
	Personality characteristics	Jackson

IPAT Anxiety Scale Questionnaire	Anxiety	Cattell & Scheier
Inventory of Beliefs	Locus of control	Rotter
Neonatal Perception Inventory	Mother's expectations	Broussard & Hartner

Maternal Attitude Scale:
Questionnaire for Mothers
  Appropriate versus
    inappropriate control
    of child's aggression
    Encouragement versus
      discouragement of reciprocity
    Acceptance versus denial of
      emotional complexity in child
      care
	Mother's attitude toward developing mother–child relationship	Cohler

Pregnancy Research
Questionnaire
  Fear for self
  Desire for pregnancy
  Dependency
  Fear for baby
  Maternal feelings
  Irritability and tension
	Mother's feelings regarding pregnancy	Schaefer & Manheimer

Knowledge of Child Care and Expectations of Child Development	Mother's knowledge	Staff
Mother's Information and Interview Sheet	General information	Staff

Birth assessment

Nurses' Ratings of Newborn	Infant temperament and characteristics	Ferreira & Staff
Hennepin County General Hospital Newborn Database	General information	Hospital Staff
Delivery room assessment of newborn	General information	Staff
Neonatal Behavioral Assessment Scale	Psychological and physiological characteristics of newborn	Brazelton
First Days Questionnaire	General information	Staff

3-month assessment

Note: All the tests given during the last trimester, with the exception of the Shipley–Hartford Vocabulary Test and Mother's Information and Interview Sheet, were also given at 3 months, plus the following:

Life Events Inventory	Amount of environmental stress on the mother	Cochrane & Robertson; Staff
Enjoyment of Baby Scale	Mother's feelings regarding infant	Staff
Carey Infant Temperament Questionnaire	Infant temperament	Carey
Observation and rating Waiting Room Rating Scale Doctor's Rating Scale Observation of Feeding	Observation of mother–infant interaction	Staff Staff Ainsworth Staff

6-month assessment

Observation of Feeding and Play	Observation of mother–infant interaction	Ainsworth; Staff

Doctor's Rating Scale	Observation of mother–infant	Staff
Waiting Room Rating Scale	Observation of mother–infant interaction	Staff
Carey Infant Temperament Questionnaire	Infant temperament	Carey

9-month assessment

Bayley Scales of Infant Development	Infant's mental and motor development	Bayley
Mother's Expectations of Child's Ability	Mother's expectation of child's performance on Bayley	Staff
Observation of mother and infant during Bayley	Mother–infant interaction	Staff

12-month assessment

Strange Situation	Security of attachment	Ainsworth & Wittig
12-Month Interview	General information	Staff
Habituation Task	Attentional development of child	Staff
Life Events Inventory	Amount of environmental stress on mother	Cochrane & Robertson; Staff
Prohibition of Forbidden Objects	Mother's style of discipline	Staff
Uzgiris and Hunt Assessment in Infancy Scale	Cognitive development	Uzgiris & Hunt

Throughout first year

| Child Care Rating Scale | Ratings of quality care | Staff |

18-month assessment

| Strange Situation | Security of attachment | Ainsworth & Wittig |
| Prohibition Task | Mother's style of discipline | Staff |

18-Month Interview	General information	Staff
Life Events Inventory	Stressful life events	Cochrane & Robertson; Staff

24-month assessment

Tool Problems	Competence, quality of play, quality of problem solving, maternal assistance and support	Matas, Arend, & Sroufe
Child Perception Inventory	Mother's expectations	Staff
Bayley Scales of Infant Development	Infant's mental, motor, and infant behavior development	Bayley
Baby's Activities at 24 Months	Mother's expectations of child's performance on Bayley Scales of Infant Development	Staff
Developmental Expectations Measure	Mother's knowledge of child development norms	Staff
Knowledge of Child Care	Knowledge of child care practices	Staff
Acquiring Child Care Information	Where mother acquires information	Staff
24-Month Interview	Mother's knowledge of children and child care practices	Staff
Child Care Rating Scale	Quality of child care	Staff

30-month assessment

Life Events Inventory	Stressful life events	Cochrane & Robertson; Staff
MacAndrew Alcoholism Scale	Tendency toward alcoholism	MacAndrew
Emotionality, Activity, Sociability, and Impulsivity Temperament Survey	Child temperament	Buss & Plomin
Sources of Information Questionnaire	Source of knowledge about child rearing	Staff

| Caldwell HOME Inventory | Social, emotional, and cognitive stimulation | Caldwell, Heider, & Kaplan |
| 30-Month Interview | General information, life circumstances | Staff |

42-month assessment

Life Events Inventory	Stressful life events	Cochrane & Robertson; Staff
Barrier Box Situation	Child's adaptation to frustration	Harrington, Block, & Block
Teaching Tasks	Child's problem solving	Staff
Preschool Language Scale	Language development	Zimmerman, Steiner, & Pond
42-Month Interview	Involvement with social agencies, child care	Staff

48-month assessment

Life Events Inventory	Stressful life events	Cochrane & Robertson; Staff
Profile of Mood States	Mother's affective mood states	McNair, Lorr, & Droppleman
Developmental Profile	Child's self-help, social, and language skills	Alpern & Boll
Center for Epidemiologic Studies Depression Scale	Mother's positive and negative feelings	Radloff
Symptom Checklist	Child behavior problems	Staff
Wechsler Adult Intelligence Scale	Intelligence	Wechsler
IPAT Anxiety Scale Questionnaire	Anxiety	Cattell & Scheier
48-Month Interview	General information, relationship status, and so forth	Staff

54-month assessment

Preschool Interpersonal Problem-Solving Test	Behavior adjustment	Shure & Spivack
Dual Focus Test	Ego resiliency	Block & Block
Curiosity Box Assessment	Involvement, quality of play	Modified version of Banta's Curiosity Box
Delay of Gratification—Gift Delivery	Child's ego control	Block & Block
Competing Set	Child's ego resiliency	Block & Block
Lowenfeld Mosaic Test	Child's playfulness and imagination	Block & Block
Overall Ratings of Child during 54-Month Assessment	Ego control, dependency, focus, positive and negative affect	Staff
Relationship status	Mother's relationship status with men; primary child caregiver	Staff
54-Month Interview	General information, life circumstances	Staff
Life Events Inventory	Stressful life events	Cochrane & Robertson; Staff
Questionnaire for Mothers	Sensitivity and empathy	Staff

Preschool assessment

Preschool Behavior Questionnaire I and II	Symptoms of emotional disturbance	Behar & Stringfield; Staff
Preschool Rating Scales	Agency and self-confidence, ego control, dependency, social skills, positive and negative affect, compliance	Staff
California Child Q-Sort	Ego resilience and control, field independence, self-esteem, social desirability	Block & Block

| School Information Form | School attendance | Staff |

64-month assessment

Child Behavior Checklist (Parent Report Form)	Parent's rating of child's behavior problems and social competence	Achenbach
64-Month Interview	Family and work status, feelings about present life situation and child, social life, and so forth	Staff
Wechsler Preschool and Primary Scale of Intelligence	Intelligence	Wechsler
Child Care Rating Scale	Quality of child care	Staff
Gender Constancy Test (gender identity)	Gender identity and stability over time, gender constancy across various situations	Slaby & Frey
Tell-A-Story	General expressive language	Staff
Draw-A-Person	General cognitive	Staff
Social Network Inventory	Social support	Staff; Belle & Longfellow; Pattison, Llamas, & Jurd
Life Events Inventory	Stressful life events	Cochrane & Robertson; Staff
16PF	Mother's personality	Cattell

Kindergarten assessment

Teacher Nomination Procedure	Peer acceptance and social competence	Staff
Devereux Elementary School Behavior Rating Scale	Classroom adjustment	Spivak & Swift
Child Behavior Checklist (Teacher Report Form)	Behavior problems	Achenbach & Edelbrock

Kindergarten Social Behaviors Scales	Agency, self-control, positive affect, negative emotional tone, dependency	Staff
Teacher Interview	Child's general adjustment, progress and behavior change	Staff
Information from School File	School attendance, referral for special programs, and so forth	Staff
Primary Grade Class Environment Form	Classroom ecology	Staff

First-grade assessment (school)

Teacher Nomination Procedure	Peer acceptance and social competence	Staff
Devereux Elementary School Behavior Rating Scale	Classroom adjustment	Spivak & Swift
Child Behavior Checklist (Teacher Report Form)	Behavior problems	Achenbach & Edelbrock
Teacher Interview	Child's general adjustment, progress, and behavior change	Staff
Teacher Rating of Actual Competence and Acceptance	Perceived competence and acceptance	Harter & Pike

First-grade assessment (home)

Peabody Individual Achievement Test	Academic achievement	Dunn & Markwardt
Pictorial Perceived Competence and Acceptance Scale for Young Children	Self-esteem	Harter & Pike
Mother Interview	Mother's feelings, expectations, and perceptions of school, mother's life circumstances	Staff
Porteus Maze Test	Playfulness and impulse control	Porteus

Life Events Inventory	Stressful life events	Cochrane & Robertson; Staff
Caldwell HOME Inventory	Environmental stimulation	Caldwell & Bradley
Child Behavior Checklist (Parent Report Form)	Parent's rating of child's behavior problems and social competence	Achenbach
Draw-A-Person	General cognitive skills	Staff
Child Care Rating Scale	Quality of child care	Staff
Relationship Status	Mother's relationship status with men; primary child caregiver	Staff

Second-grade assessment (school)

Child Behavior Checklist (Teacher Report Form)	Behavior problems	Achenbach & Edelbrock
Devereux Elementary School Behavior Rating Scale	Classroom adjustment	Spivak & Swift
Teacher Nomination Procedure (Rank Order)	Peer acceptance and social competence	Staff
Teacher Interview	Child's general adjustment, progress, and behavior change	Staff
School File Information Sheet	Attendance, referral for special programs, and so forth	Staff

Second-grade assessment (home)

Mother Interview	Mother's feelings, expectations, and perceptions of school, mother's life circumstances	Staff
Relationship Status	Mother's relationship status with men; primary child caregiver	Staff

Life Events Inventory	Stressful life events	Cochrane & Robertson; Staff
Children's Depression Rating Scale (Parent Form)	Severity of depression	Poznanski; Poznanski, Cook, & Carroll
Beck Depression Inventory	Behavioral manifestations and depth of depression in adults	Beck, Ward, Mendelson, Mock, & Erbaugh
Peabody Individual Achievement Test	Academic achievement	Dunn & Markwardt
Caldwell HOME Inventory	Environmental stimulation	Caldwell & Bradley
Pictorial Perceived Competence and Acceptance Scale for Young Children	Self-esteem	Harter & Pike
Draw-A-Person	General cognitive skills	Staff
Home Visit Ratings	Compliance, rapport with examiner, task orientation, persistence, negative and positive affect	Staff

Third-grade assessment (home)

Mother Interview	Mother's feelings, expectations, and perceptions of school, mother's life circumstances	Staff
Relationship Status	Mother's relationship status with men; primary child caregiver	Staff
Life Events Inventory	Stressful life events	Cochrane & Robertson; Staff
Children's Depression Rating Scale (Parent Form)	Severity of depression	Poznanski; Poznanski, Cook, & Carroll

Beck Depression Inventory	Behavioral manifestations and depth of depression in adults	Beck, Ward, Mendelson, Mock, & Erbaugh
Peabody Individual Achievement Test	Academic achievement	Dunn & Markwardt
Children's Depression Rating Scale (Child Form)	Severity of depression	Poznanski
Wechsler Intelligence Scale for Children—Revised	General intelligence	Wechsler
Physical Anomalies Assessment	Presence or absence of minor physical anomalies	Waldrop
Home Visit Ratings	Compliance, rapport with examiner, task orientation, persistence, negative and positive affect	Staff
Family Drawing	Perception of family	Staff

Third-grade assessment (school)

Teacher Interview	Child's general adjustment, progress and behavior change	Staff
Child Behavior Checklist (Teacher Report Form)	Behavior problems	Achenbach & Edelbrock
Devereux Elementary School Behavior Rating Scale	Classroom adjustment	Spivak & Swift
Teacher Nomination Procedure (Rank Order)	Peer acceptance and social competence	Staff
School File Information Sheet	Attendance, referral for special problems, and so forth	Staff

Sixth-grade assessment (school)

Teacher Interview	Child's general adjustment, progress, and behavior change	Staff
Child Behavior Checklist (Teacher Report Form)	Behavior problems	Achenbach & Edelbrock

Devereux Elementary School Behavior Rating Scale	Classroom adjustment	Spivak & Swift
Teacher Nomination Procedure (Rank Order)	Peer acceptance and social competence	Staff

Sixth-grade assessment (home)

Mother Interview	Mother's feelings, expectations, and perceptions of school, mother's life circumstances	Staff
Relationship Status	Mother's relationship status with men; primary child caregiver	Staff
Life Events Inventory	Stressful life events	Staff; Cochrane & Robertson
Peabody Individual Achievement Test	Academic achievement	Dunn & Markwardt
Home Visit Ratings	Compliance, rapport with examiner, task orientation, persistence, negative and positive affect	Staff
Sentence Completion	Family and peer conflict, self-concept	Staff
Fable Task	Level of moral development, care orientation	Adapted from Gilligan; Staff
Thematic Apperception Test	Intimacy motivation, conflict and aggressive imagery	McAdams; Staff
Explanatory Style Questionnaire	Attributional style	Seligman
Friendship Interview	Friendship status and friendship understanding	Staff

Seventh-grade assessment (family)

Family Observation Antismoking Campaign Object Assembly Imaginary Happenings Q-Sort Revealed Differences Plan a Holiday	Family closeness, affective tone, conflict resolution, support for autonomy	Block; Collins; Strodtbeck

16-year assessment

Mother

Mother Interview	Mother's feelings, expectations, and perceptions of school, mother's life circumstances	Staff
Life Events Scale	Stressful life events	Staff; Cochrane & Robertson
Center for Epidemiological Studies Depression Scale	Mother's positive and negative feelings	Radloff
Child Behavior Checklist (Parent Report Form)	Parent's rating of child behavior problems and social competence	Achenbach
Dissociative Experiences Scale	Frequency of dissociative experiences	Carlson & Putnam
Self-Report Family Inventory	Family health, conflict, communication, cohesion, directive leadership, and expressiveness	Beavers, Hampson, & Hulgus

Child

Adolescent Interview	Identity, friendship, school, dating	Grotevant & Cooper; Staff
Peer Relations Interview	Friendship and dating	Grotevant & Cooper; Staff
Adolescent Health Survey	Adolescent health behaviors	Resnick
Youth Self-Report	Academic, social competence, and behavior problems	Achenbach
Self-Perception Profile	Scholastic competence, athletic competence, physical appearance, social acceptance, behavioral conduct, global self-worth, job competence, close friendship, and romantic appeal	Harter
Woodcock–Johnson Psychoeducational Battery—Revised	Academic achievement	Woodcock & Johnson
Self-Report Family Inventory	Family health, conflict, family communication, family cohesion, directive leadership, and expressiveness	Beavers, Hampson, & Hulgus
Adolescent Perceived Events Scale	Stressful life events	Compas; Staff

17-½ year assessment

Mother

Mother Interview	Mother's feelings, expectations, and perceptions of school, mother's life circumstances	Staff
Life Events Scale	Stressful life events	Staff
Center for Epidemiologic Studies Depression Scale	Mother's positive and negative feelings	Radloff
Parental Influence/Child Autonomy Questionnaire	Parent's rating of amount of influence she has in child's life	Staff

Adolescent

Adolescent Interview	School, work, living situation, and dating	Staff
Schedule for Affective Disorders and Schizophrenia for School-Age Children	Presence of past and present psychiatric symptoms and disorders	Puig-Antich & Chambers

19-year assessment

Adolescent

Adolescent Sentence Completion	Inner working model of self and others	Staff
Adolescenet Health Survey	Adolescent health behaviors	Resnick; Staff
Adolescent Interview	Living arrangements, activities, education, work, religion, and politics	Staff
Dissociative Experiences Scale	Frequency of dissociative experiences	Carlson & Putnam
Adult Attachment Interview	Inner working model	Main & Hesse
Adolescent Perceived Events Scale	Stressful life events	Compas; Staff
Adjustment Scale	Global rating of functioning	Staff
Relationships Interview	Interpersonal relationships	Staff

Romantic relationship assessment: Phase I

Adolescent and partner

Current Relationships Interview	Attachment to partner	Crowell

Relationship Perceptions Battery Perceived insecurity Relationship idealization Subjective closeness and emotional tone Satisfaction Feelings of love Commitment Investment in relationship	Perception of romantic relationship	Fri & Bersheid; Attridge; Sprecher & Metts; Berscheid et al.; Hendrick; Rubin; Lund; Staff
Conflict Tactics Scales	Conflict tactics in relationship	Strauss
Relationship Problem Inventory	Relationship problems	Gottman et al.
Markman–Cox Couple Interaction Observation	Couple interaction	Markman & Cox
Ideal Couple Q-Sort	Couple interaction	Bengston & Grotevant; Staff

23-year assessment

School/Work Experience Interview	Living arrangements, education, work	Staff
Work Experience Questionnaire	Work goals, satisfaction, stress, and relationships	Staff; Mortimer
Relationships Interview	Social support, family relationships, romantic relationships, dating history, and friendships	Staff
Use of Mental Heath Services	Previous or ongoing mental health treatment	Staff; Horowitz
Adult Health Survey	General health, alcohol and drug use, sexual activity, and crime	Resnick; Staff
Young Adult Self-Report for Ages 18–30	Social competence, behavior problems, symptom checklist	Achenbach
Symptom Checklist 90—Revised	Psychopathology symptom checklist	Derogites
Life Events Schedule	Stressful life events	Staff

Romantic relationship assessment: Phase II

Adolescent and Partner		
Current Relationship Interview	Attachment to partner	Crowell
Relationship Perceptions Battery Perceived insecurity Relationship idealization Subjective closeness and emotional tone Satisfaction Feelings of love Commitment Investment in relationship	Perception of romantic relationship	Fri & Bersheid; Attridge; Sprecher & Metts; Berscheid et al.; Hendrick; Rubin; Lund; Staff
Conflict Tactics Scale	Conflict tactics in relationship	Strauss
Relationship Problem Inventory	Relationship problems	Gottman et al.
Markman–Cox Couple Interaction Observation	Couple interaction	Markman & Cox
Ideal Couple Q-Sort	Couple interaction	Bengston & Grotevant; Staff
Relationship Status Questionnaire	Describes feelings about close relationships	Staff

APPENDIX B

LIFE STRESS SCALE

1. Unemployed mother _____; husband (boyfriend) _____ (how long?)
2. Troubles with welfare (explain) _____
3. Trouble with superiors at work (explain) _____
4. New job in same line of work _____
5. New job in new line of work _____
6. Change in hours or conditions of present job _____
7. Promotion or change or responsibilities at work _____
8. Moving to different house _____ (date?)
9. Purchasing own house (taking out mortgage) _____
10. New neighbors _____
11. Quarrel with neighbors (explain) _____
12. Income decreased substantially (25%) _____
13. Getting into debt beyond means of repayment _____
14. Money problems (in debt or severe shortage) _____
15. Conviction for minor violation (e.g., traffic violation, misdemeanor) _____
16. Jail sentence (immediate family) _____ Who _____
17. Involvement in physical fight _____ Who _____
18. Immediate family member starts drinking heavily _____
19. Immediate family member attempts suicide _____
20. Death of immediate family member (what relationship?) _____
21. Death of close friend _____
22. Immediate family member seriously ill _____
23. Gain of a new family member (immediate) (birth or marriage) _____
24. Problems related to alcohol or drugs _____
25. Serious restriction of social life (explain) _____
26. Period of homelessness (no permanent residence) _____

27. Serious physical illness or injury requiring hospital treatment (explain)
    _____

28. Prolonged ill health requiring treatment by own doctor _____
29. Sudden and serious impairment of vision or hearing _____
30. Unwanted pregnancy _____
31. Miscarriage _____
32. Abortion _____
33. Marriage _____
34. Boyfriend (or girlfriend) moves in or out (explain) _____
35. Other people moving in or out _____
36. Increase in number of arguments with spouse (or boyfriend or girlfriend)
    _____

37. Increase in number of arguments with other relatives _____
38. Increase in number of serious arguments with close friend _____
39. Trouble with other relatives (e.g., in-laws) _____
40. Divorce _____
41. Marital separation or breakup _____
42. Marital reconciliation _____
43. Wife or girlfriend begins or stops work _____
44. Husband or boyfriend begins or stops work _____

Adapted from Cochrane and Robertson (1973). Copyright 1973 by Elsevier. Reprinted by permission.

APPENDIX C

12-MONTH INTERVIEW

This is a structured interview designed to elicit information on the following general areas of the mother's life and the child's development:

- Mother's attitude toward, and present enjoyment of her baby.
- Mother's expectations of the child's development.
- Mother's understanding of various aspects of child rearing (e.g., baby's crying, problems of obedience).
- Changes in mother's life following the birth of the baby (e.g., social life, beliefs, attitudes and feelings, depression or anxiety).
- Quality or extent of mother's support system (e.g., Who does mother turn to for assistance? Is the baby's father in the home and, if so, how much support does he provide?).

Name _____

Date _____

Interviewer _____

1. a. Do you feed on a regular schedule? How often?
    b. Does he still take a bottle?
    c. Is there anything unusual about the way your baby eats or what he eats?
2. Does your baby say any words yet, like "mama" or "bottle," etc.?
3. a. What specifically do you enjoy most about your child?
    b. What do you enjoy least?
    c. Do you think you will enjoy your child more when he is older? Why?
4. a. Is raising a child more or less difficult than you thought it would be? What are some specifics?
    b. Do you feel you've sacrificed much for your child? (If yes, is the sacrifice worth it?)
    c. Would you like to have more children?

5. a. What has been the biggest change in your life since having your baby?
   b. Do you have time to do the things you want to do?
   c. Have any of your relationships with husband–boyfriend, parents, relatives, friends changed? How are they now?
   d. How have you changed as a person since having your baby? (Changes in personality, beliefs, and feelings?)
   e. Are you any more or less nervous, or more or less depressed?
6. a. Does your baby have any particularly good or bad times of the day?
   b. How long does he play by himself? (Explain circumstances.)
   c. How often or how much do you play with him?
   d. How well do you and your baby get along?
7. How have your ideas about children changed in the last year?
8. a. How often do you get out of the house?
   b. Where are some of the places you like to go?
   c. Do you go with or without your baby?
   d. Is there someone you can get to stay with the child?
   e. Do you feel that you get enough rest?
   f. Do people visit you? Who?
   g. What is the longest time you have been separated from your baby? How often?
   h. Are you still able to have a social life and time for leisure activities? What do you enjoy?
9. a. Who has given you the most help in caring for your child during the first year?
   b. Is there a person always available when you need help?
   c. If you have a problem with your baby, who do you turn to?
10. a. Does the baby's father live in the home? If not, do you see him? If not, do you have a boyfriend now?
    b. Does he help in taking care of the child?
    c. Does he play with the child? (What sort of play do they enjoy?)
    d. Does your baby get along with him?
    e. Does the father like being with the baby?
    f. Who does the baby look most like?
    g. Who does the baby act most like?
    h. Do you and the father agree on how to raise the child?
11. What irritates or frustrates you the most about your child? (Describe feelings and explain how you deal with them.)
12. a. If you ask your baby to do something, does he obey?
    b. How do you get him to obey if he doesn't at first? (How about the father? If spanking, provide more information on frequency and intensity.)
13. Some mothers, when babies cry, which they all do, feel that if you pick

up a baby each time he will get spoiled. Others think you should pick
him up every time. How do you feel about this?

14. Is there anything about the baby that especially concerns you?
15. What are your hopes for your baby?
16. How did you feel about participating in this project?

(Additional question added): Do you believe you're raising your child the
same way you were raised? How were you raised?

APPENDIX D

TOOL PROBLEM-SOLVING
TASK RATINGS: 24 MONTHS

Caregiver Supportive Presence

Major criteria:
1. Secure base—helping the child feel comfortable with the task
2. Mother involvement—attentiveness to child and task

Subcriteria (components of major criteria):
   a. Focusing the child on the task when needed
   b. Tuning-in the child to reinforcing aspects of the task as needed
   c. Mood setting for a problem-solving situation as needed
   d. Helping the child achieve a sense of having solved the problem him/herself
   e. Sharing in the joy of solution
   f. Encouraging and supporting his/her efforts
   g. Physical presence when needed
   h. Anticipating frustration and taking action to help the situation
   i. Mother staying calm

Scale Points

   7. This mother meets all criteria and subcriteria. If the task is very easy for the child, he/she may not require as much support as indicated by the criteria. In this situation, it is appropriate for the mother to allow the child autonomous work. The difficulty of the task and level of comprehension and motivation of the individual child may determine how much support the mother should offer, and therefore determine how applicable the subcriteria are for the particular situation.
   6. This mother technically meets all criteria (if applicable) but is not quite able to give the child all the support required. It may be the case that the

326

mother is lacking slightly in emotional involvement, or that she may be either a bit oversupportive or overcontrolling. It may also be the case that the task is solved so quickly that it is unclear if all the subcriteria would have been met with a longer task. All subcriteria are met at least satisfactorily; however, one or two might be minimally met.

5. The mother's presence has a positive effect, but she is not as supportive and/or involved as in higher ratings. For a rating of 5, one major criterion may be minimally met. "Secure base" must be at least marginally met, as it can never receive a "no" on this scale point. There may be slight doubt about two or three subcriteria, or one or two subcriteria may not be met as long as they do not prevent the major criteria from being at least minimally met.

4. This mother is not nonsupportive, but the degree of support is not obvious or striking. She is, however, within the intermediate range of supportiveness. It may that one major criterion is not met, while the other is adequately fulfilled, or one major criterion and one subcriterion are not met, or four subcriteria are not met, resulting in one marginally met major criteria. Although the mother adds little to her child's involvement in the task, when the child directly requests aid or support, she gives it. The mother may be more directive than supportive, and try to get the child to follow her instructions rather than supporting the child's efforts. Or she may lack goal direction due to her lack of motivation or uncertainty in the situation. In this case, the child's motivation may decline.

3. The mother is lacking in areas of both major criteria and can be characterized as supportive in only a weak manner. She does have some relative strengths and may be able to fulfill two to four subcriteria. It may also be the case that one major criterion is minimally met, and at least four subcriteria are not met.

2. Most subcriteria and both major criteria are not met. The mother's support is relatively absent, although there is no distinct negative quality characterizing the interaction. The mother could not be characterized as "angry" or "cold" toward the child, but she shows very few or no strengths.

1. All criteria and subcriteria are not met, or there is a distinct negative quality to the interaction. The mother reacts to the child's performance by becoming angry, hostile, cold, and/or totally unavailable.

Caregiver Quality of Assistance

Major criteria:
1. Giving minimal assistance needed to keep the child working toward a solution, without solving it for him/her.
2. Helping the child see the relationships between actions that are required to solve the problem.

Subcriteria (components of major criteria):
a. Grading of hints
b. Clarity of hints—working in tune with the child's level
c. Flexibility—changing instructions for more effective help
d. Timing of instructions
e. Pacing of instructions
f. Cooperating—giving hints that meet the child's needs
g. Having control of the situation
h. Giving space initially
i. Comments that are helpful rather than discouraging
j. Effectiveness of instructions

Scale Points

7. The mother meets all criteria and subcriteria, or she is excellent at giving assistance. There may be some ambiguity about what is expected, or a lack of clarity at one point during the task, but, in general, the criteria and subcriteria apply, or both major and all but one subcriterion are met. The mother is sensitive to her child's schedule. This enables her to provide helpful, well-timed instructions in a clear, orderly, and understandable manner. She may be directive if it is an appropriate, nonintrusive manner.

6. This mother's assistance is quite good. The two major criteria are met but perhaps not 100%, or all but two of the subcriteria are met. Perhaps there is not quite enough focus on "helping the child see the relationships," but, otherwise, criteria and subcriteria are met. This rating may also apply to the situation in which the task is solved so quickly that it is not possible to give a lower rating.

5. This mother is moderately good at giving assistance. It may be that one major and one or two subcriteria are not met, or three subcriteria are not met. It may seem that the mother could improve on several dimensions (i.e., timing, clarity), although major criteria are met.

4. This mother's assistance to the child is moderately good to weak. She shows more than just a few strengths. Both criteria may be minimally met, but the subcriteria are generally sufficiently (but not optimally) met. Or one criterion and several subcriteria are not met.

3. The mother's assistance is weak. Neither major criterion is met, although they may be scored minimally. The mother does, however, show a few strengths meeting, or minimally meeting, three or four subcriteria.

2. This mother's assistance is very poor. Nearly all or all subcriteria are unmet. Overall, the mother contributes very little in the way of assistance, and gives little or no evidence of strengths in meeting the subcriteria.

1. The mother distracts her child, frustrates him/her, or simply provides no assistance.

Child Experience in the Session

Criteria:
1. How positive the problem-solving experience is, regardless of the degree of maternal support.
2. Extent to which the child leaves the situation with an increase belief in his/her competence, an increased positive attitude about facing challenges, and feeling good about himself.
3. In the end, is the child still OK, able to derive satisfaction from the solution?
4. Mother may enhance the experience or take away from it, or have relatively little effect.

Scale Points

5. Excellent: This child has a positive experience and will be even more confident in facing problems the next time. Tool 4, especially, may have been hard, but persistence pays off, efforts were rewarded, and satisfaction is achieved. The child feels better leaving than he felt coming in—at least about him/herself.

4. Good: A good experience, but in some minor way could be better. For example, the child gets frustrated at some point. Perhaps the mother is slightly too controlling, or perhaps the problems are solved quickly, with mother providing a bit too much of the solution.

3. Fair: This child at least feels OK. Though the experience may not have enhanced self-confidence or attitude toward facing problems, it was not a negative experience. Positive and negative experiences were relatively balanced.

2. Poor: The child has a poor experience, although not as extreme as in scale point 1.

1. Very Poor: This child has a devastating experience either due to belittling, taunting, or abuse from the mother, or breaking down himself (losing control or having to leave the scene), with the mother failing to come to the rescue. The experience may begin OK, but in the end, the child is feeling abandoned or outside of the support of mother, and impotent in the face of the task and his feelings—aggression, throwing the self about, or dejection (e.g., no interest in the reward) are signs of such an experience.

APPENDIX E

TEACHER NOMINATION PROCEDURE

The measure was developed by the Parent–Child Project staff. The purpose was to gain the teacher's general impression of the child's level of emotional health and peer acceptance in relation to the other children in the classroom. Prior to conducting the teacher interview, the teacher was asked to read the descriptions (see attached descriptions and form) of the characteristics, "emotional-health/ self-esteem" and "peer acceptance" and rank the child numerically on a scale of 1 to n, where n is the number of children in the class, and "1" is the highest rank on the characteristic (e.g., the child with the most self-esteem in the class would be ranked 1, and the child showing the least self-esteem would be ranked 30, of a class size 30). The data are scored in the form of a *percentile rank*: The score is calculated by taking the number of children below that child's ranking, divided by the number of children in the class. For example, a child ranked 12th of a class size 20 would receive a score of .40.

Emotional Health/Self-Esteem

This refers, in part, to the degree to which the child is able to take advantage of what the class has to offer. (S)he is not incapacitated by overdependency, lack of self-control, distractibility, inhibition, anxiety, or an asocial orientation. (S)he is *confident*, *curious*, *self-assured*, and *engaging*; enjoys new experiences and new challenges; and becomes involved in whatever (s)he does. This child typically enjoys social activities but can also become involved in more academic pursuits. (S)he is also usually self-directed and self-motivated. (S)he likes her/himself, and therefore brings a positive attitude to the classroom.

Peer Acceptance/Competence

A popular child is well liked by others and has clearly identifiable, mutual friends. Additionally, (s)he is respected by others, and her/his ideas and actions are followed. Criteria for a child high on popularity would include the following: (1) sociability (i.e., fairly frequent social contact with peers); (2) wide acceptance among other children; (3) friendship (i.e., one or more special companions with whom there seems to be a well-meshed relationship); (4) social skills and leadership qualities; and (5) understands another child's perspectives and desires, accepting the other child's ideas as a starting point for interaction, and uses clear, comprehensible communications toward peers. Others want to be with this child and do what (s)he is doing; and this child knows how to lead others to interesting and fun activities.

APPENDIX F

CAPACITY FOR VULNERABILITY:
CAMP REUNION RATING

Adolescence is a period of self-consciousness and, therefore, vulnerability. Yet the movement toward intimate relationships requires that the teenager be able to tolerate such vulnerability. Only by being able to experience and embrace the range of feelings attendant upon the new levels of social relatedness and self-awareness can the young person reap the benefits of a new level of emotional closeness. Teenagers differ in their capacity to risk emotionally close contact, to remain open to experiences that threaten to reveal their inner feelings, and to persist in social contacts despite intense emotions and feelings of vulnerability. Some avoid such contacts; others remain defensive in a variety of ways, even while being socially involved.

7. These individuals embrace the entire range of camp experiences. They engage in social encounters at all levels, and participate fully in the more intimate activities and those which arouse emotions (conflict, etc.). They express their opinions freely in group settings, even tolerating disagreement, and they are direct in dealing with individuals. It is not that they necessarily are always comfortable (or happy), but discomfort does not lead to defensiveness or avoidance of the situation. They allow themselves to experience the range of emotions that necessarily accompany this intense camp experience.

6. As in 7, these teens are open to the whole range of camp experiences, including clear emotional closeness with peers and tolerance of the range of feelings aroused. However, occasional signs of guardedness may be seen, or the child shows isolated examples of nonparticipation.

5. These individuals do allow themselves more generally to be vulnerable. They participate in a range of activities (though probably not the entire range), become close to other campers, and are open to a range of feelings. Still, they may not be open to certain experiences. While never marked by defensiveness, some guardedness may be present at times.

4. These individuals present a mixed picture. They may sometimes engage in emotionally arousing activities and other times not. Or they may engage such activities, but only part way. Or in some domains, they may allow themselves to be vulnerable, in others not. For example, they may form a close friendship, but they (and perhaps their friend) stay protected in broader camp activities.

3. These individuals allow themselves at times to be vulnerable, but guardedness or defensiveness still predominates. If they form a friendship, it will tend to be a safe one (a subordinate child, another child that does not seek emotional closeness, etc.). They tend to participate more fully (or less defensively) in activities that do not involve closeness or arouse emotions. They withhold opinions at times, or allow no room for disagreement.

2. These individuals only infrequently engage the more personal aspects of the camp experience, though they are not completely cut off or isolated, or uniformly defensive. They participate in social experiences and very occasionally allow themselves to be vulnerable.

1. These individuals likely avoid major aspects of the camp experience that are tinged with intensity or socially closeness; when thrust into socially intense or potentially self-revealing circumstances, they are notably defensive, subverting the activity or disowning interest.

APPENDIX G

SELECTED REFERENCES BY TOPIC

Attachment

Carlson, E. A. (1998). A prospective longitudinal study of attachment disorganization/disorientation. *Child Development, 69*(4), 1107–1128.

Carlson, E. A., Sampson, M., & Sroufe, L. A. (2003). Attachment theory and pediatric practice. *Journal of Development and Behavior Pediatrics, 24*(5), 364–379.

Carlson, E. A., & Sroufe, L. A. (1995). The contribution of attachment theory to developmental psychopathology. In D. Cicchetti & D. Cohen (Eds.), *Developmental psychopathology: Vol. 1. Theory and methods* (pp. 581–617). New York: Wiley.

Egeland, B., & Carlson, E. A. (2004). Attachment and psychopathology. In L. Atkinson & S. Goldberg (Eds.), *Clinical implications of attachment* (pp. 27–48). Mahwah, NJ: Erlbaum.

Egeland, B., & Farber, E. (1984). Infant–mother attachment: Factors related to its development and changes over time. *Child Development, 55*(3), 753–771.

Pastor, D. (1981). The quality of mother–infant attachment and its relationship to toddlers' initial sociability with peers. *Developmental Psychopathology, 17*, 326–335.

Roisman, G. I., Padron, E., Sroufe, L. A., & Egeland, B. (2002). Earned-secure attachment status in retrospect and prospect. *Child Development, 73*(4), 1204–1219.

Sroufe, L. A. (1985). Attachment classification from the perspective of infant–caregiver relationships and infant temperament. *Child Development, 56*, 1–14.

Sroufe, L. A., Carlson, E. A., Levy, A. K., & Egeland, B. (1999). Implications of attachment theory for developmental psychopathology. *Development and Psychopathology, 11*, 1–13.

Sroufe, L. A., Egeland, B., Carlson, E., & Collins, W. A. (2005). Placing early attachment experiences in developmental context: The Minnesota Longitudinal Study. In K. E. Grossmann, K. Grossmann, & E. Waters (Eds.), *Attachment from infancy to adulthood: The major longitudinal studies* (pp. 48–70). New York: Guilford Press.

Sroufe, L. A., & Fleeson, J. (1986). Attachment and the construction of relationships. In W. Hartup & Z. Rubin (Eds.), *Relationships and development* (pp. 51–71). Hillsdale, NJ: Erlbaum.

Sroufe, L. A., Fox, N., & Pancake, V. (1983). Attachment and dependency in developmental perspective. *Child Development, 54*(6), 1615–1627.

Sroufe, L. A., & Sampson, M. C. (2000). Attachment theory and systems concepts. *Human Development, 43*, 321–326.

Sroufe, L. A., & Waters, E. (1977). Attachment as an organizational construct. *Child Development, 48*, 1184–1199.

Susman-Stillman, A., Kalkoske, M., Egeland, B., & Waldman, I. (1996). Infant temperament and maternal sensitivity as predictors of attachment security. *Infant Behavior and Development, 19*(1), 33–47.

Vaughn, B., Waters, E., Egeland, B., & Sroufe, L. A. (1979). Individual differences in infant–mother attachment at 12 and 18 months: Stability and change in families under stress. *Child Development, 50*(4), 971–975.

Ward, M. J., Vaughn, B., & Robb, M. D. (1988). Attachment and adaptation in siblings: Role of the mother in cross-sibling consistency. *Child Development, 59*, 643–651.

Waters, E. (1978). The stability of individual differences in infant–mother attachment. *Child Development, 49*, 483–494.

Waters, E., Vaughn, B., & Egeland, B. (1980). Individual differences in infant–mother attachment relationships at age one: Antecedents in neonatal behavior in an urban, economically disadvantaged sample. *Child Development, 51*, 208–216.

Weinfield, N., Sroufe, L. A., & Egeland, B. (2000). Attachment from infancy to young adulthood in a high risk sample: Continuity, discontinuity, and their correlates. *Child Development, 71*, 695–702.

Weinfield, N., Whaley, G., & Egeland, B. (2004). Continuity, discontinuity, and coherence in attachment from infancy to late adolescence: Sequelae of organization and disorganization. *Attachment and Human Development, 6*, 73–97.

Infancy

Egeland, B., & Erickson, M. F. (2004). Lessons from STEEP: Linking theory, research, and practice for the well-being of infants and parents. In A. Sameroff, S. McDonough & K. Rosenblum (Eds.), *Treating parent–infant relationship problems* (pp. 213–242). New York: Guilford Press.

Egeland, B., Pianta, R. C., & O'Brien, M. A. (1993). Maternal intrusiveness in infancy and child maladaptation in early school years. *Development and Psychopathology, 5*(3), 359–370.

Pianta, R. C., & Egeland, B. (1990). Life stress and parenting outcomes in a disadvantaged sample: Results of the Mother–Child Interaction Project. *Journal of Clinical Child Psychology, 19*(4), 329–336.

Pianta, R. C., Sroufe, L. A., & Egeland, B. (1989). Continuity and discontinuity in maternal sensitivity at 6, 24, and 42 months in a high risk sample. *Child Development, 60*(2), 481–487.

Sroufe, L. A. (1996). *Emotional development: The organization of emotional life in the early years.* New York: Cambridge University Press.

Vaughn, B., Taraldson, B., Crichton, L., & Egeland, B. (1980). Relationships between neonatal behavioral organization and infant behavior during the first year of life. *Infant Behavior and Development, 3*, 47–66.

Early Childhood

Arend, R., Gove, F., & Sroufe, L. A. (1979). Continuity of individual adaptation from infancy to kindergarten: A predictive study of ego-resiliency and curiosity in preschoolers. *Child Development, 50,* 950–959.

Kestenbaum, R., Farber, E., & Sroufe, L. A. (1989). Individual differences in empathy among preschoolers: Concurrent and predictive validity. In N. Eisenberg (Ed.), *Empathy and related emotional responses* (pp. 51–56). San Francisco: Jossey-Bass.

Matas, L., Arend, R., & Sroufe, L. A. (1978). Continuity of adaptation in the second year: The relationship between quality of attachment and later competence. *Child Development, 49,* 547–556.

Sroufe, L. A. (1983). Infant–caregiver attachment and patterns of adaptation in preschool. In M. Perlmutter (Ed.), *Minnesota Symposia in Child Psychology: Vol. 16. The roots of maladaptation and competence* (pp. 129–135). Hillsdale, NJ: Erlbaum.

Sroufe, L. A., Jacobvitz, J., Mangelsdorf, S., deAngelo, E., & Ward, M. J. (1985). Generational boundary dissolution between mothers and their preschool children: A relationships systems approach. *Child Development, 56,* 317–325.

Troy, M., & Sroufe, L. A. (1987). Victimization among preschoolers: The role of attachment relationship history. *Journal of the American Academy of Child and Adolescent Psychiatry, 26*(2), 166–172.

Waters, E., Wippman, J., & Sroufe, L. A. (1979). Attachment, positive affect, and competence in the peer group: Two studies in construct validation. *Child Development, 40,* 821–829.

Middle Childhood

Collins, W. A., & van Dulmen, M. (in press). The significance of middle childhood peer competence for work and relationships in early adulthood. In A. Huston (Ed.), *Successful pathways from middle childhood to adulthood.* New York: Cambridge.

Elicker, J., Englund, M., & Sroufe, L. A. (1992). Predicting peer competence and peer relationships in childhood from early parent–child relationships. In R. Parke & G. Ladd (Eds.), *Family–peer relationships: Modes of linkage* (pp. 77–106). Hillsdale, NJ: Erlbaum.

Sroufe, L. A., Bennett, C., Englund, M., Urban, J., & Shulman, S. (1993). The significance of gender boundaries in preadolescence: Contemporary correlates and antecedents of boundary violation and maintenance. *Child Development, 64*(2), 455–466.

Adolescence and Early Adulthood

Carlson, E. A., Sroufe, L. A., Collins, W. A., Jimerson, S., Weinfield, N., Hennighausen, K., et al. (1999). Early environmental support and elementary school adjustment as predictors of school adjustment in middle adolescence. *Journal of Adolescent Research, 14*, 72–94.

Collins, W. A., Gleason, T., & Sesma, A. (1997). Internalization, autonomy, and relationships: Development during adolescence. In J. E. Grusec & L. Kuczynski (Eds.), *Parenting and children's internalization of values* (pp. 78–102). New York: Wiley.

Englund, M., Levy, A., Hyson, D., & Sroufe, L. A. (2000). Adolescent social competence: Effectiveness in a group setting. *Child Development, 71*, 1049–1060.

Hyson, D. (2002). Understanding adaptation to work in adulthood: A contextual developmental approach. *Advances in Life Course Research, 7*, 93–110.

Linder, J. R., & Collins, W. A. (in press). Parent and peer predictors of physical aggression and conflict management in romantic relationships in early adulthood. *Journal of Family Psychology.*

Siebenbruner, J., Zimmer-Gembeck, M., & Egeland, B. (2005). *Sexual partners and contraceptive use: A sixteen-year prospective study predicting abstinence and risk behavior.* Manuscript submitted for publication.

Sroufe, J. (1991). Assessment of parent–adolescent relationships: Implications for adolescent development. *Journal of Family Psychology, 5*, 21–45.

Weinfield, N. S., Ogawa, J. R., & Sroufe, L. A. (1997). Early attachment as a pathway to adolescent peer competence. *Journal of Research on Adolescence, 7*(3), 241–265.

Social Development

Collins, W. A. (1995). Relationships and development: Family adaptation to individual change. In S. Shulman (Ed.), *Close relationships and socioemotional development* (pp. 128–154). New York: Ablex.

Collins, W. A., Hennighausen, K. H., Schmit, D. T., & Sroufe, L. A. (1997). Developmental precursors of romantic relationships: A longitudinal analysis. In S. Shulman & W. A. Collins (Eds.), *Romantic relationships in adolescence: Developmental perspectives* (pp. 69–84). San Francisco: Jossey-Bass.

Collins, W. A., & Laursen, B. (2004). Family relationships and parenting influences. In R. Lerner & L. Steinberg (Eds.), *Handbook of adolescent psychology* (pp. 331–362). New York: Wiley.

Collins, W. A., & Roisman, G. I. (in press). Familial and peer influence in the development of competence during adolescence. In J. Dunn & A. Clarke-Stewart (Eds.), *Families count: Family effects on child and adolescent development.* Cambridge, UK: Cambridge University Press.

Collins, W. A., & Sroufe, L. A. (1999). Capacity for intimate relationships: A developmental construction. In W. Furman, C. Feiring & B. Brown (Eds.), *Contemporary perspectives on adolescent romantic relationships* (pp. 125–147). New York: Cambridge University Press.

Collins, W. A., & van Dulmen, M. (in press). The course of true love(s): Origins and pathways in the development of romantic relationships. In A. Booth & A. Crouter (Eds.), *Romance and sex in adolescence and emerging adulthood: Risks and opportunities*. Mahwah, NJ: Erlbaum.

Sroufe, L. A., Egeland, B., & Carlson, E. (1999). One social world: The integrated development of parent–child and peer relationships. In W. A. Collins & B. Laursen (Eds.), *Relationships as developmental context: The 30th Minnesota Symposium on Child Psychology* (pp. 241–262). Hillsdale, NJ: Erlbaum.

Sroufe, L. A., & Fleeson, J. (1988). The coherence of family relationships. In R. A. H. J. Stevenson-Hinde (Ed.), *Relationships within families: Mutual influences* (pp. 27–47). Oxford: Oxford University Press.

Sroufe, L. A., & Pierce, S. (1999). Men in the family: Associations with juvenile conduct. In G. Cunningham (Ed.), *Just in time research: Children, youth, and families* (pp. 19–26). Minneapolis: University of Minnesota Extension Services.

Representation

Carlson, E. A., Sroufe, L. A., & Egeland, B. (2004). The construction of experience: A longitudinal study of representation and behavior. *Child Development, 75*(1), 66–83.

Fury, G., Carlson, E. A., & Sroufe, L. A. (1997). Children's representations of attachment relationships in family drawings. *Child Development, 68*, 1154–1164.

McCrone, E. R., Egeland, B., Kalkoske, M., & Carlson, E. A. (1994). Relations between early maltreatment and mental representations of relationships assessed with projective storytelling in middle childhood. *Development and Psychopathology, 6*, 99–120.

Roisman, G. I., Madsen, S. D., Hennighausen, K. H., Sroufe, L. A., & Collins, W. A. (2001). The coherence of dyadic behavior across parent–child and romantic relationships as mediated by the internalized representation of experience. *Attachment and Human Development, 3*(2), 156–172.

Developmental Process

Carlson, E. A., Sroufe, L. A., & Egeland, B. (2004). The construction of experience: A longitudinal study of representation and behavior. *Child Development, 75*(1), 66–83.

Sroufe, L. A. (1979). The coherence of individual development. *American Psychologist, 34*(10), 834–841.

Sroufe, L. A. (1989). Relationships, self, and individual adaptation. In A. J.

Sameroff & R. N. Emde (Eds.), *Relationship disturbances in early childhood: A developmental approach* (pp. 70–94). New York: Basic Books.

Sroufe, L. A., Egeland, B., & Kreutzer, T. (1990). The fate of early experience following developmental change: Longitudinal approaches to individual adaptation in childhood. *Child Development, 61*, 1363–1373.

Waters, E., & Sroufe, L. A. (1983). A developmental perspective on competence. *Developmental Review, 3*, 79–97.

Maltreatment

Duggal, S., & Sroufe, L. A. (1998). Recovered memory of childhood sexual trauma: A documented case from a longitudinal study. *Journal of Traumatic Stress, 11*, 301–321.

Egeland, B. (1997). Mediators of the effects of child maltreatment on developmental adaptation in adolescence. In D. Cicchetti & S. L. Toth (Eds.), *Rochester Symposium on Developmental Psychopathology: The effects of trauma on the development process.* (Vol. 8, pp. 403–434). New York: University of Rochester Press.

Egeland, B., Jacobvitz, D., & Sroufe, L. A. (1988). Breaking the cycle of abuse. *Child Development, 59*(4), 1080–1088.

Egeland, B., & Sroufe, L. A. (1981). Developmental sequelae of maltreatment in infancy. In R. Rizley & D. Cicchetti (Eds.), *Developmental perspectives in child maltreatment* (pp. 77–92). San Francisco: Jossey Bass.

Egeland, B., Sroufe, L. A., & Erickson, M. (1983). The developmental consequences of different patterns of maltreatment. *Child Abuse and Neglect, 7*, 155–157.

Egeland, B., & Susman-Stillman, A. (1996). Dissociation as a mediator of child abuse across generations. *Child Abuse and Neglect, 20*(11), 1123–1132.

Behavior Problems

Appleyard, K., Egeland, B., van Dulmen, M., & Sroufe, L. A. (in press). When more is not better: The role of cumulative risk in child behavior outcomes. *Journal of Child Psychology and Psychiatry.*

Egeland, B., Pianta, R. C., & Ogawa, J. (1996). Early behavior problems: Pathways to mental disorder in adolescence. *Development and Psychopathology, 8*, 735–749.

Erickson, M. F., Sroufe, L. A., & Egeland, B. (1985). The relationship between quality of attachment and behavior problems in preschool in a high risk sample. *Monographs of the Society for Research in Child Development, 50* (1–2, Serial No. 209), 147–166. Chicago: University of Chicago Press.

Renken, B., Egeland, B., Marvinney, D., Sroufe, L. A., & Mangelsdorf, S. (1989). Early childhood antecedents of aggression and passive-withdrawal in early elementary school. *Journal of Personality, 57*(2), 257–281.

Psychopathology

Aguilar, B., Sroufe, L. A., Egeland, B., & Carlson, E. (2000). Distinguishing the early-onset/persistent and adolescent-onset anti-social behavior types: From birth to 16 years. *Development and Psychopathology, 12,* 109–132.

Bosquet, M., & Egeland, B. (in press). The development and maintenance of anxiety symptoms from infancy through adolescence in a longitudinal sample. *Development and Psychopathology.*

Burt, K., Carlivati, J., Sroufe, L. A., Appleyard, K., van Dulmen, M., Egeland, B., et al. (in press). Mediating links between maternal depression and offspring psychopathology: The importance of independent data. *Journal of Child Psychology and Psychiatry.*

Carlson, E. A., Jacobvitz, D., & Sroufe, L. A. (1995). A developmental investigation of inattentiveness and hyperactivity. *Child Development, 66,* 37–54.

Carlson, E. A., Yates, T. M., & Sroufe, L. A. (in press). Development of dissociation and development of the self. In P. F. Dell, J. O'Neil & E. Somer (Eds.), *Sourcebook for the dissociative disorders section of DSM-V.* Washington, DC: American Psychological Association.

Duggal, S., Carlson, E. A., Sroufe, L. A., & Egeland, B. (2001). Depressive symptomatology in childhood and adolescence. *Development and Psychopathology, 13,* 143–164.

Jacobvitz, D., & Sroufe, L. A. (1987). The early caregiver—child relationship and attention deficit disorder with hyperactivity in kindergarten: A prospective study. *Child Development, 58,* 1496–1504.

Ogawa, J. R., Sroufe, L. A., Weinfield, N. S., Carlson, E. A., & Egeland, B. (1997). Development and the fragmented self: Longitudinal study of dissociative symptomatology in a nonclinical sample. *Development and Psychopathology, 9,* 855–879.

Roisman, G. I., Aguilar, B., & Egeland, B. (2004). Antisocial behavior in the transition to adulthood: The independent and interactive roles of developmental history and emerging developmental tasks. *Development and Psychopathology, 16,* 857–872.

Sroufe, L. A., Duggal, S., Weinfield, N. S., & Carlson, E. (2000). Relationships, development, and psychopathology. In M. L. A. Sameroff (Ed.), *Handbook of developmental psychopathology* (2nd ed., pp. 75–92). New York: Kluwer Academic/Plenum Press.

Sroufe, L. A., & Rutter, M. (1984). The domain of developmental psychopathology. *Child Development, 55,* 17–29.

Warren, S., Huston, L., Egeland, B., & Sroufe, L. A. (1997). Child and adolescent anxiety disorders and early attachment. *Journal of the American Academy of Child and Adolescent Psychiatry, 36,* 637–644.

Education

Englund, M., Luckner, A., Whaley, G., & Egeland, B. (in press). Children's achievement in early elementary school: Longitudinal effects of parental involvement, expectations, and quality of assistance. *Journal of Educational Psychology.*

Jimerson, S., Egeland, B., Sroufe, L. A., & Carlson, E. A. (2000). A prospective, longitudinal study of high-school dropouts: Examining multiple predictors across development. *Journal of School Psychology, 38*(6), 525–549.

Jimerson, S., Egeland, B., & Teo, A. (1999). A longitudinal study of achievement trajectories: Factors associated with change. *Journal of Educational Psychology, 91*(1), 116–126.

Pianta, R. C., Egeland, B., & Sroufe, L. A. (1990). Maternal stress and children's development: Prediction of school outcomes and identification of protective factors. In J. Rolf, A. S. Masten, D. Cicchetti, K. H. Neuchterlein, & S. Weintraub (Eds.), *Risk and protective factors in the development of psychopathology* (pp. 215–235). New York: Cambridge University Press.

Pianta, R. C., Erickson, M. F., Wagner, N., Kreutzer, T., & Egeland, B. (1990). Early predictors of referral for special services: Child-based measures versus mother–child interaction. *School Psychological Review, 19*(2), 240–250.

Teo, A., Carlson, C., Mathieu, P., Egeland, B., & Sroufe, L. A. (1996). A prospective longitudinal study of psychosocial predictors of achievement. *Journal of School Psychology, 34*, 285–306.

References

Achenbach, T. M., & Edelbrock, C. (1986). *Manual for the Teacher's Report Form and Teacher Version of the Child Behavior Profile.* Burlington: University of Vermont, Department of Psychiatry.

Aguilar, B., Sroufe, L. A., Egeland, B., & Carlson, E. (2000). Distinguishing the early-onset/persistent and adolescent-onset antisocial behavior types: From birth to 16 years. *Development and Psychopathology, 12,* 109–132.

Ainsworth, M. D. S. (1970). *Manual for scoring maternal sensitivity.* Unpublished manuscript, Johns Hopkins University, Baltimore.

Ainsworth, M. D. S., & Bell, S. (1974). Mother–infant interaction and the development of competence. In K. Connolly & J. Bruner (Eds.), *The growth of competence* (pp. 97–118). New York: Academic Press.

Ainsworth, M. D. S., Bell, S., & Stayton, D. (1974). Infant–mother attachment and social development: Socialization as a product of reciprocal responsiveness to signals. In M. Richards (Ed.), *The integration of the child into the social world* (pp. 99–135). Cambridge, UK: Cambridge University Press.

Ainsworth, M. D. S., Blehar, M., Waters, E., & Wall, S. (1978). *Patterns of attachment.* Hillsdale, NJ: Erlbaum.

Ainsworth, M. D. S., & Wittig, B. A. (1969). Attachment and exploratory behavior of one-year-olds in a Strange Situation. In B. M. Foss (Ed.), *Determinants of infant behavior* (Vol. 4, pp. 111–136). London: Methuen.

Anderson, F. S. (1999). *The predictors and correlates of adolescent relationship identity.* Unpublished doctoral dissertation, University of Minnesota, Minneapolis.

Appleyard, K., Egeland, B., van Dulmen, M., & Sroufe, L. A. (2005). When more is not better: The role of cumulative risk in child behavior outcomes. *Journal of Child Psychology and Psychiatry.*

Appleyard, K. E. (2004). *The role of social support relationships in the lives of young high risk children.* Unpublished doctoral dissertation, University of Minnesota, Minneapolis.

Arend, R. (1984). *Preschoolers' competence in a barrier situation: Patterns of adaptation and their precursors in infancy.* Unpublished doctoral dissertation, University of Minnesota, Minneapolis.

Arend, R., Gove, F. L., & Sroufe, L. A. (1979). Continuity of individual adaptation from infancy to kindergarten: A predictive study of ego-resiliency and curiosity in preschoolers. *Child Development, 50,* 950–959.

Ashley, P. (1987). *The continuity of social adaptation from infancy through kindergarten.* Unpublished doctoral dissertation, University of Minnesota, Minneapolis.

American Psychiatric Association. (1994). *Diagnostic and statistical manual of mental disorders* (4th ed., rev.). Washington, DC: Author.

Bandura, A. (1997). *Self-efficacy: The exercise of control.* New York: Freeman.

Banta, T. (1970). Tests of the evaluation of early childhood education: The Cincinatti Autonomy Test Battery (CATB). In J. Hellmuth (Ed.), *Cognitive studies* (Vol. 1, pp. 424–490). New York: Brunner/Mazel.

Barnett, D., Hunt, K. H., Butler, C. M., McCaskill, J. W., Kaplan-Estrin, M., & Pipp-Siegel, S. (1999). Indices of attachment disorganization among toddlers with neurological and non-neurological problems. In J. Solomon & C. C. George (Eds.), *Attachment disorganization* (pp. 189–212). New York: Guilford Press.

Bates, J. (1989). Concepts and measures of temperament. In G. Kohnstamm, J. Bates, & M. Rothbart (Eds.), *Temperament in childhood* (pp. 3–26). New York: Wiley.

Bayley, N. (1969). *The Bayley Scales of Infant Development.* New York: Psychological Corporation.

Becker, W., & Krug, R. (1965). The Parent Attitude Research Instrument—a research review. *Child Development, 36,* 329–365.

Becker-Stoll, F., & Fremmer-Bombik, E. (1997, April). *Adolescent–mother interaction and attachment.* Paper presented at the meeting of the Society for Research in Child Development, Washington, DC.

Behar, L., & Stringfield, S. (1974). Behavior rating scales for the preschool child. *Developmental Psychology, 10,* 601–610.

Bell, R. (1968). A reinterpretation of the direction of effects in studies of socialization. *Psychological Review, 75,* 81–95.

Belsky, J. (1980). Child maltreatment: An ecological integration. *American Psychologist, 35,* 320–335.

Belsky, J., & Fearon, R. M. (2002). Infant–mother attachment security, contextual risk, and early development: A moderational analysis. *Development and Psychopathology, 14*(2), 293–310.

Belsky, J., Spritz, B., & Crnic, K. (1996). Infant attachment security and affective–cognitive information processing at age 3. *Psychological Science, 7,* 111–114.

Bergmann, S. (1986). *Hysteria and anorexia nervosa.* Unpublished manuscript, University of Minnesota, Minneapolis.

Bifulco, A., Moran, P. M., Ball, C., Jacobs, C., Baines, R., Bunn, A., et al. (2002).

Childhood adversity, parental vulnerability and disorder: Examining inter-generational transmission of risk. *Journal of Child Psychology and Psychiatry, 43*, 1075–1086.

Block, J. (2002). *Personality as an affect-processing system.* Mahwah, NJ: Erlbaum.

Block, J., & Block, J. H. (1973). *Ego development and the provenance of thought: A longitudinal study of ego and cognitive development in young children.* Berkeley: University of California Press.

Block, J., & Block, J. H. (1980). The role of ego-control and ego-resiliency in the organization of behavior. In W. A. Collins (Ed.), *Minnesota Symposia on Child Psychology: Vol. 13. Development of cognition, affect, and social relations* (pp. 39–101). Hillsdale, NJ: Erlbaum.

Block, J. H. (1979, August). *Personality development in males and females: The influence of different socialization.* Paper presented at the Master Lecture Series of the American Psychological Association, New York.

Blum, R. W., Resnick, M. D., & Bergeisen, L. G. (1989). *The state of adolescent health in Minnesota.* Minneapolis: University of Minnesota, Adolescent Health Program.

Borke, H. (1971). Interpersonal perception of young children: Egocentrism or empathy? *Developmental Psychology, 5*, 263–269.

Bornstein, M. H. (2002). Parenting infants. In M. H. Bornstein (Ed.), *Handbook of parenting: Vol. 1. Children and parenting* (2nd ed., pp. 3–43). Mahwah, NJ: Erlbaum.

Bosquet, M., & Egeland, B. (in press). The development and maintenance of anxiety symptoms from infancy through adolescence in a longitudinal sample. *Development and Psychopathology.*

Bowlby, J. (1982). *Attachment and loss: Vol. 1. Attachment.* New York: Basic Books. (Original work published 1969)

Bowlby, J. (1973). *Attachment and loss: Vol. 2. Separation.* New York: Basic Books.

Bowlby, J. (1988). *A secure base.* New York: Basic Books.

Brazelton, T. B. (1973). *Neonatal Behavioral Assessment Scale.* Philadelphia: Lippincott.

Brazelton, T. B., Kowslowski, B., & Main, M. (1974). The origins of reciprocity: The early mother–input interaction. In M. Lewis & L. Rosenblum (Eds.), *The effect of the infant on its caregiver* (pp. 49–76). New York: Wiley.

Breger, L. (1974). *From instinct to identity.* Englewood Cliffs, NJ: Prentice-Hall.

Bretherton, I., & Munholland, K. A. (1999). Internal working models in attachment relationships: A construct revisited. In J. Cassidy & P. R. Shaver (Eds.), *Handbook of attachment: Theory, research, and clinical applications* (pp. 89–111). New York: Guilford Press.

Bronfenbrenner, U. (1979). *The ecology of human development.* Cambridge, MA: Harvard University Press.

Broussard, E. (1976). Neonatal prediction and outcome at 10/11 years. *Child Psychiatry and Human Development, 7*(2), 85–93.

Broussard, E., & Hartner, M. S. S. (1971). Further consideration regarding maternal perception of the first born. In J. Hellmuth (Ed.), *Exceptional infant: Studies in Abnormalities* (Vol. 2, pp. 432–449). New York: Brunner/Mazel.

Brunnquell, D., Crichton, L., & Egeland, B. (1981). Maternal personality and attitude in disturbances of child-rearing. *Journal of Orthopsychiatry, 51,* 680–691.

Burt, K., Carlivati, J., Sroufe, L. A., Appleyard, K., van Dulmen, M., Egeland, B., et al. (2005). Mediating links between maternal depression and offspring psychopathology: The importance of independent data. *Journal of Child Psychology and Psychiatry.*

Buss, A. H., & Plomin, R. (1975). *Temperament theory of personal development.* New York: Wiley.

Butler, R. (1953). Discrimination learning by rhesus monkeys to visual exploration motivation. *Journal of Comparative and Physiological Psychology, 46,* 95–98.

Cadoret, R., Troughton, E., Merchant, L., & Whitters, A. (1990). Early life psychosocial events and adult psychosocial symptoms. In L. Robbins & M. Rutter (Eds.), *Straight and devious pathways from childhood to adulthood* (pp. 300–313). Cambridge, UK: Cambridge University Press.

Caldwell, B. M. (1979). *Home observation for measurement of the environment.* Little Rock: University of Arkansas, Center for Early Development and Education.

Campbell, S. (2000). Attention deficit/hyperactivity disorder. In A. Sameroff, M. Lewis, & S. Miller (Eds.), *Handbook of developmental psychology* (2nd ed., pp. 383–401). New York: Kluwer Academic/Plenum Press.

Cantwell, D. (1996). Classification of child and adolescent psychopathology. *Journal of Child Psychology and Psychiatry, 37,* 3–12.

Carey, W. B. (1970). A simplified method for measuring infant temperament. *Journal of Pediatrics, 70,* 188–194.

Carlson, E. A. (1998). A prospective longitudinal study of attachment disorganization/disorientation. *Child Development, 69*(4), 1107–1128.

Carlson, E. A., Jacobvitz, D., & Sroufe, L. A. (1995). A developmental investigation of inattentiveness and hyperactivity. *Child Development, 66,* 37–54.

Carlson, E. A., & Levy, A. K. (1999, April). *A longitudinal study of representational organization and psychopathology.* Paper presented at the meeting of the Society for Research in Child Development, Albuquerque, NM.

Carlson, E. A., Sampson, M., & Sroufe, L. A. (2003). Attachment theory and pediatric practice. *Journal of Development and Behavior Pediatrics, 24*(5), 364–379.

Carlson, E. A., & Sroufe, L. A. (1995). The contribution of attachment theory to developmental psychopathology. In D. Cicchetti & D. Cohen (Eds.), *Developmental Psychopathology: Vol. 1. Theory and methods* (pp. 581–617). New York: Wiley.

Carlson, E. A., Sroufe, L. A., Collins, W. A., Jimerson, S., Weinfield, N., Hennighausen, K., et al. (1999). Early environmental support and elementary school adjustment as predictors of school adjustment in middle adolescence. *Journal of Adolescent Research, 14,* 72–94.

Carlson, E. A., Sroufe, L. A., & Egeland, B. (2004). The construction of experience: A longitudinal study of representation and behavior. *Child Development, 75*(1), 66–83.

Carlson, E. A., Yates, T. M., & Sroufe, L. A. (in press). Development of dissociation and development of the self. In P. F. Dell, J. O'Neil, & E. Somer (Eds.), *Sourcebook for the dissociative disorders section of DSM-V*. Washington, DC: American Psychological Association.

Carlson, E. B., & Putnam, F. W. (1993). An update on the Dissociative Experiences Scale. *Dissociation, 6*(1), 16–27.

Carlson, V., Cicchetti, D., Barnett, D., & Braunwald, K. G. (1989). Disorganized/disorented attachment relationships in maltreated infants. *Developmental Psychology, 25*, 525–531.

Caron, C., & Rutter, M. (1991). Comorbidity in child psychopathology: Concepts, issues, and research strategies. *Journal of Child Psychology and Psychiatry, 32*, 1063–1079.

Caspi, A., McClay, J., Moffitt, T. E., Mill, J., Martin, J., & Craig, I. W. (2002). Role of genotype in the cycle of violence in maltreated children. *Science, 297*, 851–854.

Cattell, R. B., & Scheier, I. H. (1963). *Handbook for the IPAT Anxiety Scale Questionnaire* (2nd ed.). Champaign, IL: Institute for Personality and Ability Testing.

Charlesworth, W. (1979). An ethological approach to studying intelligence. *Human Development, 22*, 212–216.

Chi, T. C., & Hinshaw, S. P. (2002). Mother–child relationships of children with ADHD: The role of maternal depressive symptoms and depression-related distortions. *Journal of Abnormal Child Psychology, 30*, 387–400.

Cicchetti, D. (2002). How a child builds a brain: Insights from normality and psychopathology. In W. W. Hartup & R. A. Weinberg (Eds.), *Minnesota Symposia in Child Psychology: Vol. 32. Child psychology in retrospect and prospect* (pp. 23–71). Mahwah, NJ: Erlbaum.

Cicchetti, D., & Cannon, T. D. (1999). Neurodevelopmental processes in the ontogenesis and epigenesis of psychopathology. *Development and Psychopathology, 11*, 375–393.

Cicchetti, D., & Cohen, D. (1995). Perspectives on developmental psychopathology. In D. Cicchetti & D. Cohen (Eds.), *Developmental psychopathology: Vol. 1. Theory and methods* (pp. 3–17). New York: Wiley.

Cicchetti, D., Cummings, E. M., Greenberg, M. T., & Marvin, R. S. (1990). An organizational perspective on attachment beyond infancy: Implications for theory, measurement, and research. In M. T. Greenberg, D. Cicchetti, & E. M. Cummings (Eds.), *Attachment in the preschool years: Theory, research, and intervention* (pp. 3–49). Chicago: University of Chicago Press.

Cicchetti, D., & Dawson, G. (2002). Editorial: Multiple levels of analysis. *Development and Psychopathology, 14*, 417–420.

Cicchetti, D., & Rogosch, F. (1996). Equifinality and multifinality in developmental psychopathology. *Development and Psychopathology, 8*(4), 597–600.

Cicchetti, D., & Toth, S. (2000). Developmental processes in maltreated children. In D. Hansen (Ed.), *Nebraska Symposium on Motivation: Vol. 46. Child maltreatment* (pp. 85–165). Lincoln: University of Nebraska Press.

Cochrane, R., & Robertson, A. (1973). The Life Events Inventory: A measure of relative severity of psychosocial stresses. *Journal of Psychosomatic Research, 17*, 135–139.

Cohen, H., & Weil, G. R. (1971). *Tasks of Emotional Development: A projective test for children and adolescents.* Lexington, MA: Heath.

Cohler, B., Weiss, J., & Grunebaum, H. (1970). Child-care attitudes and emotional disturbance among mothers of young children. *Genetic Psychological Monograph, 82,* 3–47.

Cole, P. M., Michel, M. K., & O'Connell-Teti, L. (1994). The development of emotion regulation and dysregulation: A clinical perspective. *Monographs of the Society for Research in Child Development, 59*(2–3, Serial No. 240).

Collins, W. A. (1995). Relationships and development: Family adaptation to individual change. In S. Shulman (Ed.), *Close relationships and socioemotional development* (pp. 128–154). New York: Ablex.

Collins, W. A., Hayden, K. C., & van Dulmen, M. (2005, April). Peer competence and friendship quality: Distinct or overlapping precursors of adult romantic relationships? In C. Booth-LaForce & W. Hartup (Eds.), *New approaches to the longitudinal study of friendship.* Symposium presented at the meeting of the Society for Research in Child Development, Atlanta, GA.

Collins, W. A., Hennighausen, K. H., Schmit, D. T., & Sroufe, L. A. (1997). Developmental precursors of romantic relationships: A longitudinal analysis. In S. Shulman & W. A. Collins (Eds.), *Romantic relationships in adolescence: Developmental perspectives* (pp. 69–84). San Francisco: Jossey-Bass.

Collins, W. A., & Laursen, B. (2004). Family relationships and parenting influences. In R. Lerner & L. Steinberg (Eds.), *Handbook of adolescent psychology* (pp. 331–362). New York: Wiley.

Collins, W. A., & Madsen, S. D. (in press). Close relationships in adolescence and early adulthood. In D. Perlman & A. Vangelisti (Eds.), *Handbook of personal relationships.* New York: Cambridge University Press.

Collins, W. A., & Sroufe, L. A. (1999). Capacity for intimate relationships: A developmental construction. In W. Furman, C. Feiring, & B. Brown (Eds.), *Contemporary perspectives on adolescent romantic relationships* (pp. 125–147). New York: Cambridge University Press.

Collins, W. A., & Steinberg, L. (in press). Adolescent development in interpersonal context. In W. Damon & N. Eisenberg (Eds.), *Handbook of child psychology: Vol. 4. Socioemotional processes.* New York: Wiley.

Collins, W. A., & van Dulmen, M. (in press-a). The course of true love(s): Origins and pathways in the development of romantic relationships. In A. Booth & A. Crouter (Eds.), *Romance and sex in adolescence and emerging adulthood: Risks and opportunities.* Mahwah, NJ: Erlbaum.

Collins, W. A., & van Dulmen, M. (in press-b). The significance of middle childhood peer competence for work and relationships in early adulthood. In A. Huston (Ed.), *Successful pathways from middle childhood to adulthood.* New York: Cambridge University Press.

Compas, B. E., Davis, G. E., Forsythe, C. J., & Wagner, B. M. (1987). Assessment of major and daily stressful events during adolescence: The Adolescent Perceived Events Scale. *Journal of Clinical and Consulting Psychology, 55,* 534–541.

Cortina, M., & Marrone, M. (2003). *Attachment theory and psychoanalytic process.* London: Whurr Press.

Crockenberg, S. (1981). Infant irritability, mother responsiveness, and social support influences on the security of infant–mother attachment. *Child Development, 52,* 857–865.

Crockenberg, S., & Covey, S. L. (1991). Marital conflict and externalizing behavior in children. In D. Cicchetti & S. L. Toth (Eds.), *Rochester Symposium on Developmental Psychopathology: Vol. 3. Models and integrations* (pp. 235–260). Rochester, NY: University of Rochester Press.

Crowell, J., & Owens, G. (1996). *Current Relationships Interview.* Unpublished manuscript, State University of New York at Stony Brook.

de Wolff, M. S., & van IJzendoorn, M. H. (1997). Sensitivity and attachment: A meta-analysis on parental antecedents of infant attachment. *Child Development, 68,* 571–591.

DeHart, G. B. (1999). Conflict and averted conflict in preschoolers' interactions with siblings and friends. In W. A. Collins & B. Laursen (Eds.), *Minnesota Symposia on Child Psychology: Vol. 30. Relationships as developmental contexts: Festschrift in honor of Willard W. Hartup* (pp. 281–303). Mahwah, NJ: Erlbaum.

Dishion, T. J., & Bullock, B. M. (2002). Parenting and adolescent problem behavior: An ecological analysis of the nurturance hypothesis. In J. G. Borkowski, S. L. Ramey, & M. Bristol-Power (Eds.), *Parenting and the child's world: Influences on academic, intellectual, and social-emotional development* (pp. 215–230). Mahwah, NJ: Erlbaum.

Dodge, K. (2000). Conduct disorder. In A. J. Sameroff, M. Lewis, & S. M. Miller (Eds.), *Handbook of developmental psychopathology* (2nd ed., pp. 447–463). New York: Kluwer Academic/Plenum Press.

Dodge, K., & Frame, C. (1982). Social cognitive biases and deficits in aggressive boys. *Child Development, 53,* 620–635.

Dodge, K., Pettit, G., McClaskey, C., & Brown, M. (1986). Social competence in children. *Monographs of the Society for Research in Child Development, 51*(2, Serial No. 213).

Downey, G., & Coyne, J. (1990). Children of depressed parents: An integrative review. *Psychological Bulletin, 108,* 56–76.

Dozier, M. (1990). Attachment organization and treatment use for adults with serious psychopathological disorders. *Development and Psychopathology, 2,* 47–60.

Dozier, M., Cue, K., & Barnett, L. (1994). Clinicians as caregivers: Role of attachment organization in treatment. *Journal of Consulting and Clinical Psychology, 62,* 793–800.

Duggal, S., Carlson, E. A., Sroufe, L. A., & Egeland, B. (2001). Depressive symptomatology in childhood and adolescence. *Development and Psychopathology, 13,* 143–164.

Duggal, S., & Sroufe, L. A. (1998). Recovered memory of childhood sexual trauma: A documented case from a longitudinal study. *Journal of Traumatic Stress, 11,* 301–321.

Dunn, J., & Kendrick, C. (1982). *Siblings.* Cambridge, MA: Harvard University Press.

Dunn, L. M., & Markwardt, F. C. J. (1970). *The Peabody Individual Achievement Test (PIAT).* Circle Pines, MN: American Guidance Service..

Dunphy, D. (1963). The social structure of urban adolescent peer groups. *Sociometry, 26*, 230–246.

Eagle, M. (1995). The developmental perspectives of attachment and psychoanalytic theory. In S. Goldberg, R. Muir, & J. Kerr (Eds.), *Attachment theory: Social, developmental, and clinical perspectives* (pp. 123–153). Hillsdale, NJ: Analytic Press.

Edelman, G. (1992). *Bright air, brilliant fire.* New York: Basic Books.

Egeland, B. (1988). The consequences of physical and emotional neglect on the development of young children. In A. Cowan (Ed.), *Child neglect* (pp. D10–D22). Washington, DC: National Center on Child Abuse and Neglect.

Egeland, B. (1997). Mediators of the effects of child maltreatment on developmental adaptation in adolescence. In D. Cicchetti & S. L. Toth (Eds.), *Rochester Symposium on Developmental Psychopathology: Vol. 8. The effects of trauma on the development process* (pp. 403–434). New York: University of Rochester Press.

Egeland, B., & Abery, B. (1991). A longitudinal study of high risk children: Educational outcomes. *International Journal of Disability, Development, and Education, 38*(3), 271–287.

Egeland, B., Bosquet, M., & Levy-Chung, A. (2002). Continuities and discontinuities in the intergenerational transmission of child maltreatment: Implications for breaking the cycle of abuse. In K. D. Browne, H. Hanks, P. Stratton, & C. Hamilton (Eds.), *Early prediction and prevention of child abuse: A handbook* (pp. 217–232). Sussex, UK: Wiley.

Egeland, B., Breitenbucher, M., & Rosenberg, D. (1980). Prospective study of the significance of life stress in the etiology of child abuse. *Journal of Consulting and Clinical Psychology, 48*(2), 195–205.

Egeland, B., & Brunnquell, D. (1979). An at-risk approach to the study of child abuse: Some preliminary findings. *Journal of the American Academy of Child Psychiatry, 18*, 219–235.

Egeland, B., & Carlson, E. A. (2004). Attachment and psychopathology. In L. Atkinson & S. Goldberg (Eds.), *Clinical implications of attachment* (pp. 27–48). Mahwah, NJ: Erlbaum.

Egeland, B., Carlson, E. A., & Sroufe, L. A. (1993). Resilience as process. *Development and Psychopathology, 5*, 517–528.

Egeland, B., Deinard, A., & Brunnquell, D. (1975). *Life Stress Scale and manual.* Unpublished manuscript, University of Minnesota, Minneapolis.

Egeland, B., & Erickson, M. F. (1987). Psychologically unavailable caregiving: The effects of development of young children and the implications for intervention. In M. R. Brassard, B. R. Germain, & S. N. Hart (Eds.), *Psychological maltreatment of children and youth* (pp. 110–120). New York: Pergamon Press.

Egeland, B., & Erickson, M. F. (2004). Lessons from STEEP: Linking theory, research, and practice for the well-being of infants and parents. In A. J. Sameroff, S. C. McDonough, & K. L. Rosenblum (Eds.), *Treating parent–infant relationship problems* (pp. 213–242). New York: Guilford Press.

Egeland, B., & Farber, E. (1984). Infant–mother attachment: Factors related to its development and changes over time. *Child Development, 55*(3), 753–771.

Egeland, B., Hunt, D., & Hardt, D. (1970). College enrollment of upward bound students as a function of attitudes and motivation. *Journal of Educational Psychology, 61,* 375–379.

Egeland, B., Jacobvitz, D., & Papatola, K. (1987). Intergenerational continuity of abuse. In R. J. Gelles & J. B. Lancaster (Eds.), *Child abuse and neglect: Biosocial dimensions* (pp. 255–276). New York: Aldine de Gruyter.

Egeland, B., Jacobvitz, D., & Sroufe, L. A. (1988). Breaking the cycle of abuse. *Child Development, 59*(4), 1080–1088.

Egeland, B., Kalkoske, M., Gottesman, N., & Erickson, M. F. (1990). Preschool behavior problems: Stability and factors accounting for change. *Journal of Child Psychology and Psychiatry, 31*(6), 891–909.

Egeland, B., & Kreutzer, T. (1991). A longitudinal study of the effects of maternal stress and protective factors on the development of high risk children. In E. M. Cummings, A. L. Greene, & K. H. Karraker (Eds.), *Life-span developmental psychology: Perspectives on stress and coping* (pp. 61–85). Hillsdale, NJ: Erlbaum.

Egeland, B., Pianta, R. C., & O'Brien, M. A. (1993). Maternal intrusiveness in infancy and child maladaptation in early school years. *Development and Psychopathology, 5*(3), 359–370.

Egeland, B., Pianta, R. C., & Ogawa, J. (1996). Early behavior problems: Pathways to mental disorder in adolescence. *Development and Psychopathology, 8,* 735–749.

Egeland, B., & Sroufe, L. A. (1981). Developmental sequelae of maltreatment in infancy. In R. Rizley & D. Cicchetti (Eds.), *Developmental perspectives in child maltreatment* (pp. 77–92). San Francisco: Jossey Bass.

Egeland, B., & Sroufe, L. A. (1986, August). *Stressful life events and school outcomes: A study of protective factors.* Paper presented at the meeting of the American Psychological Association, Washington, DC.

Egeland, B., Sroufe, L. A., & Erickson, M. (1983). The developmental consequences of different patterns of maltreatment. *Child Abuse and Neglect, 7,* 155–157.

Egeland, B., & Susman-Stillman, A. (1996). Dissociation as a mediator of child abuse across generations. *Child Abuse and Neglect, 20*(11), 1123–1132.

Egeland, B., & Vaughn, B. 91981). Failure of bond formation as a cause of abuse, neglect, and maltreatment. *American Journal of Orthopsychiatry, 51,* 78–84.

Egeland, B., Weinfield, N., Bosquet, M., & Cheng, V. (2000). Remembering, repeating, and working through: Lessons from attachment-based interventions. In J. Osofsky (Ed.), *WAIMH handbook of infant mental health* (Vol. 4, pp. 35–89). New York: Wiley.

Egeland, B., Yates, T., Appleyard, K., & van Dulmen, M. (2001, August). *The long-term consequences of maltreatment in the early years: A developmental pathway model to antisocial behavior.* Paper presented at the American Psychological Association, San Francisco.

Elder, G. H., Nguyen, T. V., & Caspi, A. (1985). Linking family hardship to children's lives. *Child Development, 56,* 361–375.

Elicker, J., Englund, M., & Sroufe, L. A. (1992). Predicting peer competence and peer relationships in childhood from early parent–child relationships. In R.

Parke & G. Ladd (Eds.), *Family–peer relationships: Modes of linkage* (pp. 77–106). Hillsdale, NJ: Erlbaum.

Elmer, E. (1997). *Fragile families, troubled children*. Pittsburgh, PA: University of Pittsburgh Press.

Embry, L., & Dawson, G. (2002). Disruptions in parenting behavior related to maternal depression: Influences on children's behavioral and psychobiological development. In J. Borkowski, S. Ramey, & M. Bristol-Power (Eds.), *Parenting and your child's world* (pp. 203–214). Hillsdale, NJ: Erlbaum.

Englund, M., Forman, D., Quevedo, K., Morales, J., Johnson, L., & Sroufe, L. A. (2003, April). *Early adolescents' interactions with parents and educational outcomes in a poverty sample*. Paper presented at the meeting of the Society for Research on Adolescence, Baltimore.

Englund, M., Hudson, K., & Egeland, B. (2003, April). *Common pathways to heavy alcohol use and abstinence in adolescence*. Paper presented at the meeting of the Society for Research in Child Development, Tampa, FL.

Englund, M., Levy, A., Hyson, D., & Sroufe, L. A. (2000). Adolescent social competence: Effectiveness in a group setting. *Child Development, 71*, 1049–1060.

Englund, M., Luckner, A., Whaley, G., & Egeland, B. (2005). Children's achievement in early elementary school: Longitudinal effects of parental involvement, expectations, and quality of assistance. *Journal of Educational Psychology.*

Epstein, S. (1979). The stability of behavior: On predicting most of the people much of the time. *Journal of Personality and Social Psychology, 37*, 1097–1126.

Erez, T. (1987). *Individual patterns of coping*. Unpublished doctoral dissertation, University of Minnesota, Minneapolis.

Erickson, M. F., & Egeland, B. (1987). A developmental view of the psychological consequences of maltreatment. *School Psychological Review, 16*(2), 156–168.

Erickson, M. F., & Egeland, B. (1999). The STEEP program: Linking theory and research to practice. *Zero to Three, 20*(2), 11–16.

Erickson, M. F., Egeland, B., & Pianta, R. (1989). The effects of maltreatment on the development of young children. In D. Cicchetti & V. Carlson (Eds.), *Child maltreatment: Theory and research on the causes and consequences of child abuse and neglect* (pp. 647–684). Cambridge, MA: Harvard University Press.

Erickson, M. F., Sroufe, L. A., & Egeland, B. (1985). The relationship between quality of attachment and behavior problems in preschool in a high risk sample. *Monographs of the Society for Research in Child Development, 50*(1–2, Serial No. 209), 147–166.

Erikson, E. (1963). *Childhood and society*. New York: Norton. (Original work published 1950)

Eron, L., & Huesman, L. (1990). The stability of aggressive behavior—even into the third generation. In M. Lewis & S. Miller (Eds.), *Handbook of developmental psychopathology* (pp. 147–156). New York: Plenum Press.

Faraone, S., & Tsuang, M. (1988). Family links between schizophrenia and other disorders: Psychopathology in offspring. *Psychiatry, 51*, 37–47.

Farrington, D. (1995). The twelfth Jack Tizard Memorial Lecture: The development of offending and antisocial behavior in childhood: Key findings from the Cambridge Study of Delinquent Development. *Journal of Child Psychology and Psychiatry, 36,* 929–964.

Farrington, D., Ohlin, L., & Wilson, J. (1986). *Understanding and controlling crime.* New York: Springer-Verlag.

Fergusson, D., Swain-Campbell, N., & Horwood, J. (2004). How does childhood economic disadvantage lead to crime? *Journal of Child Psychology and Psychiatry, 45,* 956–966.

Flavell, J. (1963). *The developmental psychology of Jean Piaget.* New York: Van Nostrand.

Fleeson, W. (2001). Toward a structure-and-process-integrated view of personality: Traits as density distributions of states. *Journal of Personality and Social Psychology, 80*(6), 1011–1027.

Fogel, A. (1993). *Developing through relationships: Origins of communication, self, and culture.* Chicago: University of Chicago Press.

Fonagy, P. (1999). Psychoanalytic theory from the viewpoint of attachment theory and research. In J. Cassidy & P. R. Shaver (Eds.), *Handbook of attachment* (pp. 595–624). New York: Guilford Press.

Fonagy, P., Steele, M., Steele, H., Leigh, T., Kennedy, R., Mattoon, G., et al. (1995). Attachment, the reflective self, and borderline states: The predictive specificity of the Adult Attachment Interview and pathological emotional development. In S. Goldberg, R. Muir, & J. Kerr (Eds.), *Attachment theory: Social, developmental, and clinical perspective* (pp. 233–279). Hillsdale, NJ: Analytic Press.

Fox, N., Kimmerly, N., & Schafer, W. (1991). Attachment to mother/attachment to father: A meta-analysis. *Developmental Psychology, 62,* 210–225.

Fraiberg, S., Adelson, E., & Shapiro, V. (1975). Ghosts in the nursery: A psychoanalytic approach to the problems of impaired infant–mother relationships. *Journal of the American Academy of Child Psychiatry, 14,* 387–421.

Freud, A., & Dann, S. (1951). An experiment in group upbringing. *Psychoanalytic Study of the Child, 6,* 127–168.

Freud, S. (1926). Inhibitions, symptoms, and anxiety. In J. Strachey (Ed. & Trans.), *Standard edition of the complete psychological works of Sigmund Freud* (pp. 87–174). London: Hogarth Press.

Freud, S. (1964). An outline of psychoanalysis. In J. Strachey (Ed. & Trans.), *Standard edition of the complete psychological works of Sigmund Freud* (Vol. 23, pp. 137–207). London: Hogarth Press. (Original work published 1940)

Frick, P. J., & Lahey, B. B. (1991). The nature and characteristics of attention-deficit hyperactivity disorder. *School Psychological Review, 20,* 163–173.

Fury, G., Carlson, E. A., & Sroufe, L. A. (1997). Children's representations of attachment relationships in family drawings. *Child Development, 68,* 1154–1164.

Garmezy, N. (1971). Vulnerability research and the issue of primary prevention. *American Journal of Orthopsychiatry, 41*(1), 101–116.

Garmezy, N. (1975). The experimental study of children vulnerable to psychopathology. In A. Davids (Ed.), *Child personality and psychopathology: Current trends* (pp. 171–216). New York: Wiley.

Gelles, R. (1973). Child abuse or psychopathology: A sociological critique and reformulation. *American Journal of Orthopsychiatry, 43*, 611–621.

George, C., Kaplan, N., & Main, M. (1985). *Adult Attachment Interview protocol.* Unpublished manuscript, University of California, Berkeley.

Gilliom, M., & Shaw, D. (2004). Codevelopment of externalizing and internalizing problems in early childhood. *Development and Psychopathology, 16*, 313–334.

Goldsmith, H., Buss, A., Plomin, R., Rothbart, M., Thomas, A., Chess, S., et al. (1987). What is temperament? Four approaches. *Child Development, 58*, 505–529.

Goodwin, B. (1994). *How the leopard changed its spots.* New York: Touchstone.

Gottesman, I., & Hanson, D. (in press). Human development: Biological and genetic processes. *Annual Review of Psychology.*

Gottfried, A. W. (1973). Intellectual consequences of perinatal anoxia. *Psychological Bulletin, 80*, 231–242.

Gottlieb, G. (1971). *Development of species identification in birds: An inquiry into the prenatal determinants of perception.* Chicago: University of Chicago Press.

Gottlieb, G., Gilbert, & Halpern, C. T. (2002). A relational view of causality in normal and abnormal development. *Development and Psychopathology, 14*(3), 421–435.

Gove, F. (1983). *Patterns and organizations of behavior and affective expression during the second year of life.* Unpublished doctoral dissertation, University of Minnesota, Minneapolis.

Greenspan, S., & Wieder, S. (1994, June–July). Diagnostic classifications of mental health and developmental disorders of infancy and early childhood. *Zero to Three*, pp. 34–41.

Grossmann, A., Churchill, J., McKinney, B., Kodish, I., Otte, S., & Greenough, W. (2003). Experience effects on brain development: Possible contributions to psychopathology. *Journal of Child Psychology and Psychiatry, 44*, 33–63.

Grossmann, K., Grossmann, K., Spangler, G., Seuss, G., & Unzer, L. (1985). Maternal sensitivity and newborns' orientation responses as related to quality of attachment in northern Germany. *Monographs of the Society for Research in Child Development, 50*(1–2, Serial No. 209), 233–256.

Gunnar, M. (2001). Effects of early deprivation: Findings from orphanage-reared infants and children. In C. Nelson & M. Luciana (Eds.), *Handbook of developmental cognitive neuroscience* (pp. 617–629). Cambridge, MA: MIT Press.

Gunnar, M., Mangelsdorf, S., Larson, M., & Hertsgaard, L. (1989). Attachment, temperament, and adrenocortical activity in infancy: A study of psychoendocrine regulation. *Developmental Psychology, 25*, 355–363.

Hamilton, C. (2000). Continuity and discontinuity of attachment from infancy through adolescence. *Child Development, 71*, 690–694.

Harlow, H. (1966). Learning to love. *American Scientist, 54*, 244–272.

Harrington, R., Rutter, M., & Fombonne, E. (1996). Developmental pathways in depression: Multiple meanings, antecedents, and endpoints. *Development and Psychopathology, 8*, 601–618.

Harris, J. (1998). *The nurture assumption: Why children turn out the way they do.* New York: Free Press.

Harter, S. (1979). *Perceived Competence Scale for Children: Manual Form O.* Denver, CO: University of Denver Press.

Harter, S. (1998). The development of self-representations. In W. Damon & N. Eisenberg (Eds.), *Handbook of child psychology: Vol. 3. Social, emotional, and personality develeopment* (5th ed., pp. 553–617). New York: Wiley.

Hatem, M. (1996). *Quality of attachment and later use of mother as a resource.* Unpublished doctoral dissertation, University of Minnesota, Minneapolis.

Havighurst, R. J. (1972). *Developmental tasks and education.* London: Longman. (Original work published in 1948)

Hendrick, S. (1988). A generic measure of relationship satisfaction. *Journal of Marriage and the Family, 50*, 93–98.

Hennighausen, K. H. (1996). *Connecting preadolescent gender boundary behavior to adolescent dating and sexual activity.* Unpublished manuscript, University of Minnesota, Minneapolis.

Hennighausen, K. H. (1999). *Developmental antecedents of young adult romantic relationships.* Unpublished doctoral dissertation, University of Minnesota, Minneapolis.

Hesse, E. (1999). The Adult Attachment Interview: Historical and current perspectives. In J. Cassidy & P. R. Shaver (Eds.), *Handbook of attachment* (pp. 395–433). New York: Guilford Press.

Hiester, M. (1993). *Generational boundary dissolution between mothers and children in early childhood and early adolescence: A longitudinal study.* Unpublished doctoral dissertation, University of Minnesota, Minneapolis.

Hill, J., & Lynch, M. (1983). The intensification of gender-related role expectations during early adolescence. In J. Brooks-Gunn & A. Peterson (Eds.), *Girls at puberty: Biological and psychosocial perspectives* (pp. 201–228). New York: Plenum Press.

Hinde, R., & Bateson, P. (1984). Discontinuities versus continuities in behavioral development and the neglect of process. *International Journal of Behavioral Development, 7*, 129–143.

Holmes, J. (1998). Defensive and creative uses of narrative psychotherapy: An attachment perspective. In G. Roberts & J. Holmes (Eds.), *Narrative in psychotherapy and psychiatry* (pp. 49–68). Oxford, UK: Oxford University Press.

Homan, K. J. (1990). *A longitudinal analysis of learned helplessness in school children.* Unpublished doctoral dissertation, University of Minnesota, Minneapolis.

Huston, L. (2001). *Consequences of using different child maltreatment sampling methodologies: A comparative study of a prospective sampling approach and a self-report sampling approach.* Unpublished doctoral dissertation, University of Minnesota, Minneapolis.

Hyson, D. (2002). Understanding adaptation to work in adulthood: A contextual developmental approach. *Advances in Life Course Research, 7*, 93–110.

Isabella, R. (1993). Origins of attachment: Maternal interactive behavior across the first year. *Developmental Psychology, 64*, 605–621.

Jackson, D. N. (1974). *Personality Research Form manual.* Goshen, NY: Research Psychological Press.

Jacobvitz, D., Hazen, N., Curran, M., & Hitchens, K. (2004). Observations of early triadic family interactions: Boundary disturbances in the family predict symptoms of depression, anxiety, and attention deficit/hyperactivity disorder in middle childhood. *Development and Psychopathology, 16,* 577–592.

Jacobvitz, D., Hazen, N., & Riggs, S. (1997, April). *Disorganized mental processes in mothers, frightened/frightening caregiving, and disorganized/disoriented behavior in infancy.* Paper presented at the meeting of the Society for Research in Child Development, Washington, DC.

Jacobvitz, D., & Sroufe, L. A. (1987). The early caregiver–child relationship and attention deficit disorder with hyperactivity in kindergarten: A prospective study. *Child Development, 58,* 1496–1504.

Jessor, R. (1984). Adolescent development and behavioral health. In J. Matarazzo, S. Weiss, J. Herd, N. Miller, & S. Weiss (Eds.), *Behavioral health* (pp. 69–90). New York: Wiley.

Jimerson, S., Egeland, B., Sroufe, L. A., & Carlson, E. A. (2000). A prospective, longitudinal study of high-school dropouts: Examining multiple predictors across development. *Journal of School Psychology, 38*(6), 525–549.

Jimerson, S., Egeland, B., & Teo, A. (1999). A longitudinal study of achievement trajectories: Factors associated with change. *Journal of Educational Psychology, 91*(1), 116–126.

Johnson, J. G., Cohen, P., Kasen, S., Smailes, E., & Brook, J. S. (2001). Association of maladaptive parental behavior with psychiatric disorder among parents and their offspring. *Archives of General Psychiatry, 58,* 453–460.

Johnston, D. (1988). Adolescents' solutions to dilemmas in fables: Two moral orientations—two problem-solving strategies. In C. Gilligan, J. Ward, & J. Taylor (Eds.), *Mapping the moral domain: A contribution of women's thinking to psychological theory and education* (pp. 49–71). Cambridge, MA: Harvard University Press.

Kagan, J. (1971). *Change and continuity in infancy.* New York: Wiley.

Kagan, J. (1984). *The nature of the child.* New York: Basic Books.

Kagan, J., & Moss, H. (1962). *Birth to maturity.* New York: Wiley.

Kalsched, D. (1996). *The inner world of trauma: Archetypal defenses of the personal spirit.* London: Routledge.

Kaplan, N., & Main, M. (1986). *Instructions for the classification of children's family drawings in terms of representation and attachment.* Unpublished manuscript, University of California, Berkeley.

Kaufman, J., & Zigler, E. (1987). Do abused children become abusive parents? *American Journal of Orthopsychiatry, 57,* 186–192.

Kestenbaum, R., Farber, E., & Sroufe, L. A. (1989). Individual differences in empathy among preschoolers: Concurrent and predictive validity. In N. Eisenberg (Ed.), *Empathy and related emotional responses* (pp. 51–56). San Francisco: Jossey-Bass.

Kim, J., & Cicchetti, D. (2004). A longitudinal study of maltreatment, mother–child relationship quality and maladjustment: The role of self-esteem and social competence. *Journal of Abnormal Child Psychology, 32*(4), 341–354.

Kirsch, I., Jungeblut, A., Jenkins, L., & Kolstad, A. (1993). *Adult literacy in America: A first look at the results of the National Adult Literacy Survey*. Washington, DC: National Center for Education Statistics.

Klein, G. S. (1976). *Psychoanalytic theory: An exploration of essentials*. New York: International Universities Press.

Kobak, R. (1999). The emotional dynamics of disruptions in attachment relationships: Implications for theory, research, and clinical intervention. In J. Cassidy & P. Shaver (Eds.), *Handbook of attachment: Theory, research, and clinical applications* (pp. 21–43). New York: Guilford Press.

Kobak, R., Ruckdeschel, K., & Hazan, C. (1994). From symptom to signal: An attachment view of emotion in marital therapy. In S. M. Johnson & L. S. Greenberg (Eds.), *The heart of the matter: Perspectives on emotion in marital therapy* (pp. 46–71). Philadelphia: Brunner/Mazel.

Kochanska, G. (1993). Toward a synthesis of parental socialization and child temperament in the early development of conscience. *Child Development, 62*, 325–347.

Kochanska, G. (1997). Multiple pathways to conscience for children with different temperaments: From toddlerhood to age 5. *Developmental Psychology, 33*, 228–240.

Kochanska, G., Aksan, N., Knaack, A., & Rhines, H. (2004). Maternal parenting and children's conscience: Early security as moderator. *Child Development, 75*, 1229–1242.

Korfmacher, J., Adam, E., Ogawa, J., & Egeland, B. (1997). Adult attachment: Implication for the therapeutic process in a home intervention. *Applied Developmental Science, 1*, 43–52.

Kovan, N., Kempner, S., & Carlson, E. A. (2004, August). *Continuity of parenting toddlers across two generations*. Paper presented at the meeting of the American Psychological Association, Honolulu, HI.

Kuo, Z. (1967). *The dynamics of behavior development*. New York: Random House.

Ladd, G. (1983). Social networks of popular, average, and rejected children in school settings. *Merrill–Palmer Quarterly, 29*, 283–307.

LaFreniere, P. J., & Sroufe, L. A. (1985). Profiles of peer competence in the preschool: Interrelations among measures, influence of social ecology, and relation to attachment history. *Developmental Psychology, 21*, 56–66.

Lazare, A. (1973). Hidden conceptual models in clinical psychiatry. *New England Journal of Medicine, 288*, 345–350.

Lenneberg, E. (1967). *Biological foundations of language*. New York: Wiley.

Levy, A. (1998, April). *Longitudinal predictors of adolescent pregnancy and impregnation*. Paper presented at the meeting of the Society for Research on Adolescence, San Diego, CA.

Lewis, M. (1992). The self in self-conscious emotions: Commentary on Stipek et al. *Monographs of the Society for Research in Child Development, 57*, 85–95.

Lewis, M. (1998). *Altering fate: Why the past does not predict the future*. New York: Guilford Press.

Lewis, M., & Brooks, J. (1978). Self-knowledge and emotional development. In

M. Lewis & L. Rosenblum (Eds.), *The development of affect* (pp. 205–226). New York: Plenum Press.

Lewis, M., Feiring, C., & Rosenthal, S. (2000). Attachment over time. *Child Development, 71,* 707–720.

Lieberman, A. (1977). Preschoolers' competence with a peer: Relations with attachment and peer experience. *Child Development, 48,* 1277–1287.

Lieberman, A. (1991). Attachment theory and infant–parent psychotherapy: Some conceptual, clinical, and research considerations. In D. Cicchetti & S. Toth (Eds.), *Rochester Symposium on Developmental Psychopathology: Vol. 3. Models and integrations* (pp. 375–398). Hillsdale, NJ: Erlbaum.

Lieberman, A. (1992). Infant–parent psychotherapy with toddlers. *Development and Psychopathology, 4,* 559–574.

Lieberman, A. (1993). *The emotional life of a toddler.* New York: Free Press.

Lieberman, A. F., & Zeanah, C. H. (1999). Contributions of attachment theory to infant–parent psychotherapy and other interventions with infants and young children. In J. Cassidy & P. R. Shaver (Eds.), *Handbook of attachment: Theory, research, and clinical applications* (pp. 555–574). New York: Guilford Press.

Linder, J. R., & Collins, W. A. (in press). Parent and peer predictors of physical aggression and conflict management in romantic relationships in early adulthood. *Journal of Family Psychology.*

Liotti, G. (1992). Disorganized/disoriented attachment in the etiology of the dissociative disorders. *Dissociation, 4,* 196–204.

Loeber, R., Wang, P., Keenan, K., Giroux, B., Stouthamer-Loeber, M., van Kammen, W., et al. (1993). Developmental pathways in disruptive child behaviors. *Development and Psychopathology, 5,* 103–134.

Loevinger, J. (1976). *Ego development.* San Francisco: Jossey-Bass.

Loewen, G. (2004). [Attachment predictors of teacher social competence judgments]. Unpublished data, University of Minnesota, Minneapolis.

Lojkasek, M., Cohen, N., & Muir, E. (1994). Where is the infant in infant intervention?: A review of the literature on changing troubled mother–infant relationships. *Psychotherapy, 31,* 208–220.

Lyons-Ruth, K., Bronfman, E., & Parsons, E. (1999). Maternal disruptive affective communication, maternal frightened or frightening behavior, and disorganized infant attachment strategies. *Monographs of the Society for Research in Child Development, 64*(3), 67–96.

Lyons-Ruth, K., & Jacobvitz, D. (1999). Attachment disorganization: Unresolved loss, relational violence, and lapses in behavioral and attentional strategies. In J. Cassidy & P. R. Shaver (Eds.), *Handbook of attachment theory and research* (pp. 520–554). New York: Guilford Press.

Lyons-Ruth, K., Repacholi, B., McLeod, S., & Silva, E. (1991). Disorganized attachment behavior in infancy: Short-term stability, maternal and infant correlates and risk-related subtypes. *Development and Psychopathology, 3,* 377–396.

Maccoby, E. (1992). The role of parents in the socialization of children: A historical overview. *Development and Psychopathology, 28,* 1006–1017.

Madsen, M. (1971). Development and cross-cultural differences in cooperative and competitive behavior of young children. *Journal of Cross-Cultural Psychology, 2,* 365–371.

Mahler, M., Pine, F., & Bergman, A. (1975). *The psychological birth of the human infant.* New York: Basic Books.

Main, M. (1995). Recent studies in attachment: Overview with selected implications for clinical work. In S. Goldberg, R. Muir, & J. Kerr (Eds.), *Attachment theory: Social, developmental, and clinical perspectives* (pp. 407–475). Hillsdale, NJ: Analytic Press.

Main, M., & Goldwyn, R. (1998). *Adult Attachment Interview scoring and classification manual—6th version.* Unpublished manuscript, University of California, Berkeley.

Main, M., & Hesse, E. (1990). Parents' unresolved traumatic experiences are related to infant disorganized attachment status: Is frightened or frightening parental behavior the linking mechanism? In M. Greenberg, D. Cicchetti, & E. M. Cummings (Eds.), *Attachment in the preschool years* (pp. 161–182). Chicago: University of Chicago Press.

Main, M., Hesse, E., & Kaplan, N. (2005). Predictability of attachment behavior at 1, 6, and 19 years of age: The Berkeley Longitudinal Study. In K. E. Grossmann, K. Grossmann, & E. Waters (Eds.), *Attachment from infancy to adulthood: The major longitudinal studies* (pp. 245–304). New York: Guilford Press.

Main, M., Kaplan, N., & Cassidy, J. (1985). Security in infancy, childhood, and adulthood: A move to the level of representation. *Monographs of the Society for Research in Child Development, 50*(1–2, Serial No. 209), 66–104.

Main, M., & Solomon, J. (1990). Procedures for identifying infants as disorganized/disoriented during the Ainsworth Strange Situation. In M. T. Greenberg, D. Cicchetti, & E. M. Cummings (Eds.), *Attachment in the preschool years* (pp. 121–160). Chicago: University of Chicago Press.

Main, M., & Weston, D. (1981). The quality of the toddlers' relationship to mother and to father: Related to conflict behavior and the readiness to establish new relationships. *Child Development, 52,* 932–940.

Mangelsdorf, S., Gunnar, M., Kestenbaum, R., Lang, S., & Andreas, D. (1990). Infancy proneness-to-distress temperament, maternal personality, and mother–infant attachment: Associations and goodness of fit. *Child Development, 61,* 820–831.

Mans, L., Cicchetti, D., & Sroufe, L. A. (1978). Mirror reactions of Down syndrome infants and toddlers: Cognitive underpinnings of self-recognition. *Child Development, 49,* 1247–1250.

Marvin, R., Cooper, C., Hoffman, K., & Powell, B. (2002). The Circle of Security project: Attachment-based intervention with caregiver–preschool child dyads. *Attachment and Human Development, 4*(1), 107–124.

Marvinney, D. (1988). *Sibling relationships in middle childhood: Implications for social–emotional development.* Unpublished doctoral dissertation, University of Minnesota, Minneapolis.

Mash, E., & Wolfe, D. (2002). *Abnormal child psychology.* New York: Wadsworth.

Masten, A. S. (2001). Ordinary magic: Resilience processes in development. *American Psychologist, 56*(3), 227–238.

Masten, A. (Ed.). (in press). *Minnesota Symposium on Child Psychology: Vol. 33. Multilevel dynamics in developmental psychopathology: Pathways to the future*. Hillsdale, NJ: Erlbaum.

Masters, J., & Wellman, H. (1974). Human infant attachment: A procedural critique. *Psychological Bulletin, 81*, 218–237.

Matas, L., Arend, R., & Sroufe, L. A. (1978). Continuity of adaptation in the second year: The relationship between quality of attachment and later competence. *Child Development, 49*, 547–556.

Mathieu, P. (1990). *Developmental antecedents of school achievement: The influence of developmental history*. Unpublished doctoral dissertation, University of Minnesota, Minneapolis.

McCrone, E. R., Egeland, B., Kalkoske, M., & Carlson, E. A. (1994). Relations between early maltreatment and mental representations of relationships assessed with projective storytelling in middle childhood. *Development and Psychopathology, 6*, 99–120.

McDonough, S. C. (1999). Interaction guidance: An approach for difficult-to-engage families. In C. H. Zeanah (Ed.), *Handbook of infant mental health* (2nd ed., pp. 485–493). New York: Guilford Press.

McKinney, W. (1977). Animal behavioral/biological models relevant to depression and affective disorders in humans. In J. Schulterbrandt & A. Raskin (Eds.), *Depression in childhood* (pp. 117–144). New York: Raven Press.

Minde, K., & Hesse, E. (1996). The role of the Adult Attachment Interview in parent–infant psychotherapy: A case presentation. *Infant Mental Health Journal, 17*, 115–126.

Mischel, W. (1968). *Personality and assessment*. New York: Wiley.

Mischel, W. (1973). Toward a cognitive social learning re-conceptualization of personality. *Psychological Bulletin, 80*, 252–283.

Mischel, W., Shoda, Y., & Rodriguez, M. (1989). Delay of gratification in children. *Science, 244*, 933–937.

Moffitt, T. (1993). Adolescence-limited and life-course-persistent antisocial behavior: A developmental taxonomy. *Psychological Review, 100*, 674–701.

Molitor, N., Jaffe, L., Barglow, P., Benveniste, R., & Vaughn, B. (1984, April). *Biochemical and psychological antecedents of newborn performance on the Neonatal Behavioral Assessment Scale*. Paper presented at the annual meeting of the International Conference on Infant Studies, New York.

Morris, D. (1980). *Infant attachment and problem solving in the toddler: Relations to mother's family history*. Unpublished doctoral dissertation, University of Minnesota, Minneapolis.

Motti, E. (1986). *Patterns of behaviors of preschool teachers with children of varying developmental histories*. Unpublished doctoral dissertation, University of Minnesota, Minneapolis.

Muir, E. (1992). Watching, waiting, and wondering: Applying psychoanalytic principles to mother–infant intervention. *Infant Mental Health Journal, 13*(4), 319–328.

Murray, H. A. (1938/1943). *Thematic Apperception Test and manual*. Cambridge, MA: Harvard University Press.

Nachmias, M., Gunnar, M., Mangelsdorf, S., Parritz, R. H., & Buss, K. (1996). Behavioral inhibition and stress reactivity: The moderating role of attachment security. *Child Development, 67*, 508–522.

Nelson, C. A. (2000). Neural plasticity and human development: The role of early experience in sculpting memory systems. *Developmental Science, 3*, 115–130.

Nelson, C. A. (2002). Neural development and life-long plasticity. In R. M. Lerner, F. Jacobs, & D. Wetlieb (Eds.), *Promoting positive child, adolescent, and family development: Handbook of program and policy interventions* (pp. 31–60). Thousand Oaks, CA: Sage.

Nelson, C. A., de Haan, M., & Thomas, K. M. (in press). Neural bases of cognitive development. In W. Damon, R. Lerner, D. Kuhn, & R. Siegler (Vol. Eds.), *Handbook of child psychology: Vol. 2. Cognition, perception, and language* (6th ed.). New York: Wiley.

Nelson, K. (1999). Levels and modes of representation: Issues for the theory of conceptual change and development. In E. K. Scholnick, K. Nelson, S. Gelman, & P. H. Miller (Eds.), *Conceptual development: Piaget's legacy* (pp. 269–291). Mahwah, NJ: Erlbaum.

Nelson, K., & Gruendel, J. (1979). At morning it's lunchtime: A scriptal view of children's dialogues. *Discourse Processes, 2*, 73–94.

Nelson, N. (1994). *Predicting adolescent behavior problems in late adolescence from parent–child interactions in early adolescence.* Unpublished doctoral dissertation, University of Minnesota, Minneapolis.

Nezworski, T. (1983). *Continuity of adaptation into the fourth year: Individual differences in curiosity and exploratory behavior of preschool children.* Unpublished doctoral dissertation, University of Minnesota, Minneapolis.

NICHD Early Child Care Research Network. (1997). The effects of infant child care on infant–mother attachment security: Results of the NICHD study of early child care. *Child Development, 68*, 860–879.

NICHD Early Child Care Research Network. (2001). Nonmaternal care and family factors in early development. *Journal of Applied Developmental Psychology, 22*, 457–492.

NICHD Early Child Care Research Network. (2004). Affect dysregulation in the mother–child relationship in the toddler years: Antecedents and consequences. *Development and Psychopathology, 16*, 43–68.

Novak, M., O'Neill, P., Beckley, S., & Suomi, S. (1992). Naturalistic environments for captive primates. In E. Gibbons, E. Wyers, & E. Waters (Eds.), *Naturalistic habitats in captivity* (pp. 236–258). New York: Academic Press.

O'Brien, L., Huston, L., Egeland, B., & Duggal, S. (1998, April). *A longitudinal study of participation in criminal activity in late adolescence.* Paper presented at the annual meeting of the Society for Research on Adolescence, San Diego, CA.

O'Connor, M. J., Sigman, M., & Brill, N. (1987). Disorganization of attachment in relation to maternal alcohol consumption. *Journal of Consulting and Clinical Psychology, 55*, 831–836.

O'Connor, T. G., & Plomin, R. (2000). Developmental behavioral genetics. In A. Sameroff, M. Lewis, & S. M. Miller (Eds.), *Handbook of developmental psychopathology* (pp. 217–235). New York: Plenum Press.

Ogawa, J. R., Sroufe, L. A., Weinfield, N. S., Carlson, E. A., & Egeland, B. (1997).

Development and the fragmented self: Longitudinal study of dissociative symptomatology in a nonclinical sample. *Development and Psychopathology, 9*, 855–879.

Ostoja-Starzewska, E. (1996). *Developmental antecedents of friendship competence in adolescence: The roles of early adaptational history and middle childhood peer competence.* Unpublished doctoral dissertation, University of Minnesota, Minneapolis.

Pancake, V. (1988). *Quality of attachment in infancy as a predictor of hostility and emotional distance in preschool peer relationships.* Unpublished doctoral dissertation, University of Minnesota, Minneapolis.

Pastor, D. (1981). The quality of mother–infant attachment and its relationship to toddlers' initial sociability with peers. *Developmental Psychopathology, 17*, 326–335.

Patterson, G., Capaldi, D., & Bank, L. (1991). An early starter model for predicting delinquency. In D. Pepler & K. Rubin (Eds.), *The development and treatment of aggression* (pp. 139–168). Hillsdale, NJ: Erlbaum.

Patterson, G., & Dishion, T. (1988). A mechanism for transmitting the antisocial trait across generations. In R. Hinde & J. Stevenson-Hinde (Eds.), *Relations between relationships within families* (pp. 283–310). Oxford, UK: Oxford University Press.

Pederson, D., Gleason, K., Moran, G., & Bento, S. (1998). Maternal attachment representations, maternal sensitivity, and the infant–mother attachment relationship. *Developmental Psychology, 34*, 925–933.

Pettit, G., Bates, J., Dodge, K., & Meece, D. (1999). The impact of after-school peer contact on early adolescent externalizing problems is moderated by parental monitoring, perceived neighborhood safety, and prior adjustment. *Child Development, 70*, 768–778.

Piaget, J. (1952). *The origins of intelligence in children.* New York: Norton.

Pianta, R. C., & Egeland, B. (1990). Life stress and parenting outcomes in a disadvantaged sample: Results of the Mother–Child Interaction Project. *Journal of Clinical Child Psychology, 19*(4), 329–336.

Pianta, R. C., & Egeland, B. (1994). Predictors of instability in children's mental test performance at 24, 48, and 96 months. *Intelligence, 18*(2), 145–163.

Pianta, R. C., Egeland, B., & Erickson, M. F. (1989). The antecedents of child maltreatment: The results of the Mother–Child Interaction Research Project. In D. Cicchetti & V. Carlson (Eds.), *Child maltreatment: Theory and research on the causes and consequences of child abuse and neglect* (pp. 203–253). Boston: Harvard University Press.

Pianta, R. C., Egeland, B., & Sroufe, L. A. (1990). Maternal stress and children's development: Prediction of school outcomes and identification of protective factors. In J. Rolf, A. S. Masten, D. Cicchetti, K. H. Neuchterlein, & S. Weintraub (Eds.), *Risk and protective factors in the development of psychopathology* (pp. 215–235). New York: Cambridge University Press.

Pianta, R. C., Erickson, M. F., Wagner, N., Kreutzer, T., & Egeland, B. (1990). Early predictors of referral for special services: Child-based measures versus mother–child interaction. *School Psychological Review, 19*(2), 240–250.

Pianta, R. C., Hyatt, A., & Egeland, B. (1986). Maternal relationship history as an indicator of developmental risk. *American Journal of Orthopsychiatry, 56*(2), 385–398.

Pianta, R. C., Sroufe, L. A., & Egeland, B. (1989). Continuity and discontinuity in maternal sensitivity at 6, 24, and 42 months in a high risk sample. *Child Development, 60*(2), 481–487.

Pierce, S. (1999). *The role of fathers and men in the development of child and adolescent externalizing behavior.* Unpublished doctoral dissertation, University of Minnesota, Minneapolis.

Pope, A. (Ed.). (1961). *Epistles to several persons: Moral essays.* London: Methuen. (Original work published 1731)

Porteus, S. D. (1965). *The Maze Test: Recent advances.* Palo Alto, CA: Pacific Books.

Posada, G., Jacobs, A., Carbonell, O. A., Alzate, G., Bustamante, M., & Arenas, A. (1999). Maternal care and attachment security in ordinary and emergency contexts. *Developmental Psychopathology, 35,* 1379–1388.

Poznanski, E. D., Cook, S. C., & Carroll, B. J. (1979). A depression rating scale for children. *Pediatrics, 64,* 442–450.

Puig-Antich, J., & Chambers, W. (1978). *The Schedule for Affective Disorders and Schizophrenia for School-Age Children.* New York: New York Psychiatric Institute.

Radke-Yarrow, M., Cummings, E. M., Kuczynski, L., & Chapman, M. (1985). Patterns of attachment in 2- and 3-year olds in normal families with parental depression. *Child Development, 56,* 884–893.

Radke-Yarrow, M., Richters, J., & Wilson, W. (1988). Child development in the network of relationships. In R. A. Hinde & J. Stevenson-Hinde (Eds.), *Relationships within families: Mutual influences* (pp. 48–67). Oxford, UK: Oxford University Press.

Rahe, D. (1984). *Interaction patterns between children and mothers on teaching tasks at age 42 months: Antecedents in attachment history, intellectual correlates, and consequences of children's socio-emotional functioning.* Unpublished doctoral dissertation, University of Minnesota, Minneapolis.

Ramirez, M. L., Carlson, E. A., Gest, S., & Egeland, B. (1991, July). *The relationship between children's behavior at school and internal representations of their relationships as measured by the sentence completion method.* Poster presented at the annual meeting of the International Society for the Study of Behavioral Development, Minneapolis, MN.

Renken, B., Egeland, B., Marvinney, D., Sroufe, L. A., & Mangelsdorf, S. (1989). Early childhood antecedents of aggression and passive-withdrawal in early elementary school. *Journal of Personality, 57*(2), 257–281.

Robins, L., & Price, R. (1991). Adult disorders predicted by childhood conduct problems: Results from the NIMH Epidemiological Catchment Area Project. *Psychiatry, 54,* 116–132.

Rodning, C., Beckwith, L., & Howard, J. (1991). Quality of attachment and home environments in children prenatally exposed to PCP and cocaine. *Development and Psychopathology, 3,* 351–366.

Rogoff, B. (1990). *Apprenticeship in thinking: Cognitive development in social context.* New York: Oxford University Press.

Roisman, G. I., Aguilar, B., & Egeland, B. (2004). Antisocial behavior in the transition to adulthood: The independent and interactive roles of developmental history and emerging developmental tasks. *Development and Psychopathology, 16,* 857–872.

Roisman, G. I., Collins, W. A., Sroufe, L. A., & Egeland, B. (in press). Predictors of young adults, security in their current romantic relationship: A prospective test of the prototype hypothesis. *Attachment and Human Development.*

Roisman, G. I., Madsen, S. D., Hennighausen, K. H., Sroufe, L. A., & Collins, W. A. (2001). The coherence of dyadic behavior across parent–child and romantic relationships as mediated by the internalized representation of experience. *Attachment and Human Development, 3*(2), 156–172.

Roisman, G. I., Padron, E., Sroufe, L. A., & Egeland, B. (2002). Earned-secure attachment status in retrospect and prospect. *Child Development, 73*(4), 1204–1219.

Rosenberg, D. (1984). *The quality and content of preschool fantasy play: Correlates in concurrent social–personality functioning and early mother–child attachment relationships.* Unpublished doctoral dissertation, University of Minnesota, Minneapolis.

Rotter, J. (1966). Generalized expectancies for internal versus external control of reinforcement. *Psychological Monographs, 80*(1), 1–28.

Rubin, K. H., Bukowski, W., & Parker, J. G. (1998). Peer interactions, relationships, and groups. In W. Damon (Series Ed.) & R. M. Lerner (Vol. Ed.), *Handbook of child psychology: Vol. 1. Theoretical models of human development* (5th ed., pp. 619–700). New York: Wiley.

Rutter, M. (1980). Introduction. In M. Rutter (Ed.), *Scientific foundations of developmental psychiatry* (pp. 1–8). London: Heinemann.

Rutter, M. (1997). Antisocial behavior: Developmental psychopathology perspectives. In D. M. Stoff, J. Breiling, & J. Maser (Eds.), *Handbook of antisocial behavior* (pp. 115–124). New York: Wiley.

Rutter, M., & Sroufe, L. A. (2000). Developmental psychopathology: Concepts and challenges. *Development and Psychopathology, 12,* 265–296.

Sable, P. (1992). Attachment theory: Application to clinical practice with adults. *Clinical Social Work Journal, 20,* 271–283.

Sackett, J., Sameroff, A., Cairns, R., & Suomi, S. (1981). Continuity in behavioral development. In K. Immelman, G. Barlow, I. Petrinovitch, & M. Main (Eds.), *Behavioral development* (pp. 23–57). Cambridge, UK: Cambridge University Press.

Sameroff, A. (1983). Developmental systems: Context and evolution. In W. Kessen (Ed.), *Handbook of child psychology: Vol. 1. History, theories, and methods* (pp. 327–394). New York: Wiley.

Sameroff, A. (2000). Dialectical processes in developmental psychopathology. In A. Sameroff, M. Lewis, & S. Miller (Eds.), *Handbook of developmental psychopathology* (2nd ed., pp. 23–40). New York: Plenum Press.

Sameroff, A., & Chandler, M. J. (1975). Reproductive risk and the continuum of caretaking casualty. In F. D. Horowitz, M. Hetherington, S. Scarr-Salapatek, & G. Siegel (Eds.), *Review of child development research* (Vol. 4, pp. 187–243). Chicago: Chicago University Press.

Sameroff, A., & Emde, R. (1989). *Relationship disturbances in early childhood.* New York: Basic Books.

Sameroff, A., & Fiese, B. (2000). Transactional regulation: The developmental ecology of early intervention. In J. Shonkoff & S. Meisels (Eds.), *Handbook of early childhood intervention* (pp. 135–139). New York: Cambridge University Press.

Sampson, M. (2004). *Continuity and change in patterns of attachment between infancy, adolescence, and early adulthood in a high risk sample.* Unpublished doctoral dissertation, University of Minnesota, Minneapolis.

Sanchez, M., Ladd, C., & Plotsky, P. (2003). Early adverse experience as a developmental risk factor for later psychopathology: Evidence from rodent and primate models. *Development and Psychopathology, 13,* 419–449.

Sander, L. (1962). Issues in early mother–child interaction. *Journal of the American Academy of Child Psychiatry, 1,* 141–166.

Sander, L. (1975). Infant and caretaking environment. In E. J. Anthony (Ed.), *Explorations in child psychiatry* (pp. 129–165). New York: Plenum Press.

Schaefer, E. S., & Manheimer, H. (1960, May). *Dimensions of perinatal adjustment.* Paper presented at the annual meeting of the Eastern Psychological Association, New York.

Schmit, D. (1995). *Continuity and change in heterosexual relations from middle childhood to adolescence: Evidence from a longitudinal study.* Unpublished doctoral dissertation, University of Minnesota, Minneapolis.

Schneider, B. H., Atkinson, L., & Tardif, C. (2001). Child–parent attachment and children's peer relations: A quantitative review. *Developmental Psychology, 37,* 86–100.

Schneider, M., & Moore, C. (2000). Effect of prenatal stress on development: A non-human primate model. In C. A. Nelson (Ed.), *Minnesota Symposia on Child Psychology: Vol. 31. The effect of early adversity on neurobehavioral development* (pp. 201–244). Mahwah, NJ: Erlbaum.

Schore, A. N. (1994). *Affect regulation and the origin of the self: The neurobiology of emotional development.* Hillsdale, NJ: Erlbaum.

Schore, A. N. (2002). Dysregulation of the right brain: A fundamental mechanism of traumatic attachment and the psychopathogenesis of posttraumatic stress disorder. *Australian and New Zealand Journal of Psychiatry, 36,* 9–30.

Schuengel, C., Bakermans-Kranenburg, M. J., van IJzendoorn, M. H., & Blom, M. (1999). Unresolved loss and infant disorganization: Links to frightening maternal behavior. In J. Solomon & C. C. George (Eds.), *Attachment disorganization* (pp. 71–94). New York: Guilford Press.

Segal, J., & Yahres, H. (1978, November). Bringing up mother. *Psychology Today,* pp. 92–96.

Seligman, M. E. P., Peterson, C., Kaslow, N. J., Tannebaum, R. L., Alloy, L. B., & Abramson, L. Y. (1984). Attributional style and depressive symptoms among children. *Journal of Abnormal Child Psychology, 83,* 235–238.

Shaffer, A., & Sroufe, L. A. (in press). The developmental and adaptational implications of generational boundary dissolution: Findings from a prospective longitudinal study. *Journal of Emotional Abuse.*

Shane, M., Shane, E., & Gales, M. (1997). *Intimate attachments: Toward a new self psychology.* New York: Guilford Press.

Shaw, D., Owens, E., Vondra, I. J., Keenan, K., & Winslow, E. (1996). Early risk factors and pathways in the development of early disruptive behavior problems. *Development and Psychopathology, 8,* 679–699.

Shelder, J., & Block, J. (1990). Adolescent drug use and psychological health: A longitudinal inquiry. *American Psychologist, 45,* 612–630.

Shulman, S., Elicker, J., & Sroufe, L. A. (1994). Stages of friendship growth in preadolescence as related to attachment history. *Journal of Social and Personal Relationships, 11,* 341–361.

Shure, M. B., & Spivak, G. (1970). *Preschool Interpersonal Problem-Solving manual.* Philadelphia: Hahnemann Medical College and Hospitals.

Siebenbruner, J., Zimmer-Gembeck, M., & Egeland, B. (2005). *Sexual partners and contraceptive use: A sixteen-year prospective study predicting abstinence and risk behavior.* Manuscript submitted for publication.

Siegel, D. J. (1999). *The developing mind: How relationships and the brain interact to shape who we are.* New York: Guilford Press.

Slaby, R., & Frey, K. (1975). Development of gender constancy and selective attention to same-sex models. *Child Development, 46,* 849–856.

Slade, A. (1999). Attachment theory and research: Implications for the theory and practice of individual psychotherapy with adults. In J. Cassidy & P. R. Shaver (Eds.), *Handbook of attachment: Theory, research, and clinical applications* (pp. 575–594). New York: Guilford Press.

Solomon, J., & George, C. C. (1999). *Attachment disorganization.* New York: Guilford Press.

Sorce, J. F., Emde, R. N., Campos, J. J., & Klinnert, M. D. (1985). Maternal emotional signaling: Its effect on the visual cliff behavior of one-year-olds. *Developmental Psychology, 21,* 195–200.

Spangler, G., & Grossmann, K. E. (1993). Biobehavioral organization in securely and insecurely attached infants. *Child Development, 64,* 1439–1450.

Spitz, R., Emde, R., & Metcalf, D. (1970). Further prototypes of ego formation. *Psychoanalytic Study of the Child, 25,* 417–444.

Spivak, G., & Swift, M. (1982). *Devereux Elementary School Behavior Rating Scale.* Devon, PA: Devereux Foundation.

Sroufe, J. (1991). Assessment of parent–adolescent relationships: Implications for adolescent development. *Journal of Family Psychology, 5,* 21–45.

Sroufe, J. (2003). Applications of attachment theory to the treatment of latency age children. In M. Cortina & M. Marrone (Eds.), *Attachment theory and the psychoanalytic process* (pp. 204–226). London: Whurr Press.

Sroufe, L. A. (1978). Attachment and the roots of competence. *Human Nature, 1,* 50–57.

Sroufe, L. A. (1979). The coherence of individual development. *American Psychologist, 34*(10), 834–841.

Sroufe, L. A. (1983). Infant–caregiver attachment and patterns of adaptation in preschool. In M. Perlmutter (Ed.), *Minnesota Symposia on Child Psychology: Vol. 16. The roots of maladaptation and competence* (pp. 129–135). Hillsdale, NJ: Erlbaum.

Sroufe, L. A. (1985). Attachment classification from the perspective of infant–caregiver relationships and infant temperament. *Child Development, 56,* 1–14.

Sroufe, L. A. (1986). Appraisal: Bowlby's contribution to psychoanalytic theory and developmental psychology— attachment, separation, loss. *Journal of Child Psychology and Psychiatry, 27,* 841–849.

Sroufe, L. A. (1989). Relationships, self, and individual adaptation. In A. J. Sameroff & R. N. Emde (Eds.), *Relationship disturbances in early childhood: A developmental approach* (pp. 70–94). New York: Basic Books.

Sroufe, L. A. (1996). *Emotional development: The organization of emotional life in the early years.* New York: Cambridge University Press.

Sroufe, L. A. (1997). Psychopathology as an outcome of development. *Development and Psychopathology, 9,* 251–268.

Sroufe, L. A. (1999, February). *Changing the odds: The development of resilience.* Paper presented at the annual meeting of the American Association for the Advancement of Science, Anaheim, CA.

Sroufe, L. A., Bennett, C., Englund, M., Urban, J., & Shulman, S. (1993). The significance of gender boundaries in preadolescence: Contemporary correlates and antecedents of boundary violation and maintenance. *Child Development, 64*(2), 455–466.

Sroufe, L. A., Carlson, E. A., Levy, A. K., & Egeland, B. (1999). Implications of attachment theory for developmental psychopathology. *Development and Psychopathology, 11,* 1–13.

Sroufe, L. A., Cooper, R., & DeHart, G. (1992). *Child development: Its nature and course* (2nd ed.). New York: McGraw-Hill.

Sroufe, L. A., Duggal, S., Weinfield, N. S., & Carlson, E. (2000). Relationships, development, and psychopathology. In A. Sameroff, M. Lewis, & S. Miller (Eds.), *Handbook of developmental psychopathology* (2nd ed., pp. 75–92). New York: Kluwer Academic/Plenum Press.

Sroufe, L. A., & Egeland, B. (1991). Illustrations of person and environment interaction from a longitudinal study. In T. Wachs & R. Plomin (Eds.), *Conceptualization and measurement of organism–environment interaction* (pp. 68–84). Washington, DC: American Psychological Association.

Sroufe, L. A., Egeland, B., & Carlson, E. (1999). One social world: The integrated development of parent–child and peer relationships. In W. A. Collins & B. Laursen (Eds.), *Relationships as developmental context: The 30th Minnesota Symposium on Child Psychology* (pp. 241–262). Hillsdale, NJ: Erlbaum.

Sroufe, L. A., Egeland, B., Carlson, E., & Collins, W. A. (2005). Placing early attachment experiences in developmental context: The Minnesota Longitudinal Study. In K. E. Grossmann, K. Grossmann, & E. Waters (Eds.), *Attachment from infancy to adulthood: The major longitudinal studies* (pp. 48–70). New York: Guilford Press.

Sroufe, L. A., Egeland, B., & Kreutzer, T. (1990). The fate of early experience following developmental change: Longitudinal approaches to individual adaptation in childhood. *Child Development, 61,* 1363–1373.

Sroufe, L. A., & Fleeson, J. (1986). Attachment and the construction of relationships. In W. Hartup & Z. Rubin (Eds.), *Relationships and development* (pp. 51–71). Hillsdale, NJ: Erlbaum.

Sroufe, L. A., & Fleeson, J. (1988). The coherence of family relationships. In R. A. Hinde & J. Stevenson-Hinde (Ed.), *Relationships within families: Mutual influences* (pp. 27–47). Oxford, UK: Clarendon.

Sroufe, L. A., Fox, N., & Pancake, V. (1983). Attachment and dependency in developmental perspective. *Child Development, 54*(6), 1615–1627.

Sroufe, L. A., & Jacobvitz, D. (1989). Diverging pathways, developmental transformation, multiple etiologies and the problem of continuity in development. *Human Development, 32*(3–4), 196–203.

Sroufe, L. A., Jacobvitz, J., Mangelsdorf, S., DeAngelo, E., & Ward, M. J. (1985). Generational boundary dissolution between mothers and their preschool children: A relationships systems approach. *Child Development, 56*, 317–325.

Sroufe, L. A., & Pierce, S. (1999). Men in the family: Associations with juvenile conduct. In G. Cunningham (Ed.), *Just in time research: Children, youth, and families* (pp. 19–26). Minneapolis: University of Minnesota Extension Services.

Sroufe, L. A., & Rutter, M. (1984). The domain of developmental psychopathology. *Child Development, 55*, 17–29.

Sroufe, L. A., & Sampson, M. C. (2000). Attachment theory and systems concepts. *Human Development, 43*, 321–326.

Sroufe, L. A., Schork, E., Motti, F., Lawroski, N., & LaFreniere, P. (1984). The role of affect in social competence. In C. E. Izard, J. Kagan, & R. Zajonc (Eds.), *Emotions, cognition, and behavior* (pp. 289–319). New York: Plenum Press.

Sroufe, L. A., & Ward, M. J. (1980). Seductive behavior of mothers of toddlers: Occurrence, correlates, and family origins. *Child Development, 51*, 1222–1229.

Sroufe, L. A., & Waters, E. (1977a). Attachment as an organizational construct. *Child Development, 48*, 1184–1199.

Sroufe, L. A., & Waters, E. (1977b). Heart rate as a convergent measure in clinical and developmental research. *Merrill–Palmer Quarterly, 23*, 3–27.

Sroufe, L. A., Waters, E., & Matas, L. (1974). Contextual determinants of infant affective response. In M. Lewis & L. Rosenblum (Eds.), *Origins of fear* (pp. 49–72). New York: Wiley.

Stechler, G., & Carpenter, G. (1967). A viewpoint on early affective development. In J. Hellmuth (Ed.), *The exceptional infant* (Vol. 1, pp. 163–190). Seattle, WA: Special Child Publications.

Steinberg, L., & Morris, A. (2001). Adolescent development. *Annual Review of Psychology, 52*, 83–110.

Steinhausen, H. (1994). Anorexia and bulimia nervosa. In M. Rutter, E. Taylor, & L. Hersov (Eds.), *Child and adolescent psychiatry* (pp. 425–440). London: Blackwell.

Stern, D. (1985). *The interpersonal world of the infant: A view from psychoanalysis and developmental psychology.* New York: Basic Books.

Stevens, G., & Featherman, D. L. (1981). A revised socioeconomic index of occupational status. *Social Science Research, 10*, 364–393.

Stouthamer-Loeber, M., Loeber, R., Farrington, D. P., Zhang, Q., van Kammen, W., & Maguin, E. (1993). The double edge of protective and risk factors for delinquency: Interrelations and developmental patterns. *Development and Psychopathology, 5,* 683–701.

Stovall-McClough, K. C., & Dozier, M. (2004). Forming attachments in foster care: Infant attachment behaviors during the first 2 months of placement. *Development and Psychopathology, 16,* 253–271.

Strauss, M. A. (1990). The Conflict Tactics Scales and its critics: An evaluation and new data validity and reliability. In M. A. Strauss & J. Gelles (Eds.), *Physical violence in American families: Risk factors and maladaptations to violence in 8,145 families.* New Brunswick, NJ: Transaction.

Suess, G. J., Grossmann, K. E., & Sroufe, L. A. (1992). Effects of infant attachment to mother and father on quality of adaptation in preschool: From dyadic to individual organization of self. *International Journal of Behavioural Development, 15,* 43–65.

Sullivan, H. S. (1953). *The interpersonal theory of psychiatry.* New York: Norton.

Suomi, S. (2002). Parents, peers, and the process of socialization in primates. In J. Borkowski, S. Ramey, & M. Bristol-Power (Eds.), *Parenting and your child's world* (pp. 265–282). Hillsdale, NJ: Erlbaum.

Susman-Stillman, A., Kalkoske, M., Egeland, B., & Waldman, I. (1996). Infant temperament and maternal sensitivity as predictors of attachment security. *Infant Behavior and Development, 19*(1), 33–47.

Taraldson, B., Brunnquell, D., Deinard, A., & Egeland, B. (1977, April). *Psychometric and theoretical credibility of three measures of infant temperament.* Paper presented at the meeting of the Society for Research in Child Development, New Orleans, LA.

Teo, A., Carlson, C., Mathieu, P., Egeland, B., & Sroufe, L. A. (1996). A prospective longitudinal study of psychosocial predictors of achievement. *Journal of School Psychology, 34,* 285–306.

Thelen, E. (1989). Self-organization in developmental processes: Can a systems approach work? In M. Gunnar & L. A. Sroufe (Eds.), *Minnesota Symposia in Child Psychology: Vol. 22. Systems and development* (pp. 77–117). Hillsdale, NJ: Erlbaum.

Thomas, A., Chess, S., & Birch, H. G. (1968). *Temperament and behavior disorders in children.* New York: New York University Press.

Thompson, R. (1998). Early sociopersonality development. In W. Damon (Ed.), *Handbook of child psychology: Vol. 3. Social, emotional, and personality development* (5th ed., pp. 25–104). New York: Wiley.

Thompson, R. (2003, October). *Early social attachment and its consequences: The dynamics of a developing relationship.* Report from the Dahlem Workshop on Attachment and Bonding: A New Synthesis, Berlin.

Thorne, B. (1986). Girls and boys together . . . but mostly apart: Gender arrangements in elementary schools. In W. H. Z. Rubin (Ed.), *Relationships and development* (pp. 167–184). Hillsdale, NJ: Erlbaum.

Tienari, P., Lahti, I., Sorri, A., Naarala, M., Moring, J., Kaleva, M., et al. (1990). Adopted-away offspring of schizophrenics and controls: The Finnish Adoptive Family Study of Schizophrenia. In L. Robins & M. Rutter (Eds.), *Straight and devious pathways from childhood to adulthood* (pp. 365–379). Cambridge, UK: Cambridge University Press.

Toth, S., Manly, J., & Cicchetti, D. (1992). Child maltreatment and vulnerability to depression. *Development and Psychopathology, 4*, 97–112.

Trickett, P. K., & Putnam, F. W. (1993). Impact of child sexual abuse on females: Toward a developmental, psychobiological integration. *Psychological Science, 4*(2), 81–87.

Tronick, E. (1989). Emotions and emotional communication in infants. *American Psychologist, 44*, 112–119.

Troy, M. (1988). *Antecedents, correlates, and continuity of ego-control and ego-resiliency in a high risk sample of preschool children.* Unpublished doctoral dissertation, University of Minnesota, Minneapolis.

Troy, M., & Sroufe, L. A. (1987). Victimization among preschoolers: The role of attachment relationship history. *Journal of the American Academy of Child and Adolescent Psychiatry, 26*(2), 166–172.

Urban, J., Carlson, E., Egeland, B., & Sroufe, L. A. (1991). Patterns of individual adaptation across childhood. *Development and Psychopathology, 3*, 445–460.

Uzgiris, I. C., & Hunt, J. (1975). *Assessment in infancy: Ordinal scales of psychological development.* Urbana: University of Illinois Press.

van den Boom, D. C. (1989). Neonatal irritability and the development of attachment. In G. Kohnstamm, J. Bates, & M. Rothbart (Eds.), *Temperament in childhood* (pp. 299–318). New York: Wiley.

van den Boom, D. C. (1995). Do first-year interventions endure? Follow-up during toddlerhood of a sample of Dutch irritable infants. *Child Development, 66*(6), 1798–1816.

Vaughn, B. E., & Bost, K. K. (1999). Attachment and temperament: Redundant, independent, or interacting influences on interpersonal adaptation and personality development? In J. Cassidy & P. R. Shaver (Ed.), *Handbook of attachment: Theory, research, and clinical applications* (pp. 198–225). New York: Guilford Press.

Vaughn, B. E., Colvin, T. N., Azria, M. R., Caya, L., & Krzysik, L. (2001). Dyadic analyses of friendship in a sample of preschool-age children attending Head Start: Correspondence between measures and implications for social competence. *Child Development, 72*(3), 862–878.

Vaughn, B., Taraldson, B., Crichton, L., & Egeland, B. (1980). Relationships between neonatal behavioral organization and infant behavior during the first year of life. *Infant Behavior and Development, 3*, 47–66.

Vaughn, B., & Waters, E. (1981). Attention structure, sociometric status, and dominance: Interrelations, behavioral correlates, and relationships to social competence. *Developmental Psychology, 17*, 275–288.

Vaughn, B., Waters, E., Egeland, B., & Sroufe, L. A. (1979). Individual differences in infant–mother attachment at 12 and 18 months: Stability and change in families under stress. *Child Development, 50*(4), 971–975.

von Bertalanffy, L. (1952). *Problems of life: An evaluation of modern biological thought.* Oxford, UK: Wiley.

Vygotsky, L. (1962). *Thought and language.* Cambridge, MA: MIT Press.

Vygotsky, L. (1978). *Mind and society.* Cambridge, MA: Harvard University Press.

Waddington, C. (1957). *The strategy of the genes.* London: Allen & Unwin.

Waldrop, M. F., Pedersen, F. A., & Bell, R. Q. (1968). Minor physical anomalies and behavior in preschool children. *Child Development, 39*(2), 391–400.

Waldrop, W. M. (1992). *Complexity.* New York: Simon & Schuster.

Ward, M. J., Vaughn, B., & Robb, M. D. (1988). Attachment and adaptation in siblings: Role of the mother in cross-sibling consistency. *Child Development, 59*, 643–651.

Warren, S., Huston, L., Egeland, B., & Sroufe, L. A. (1997). Child and adolescent anxiety disorders and early attachment. *Journal of the American Academy of Child and Adolescent Psychiatry, 36*, 637–644.

Waters, E. (1978). The stability of individual differences in infant–mother attachment. *Child Development, 49*, 483–494.

Waters, E., Kondo-Ikemura, K., & Richters, J. (1990). Learning to love: Milestones and mechanisms in attachment, identity, and identification. In M. Gunnar & L. A. Sroufe (Eds.), *Minnesota Symposia on Child Psychology: Vol. 23. Self-processes in development* (pp. 217–255). Hillsdale, NJ: Erlbaum.

Waters, E., Merrick, S., Treboux, D., Crowell, J., & Albersheim, L. (2000). Attachment security in infancy and early adulthood. *Child Development, 71*, 684–689.

Waters, E., & Sroufe, L. A. (1983). A developmental perspective on competence. *Developmental Review, 3*, 79–97.

Waters, E., Vaughn, B., & Egeland, B. (1980). Individual differences in infant–mother attachment relationships at age one: Antecedents in neonatal behavior in an urban, economically disadvantaged sample. *Child Development, 51*, 208–216.

Waters, E., Wippman, J., & Sroufe, L. A. (1979). Attachment, positive affect, and competence in the peer group: Two studies in construct validation. *Child Development, 40*, 821–829.

Waters, H., Rodrigues, L., & Ridgeway, D. (1998). Cognitive underpinnings of narrative attachment assessment. *Journal of Experimental Child Psychology, 71*, 211–234.

Wechsler, D. (1955). *Wechsler Adult Intelligence Scale.* New York: Psychological Corporation.

Wechsler, D. (1967). *Wechsler Preschool and Primary Scale of Intelligence.* New York: Psychological Corporation.

Wechsler, D. (1974). *Wechsler Intelligence Scale for Children—Revised (WISC-R).* New York: Psychological Corporation.

Weinfield, N., Ogawa, J. R., & Sroufe, L. A. (1997). Early attachment as a pathway to adolescent peer competence. *Journal of Research on Adolescence, 7*(3), 241–265.

Weinfield, N., Sroufe, L. A., & Egeland, B. (2000). Attachment from infancy to young adulthood in a high risk sample: Continuity, discontinuity, and their correlates. *Child Development, 71*, 695–702.

Weinfield, N., Whaley, G., & Egeland, B. (2004). Continuity, discontinuity, and coherence in attachment from infancy to late adolescence: Sequelae of organization and disorganization. *Attachment and Human Development, 6,* 73–97.

Weiss, P. (1949). The biological basis of adaptation. In J. Romano (Ed.), *Adaptation* (pp. 1–22). Ithaca, NY: Cornell University Press.

Weiss, P. (1961). Deformities as cues to understanding development of form. *Perspectives in Biology and Medicine, 4,* 133–151.

Werner, E. E., Bierman, J. H., & French, F. E. (1971). *The children of Kauai.* Honolulu: University of Hawaii.

Werner, E. E., & Smith, R. S. (1992). *Overcoming the odds.* New York: Cornell University Press.

Werner, H. (1948). *The comparative psychology of mental development.* New York: International Universities Press.

Wiens, M., & Collins, W. A. (1983). *The blind-folded partner task: Assessing dyadic collaboration under stress.* Unpublished manuscript, University of Minnesota, Minneapolis.

Winnicott, D. W. (1965). *The family and individual development.* London: Tavistock.

Woodcock, R. W., & Mather, N. (1989/1990). WJ-R Tests of Achievement: Examiner's Manual. In R. W. Woodcock & M. B. Johnson (Eds.), *Woodcock–Johnson Psychoeducational Battery—Revised.* Allen, TX: DLM Teaching Resources.

Wordsworth, W. (1940). *The poetical works of William Wordsworth.* Oxford, UK: Clarendon Press. (Original work published 1807)

Yates, T. M. (2004). *A longitudinal study of self-injurious behavior in a community sample.* Unpublished doctoral dissertation, University of Minnesota, Minneapolis.

Yates, T. M., Dodds, M. F., Sroufe, L. A., & Egeland, B. (2003). Exposure to partner violence and child behavior problems: A prospective study controlling for child physical abuse and neglect, child cognitive ability, socioeconomic status, and life stress. *Development and Psychopathology, 15*(1), 199–218.

Yates, T. M., Egeland, B., & Sroufe, L. A. (2003). Rethinking resilience: A developmental process perspective. In S. S. Luthar (Ed.), *Resilience and vulnerabilities: Adaptation in the context of childhood adversities* (pp. 243–266). New York: Cambridge University Press.

Zahn-Waxler, C., Radke-Yarrow, M., Wagner, E., & Chapman, M. (1992). Development of concern for others. *Developmental Psychology, 28,* 126–136.

Zeanah, C., Boris, N. W., Heller, S. S., Hinshaw-Fuselier, S., Larrieu, J. A., Lewis, M., et al. (1997). Relationship assessment in infant and mental health. *Infant Mental Health Journal, 18*(2), 182–197.

Zeanah, C., Boris, N., & Lieberman, A. (2000). Attachment disorders in infancy. In A. J. Sameroff, M. Lewis & S. M. Miller (Eds.), *Handbook of developmental psychopathology* (2nd ed., pp. 293–307). New York: Plenum Press.

Zimmerman, I., Steiner, V., & Pond, R. (1979). *Preschool language scale.* Columbus, OH: Merrill.

Zimmerman, P. (1994). *Attachment in adolescence: Development while coping with actual challenges.* Unpublished doctoral dissertation, University of Regensberg, Germany.

Index

Page numbers followed by an *f* indicate figure; *t*, table.

373